Health and Public Health Applications for Decision Support Using Machine Learning

Health and Public Health Applications for Decision Support Using Machine Learning

Editors

Pedro Miguel Rodrigues
João Alexandre Lobo Marques
João Paulo do Vale Madeiro

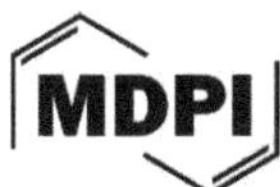

Basel • Beijing • Wuhan • Barcelona • Belgrade • Novi Sad • Cluj • Manchester

Editors

Pedro Miguel Rodrigues
Escola Superior de
Biotecnologia
Universidade Católica
Portuguesa
Porto
Portugal

João Alexandre Lobo
Marques
Laboratory of Applied
Neurosciences - LAN
University of Saint Joseph
Macau
Macau

João Paulo do Vale Madeiro
Departamento de
Computação
Universidade Federal do
Ceará
Fortaleza
Brazil

Editorial Office
MDPI
St. Alban-Anlage 66
4052 Basel, Switzerland

This is a reprint of articles from the Special Issue published online in the open access journal *Bioengineering* (ISSN 2306-5354) (available at: www.mdpi.com/journal/bioengineering/special_issues/public_health_decision).

For citation purposes, cite each article independently as indicated on the article page online and as indicated below:

Lastname, A.A.; Lastname, B.B. Article Title. *Journal Name* **Year**, *Volume Number*, Page Range.

ISBN 978-3-0365-8549-9 (Hbk)
ISBN 978-3-0365-8548-2 (PDF)
doi.org/10.3390/books978-3-0365-8548-2

Contents

About the Editors

Pedro Miguel Rodrigues

Pedro Miguel de Luís Rodrigues is an Assistant Professor at the Faculty of Biotechnology - Universidade Católica Portuguesa (ESB-UCP) and an integrated member of the Research Centre for Biotechnology and Fine Chemistry (CBQF-UCP), Porto, Portugal. He holds B.Sc., M.Sc., and Ph.D. degrees in Biomedical Engineering. He is the Co-coordinator of the Bioengineering Degree and the Coordinator of the Data Science in Biotechnology Post-graduation Program at ESB-UCP. As the main responsible teacher, he lectures signal and image processing, computer programming, imaging, artificial intelligence, machine learning, and waves and electromagnetism disciplines. He has published over 70 international peer-reviewed articles, book chapters, and conference papers in the field of the interface between artificial intelligence and medicine, having already been recognized by the Health INNOVATION Awards and the HiTech international programs. The innovation in his work generates one patent. He has been participating as a researcher in 10 international co-financed projects, 1 of them as principal investigator. He is a scientific reviewer for several scientific journals and conferences. He has participated in more than 10 scientific committees of international conferences. He is highly skilled in software design and development in different platforms such as Python, C++, R, Matlab, and others. His research focuses on (i) early detection of neurodegenerative illnesses through EEG signals (e.g. Alzheimer's, Parkinson's, Schizophrenia); (ii) detection of cardiac diseases by ECG signal analysis; (iii) voice diseases detection using speech signal analysis and machine learning algorithms; (iv) and on the development of biosensors, electronic instrumentation tools, micro-controllers, and smart-tools for fast controlling and monitoring living cities and spaces, and agri-food and biological/biomedical systems.

João Alexandre Lobo Marques

João Alexandre Lobo Marques, Associate Professor, Head of the Laboratory of Applied Neurosciences and Head of the Department of Business Administration at the University of Saint Joseph/USJ, Macau SAR, China. Visiting Associate Professor at the Chinese Academy of Sciences (CAS) - Shenzhen Institutes of Advanced Technologies (SIAT). Member of the Board of Advisors - Master in Global MarketingManagement - Boston University Metropolitan College (BU-MET) –USA. Visiting Researcher at Catolica Porto Business School. PhD in Engineering from the Federal University of Ceara, Brazil, with an exchange period at Trium Analysis Online, GmBH, Munich. Post-doctorate and Honorary Research Fellow from the University of Leicester-UK. More than 20 years of experience leading and managing international/multi-cultural teams as Head of Department, Director of Research, Undergraduate, and Post-graduate Programs Coordinator and Head of Institutional/Program Accreditation and Review with international agencies (A3ES-Portugal, BAC-UK, ME-China, INEP-Brazil). Managed more than USD 6 million in applied research and product development grants. Has large experience in Artificial Intelligence, Data Sciences, Big Data, Business Analytics, and Applied Mathematics. Highly skilled in software design and development in different platforms such as Python, C++, R, Matlab, and others. Specialist in Project Management frameworks application in international projects, including PMBOK and Agile. Trained 2,600+ professionals from 35+ different countries. Author of multiple books and scientific papers published in high-impact journals and relevant international conferences.

João Paulo do Vale Madeiro

João Paulo do Vale Madeiro is currently an Effective Professor, Adjunct A class, at the Federal University of Ceará, Campus do Pici, in Fortaleza, Ceará, assigned to the Department of Computing. He is also an Effective Member of the Master's and Doctorate Graduate Program in Computer Science at the Federal University of Ceará and the Graduate Program in Energy and Environment at the University for the International Integration of Afro-Brazilian Lusophony. He completed his Doctorate program in Teleinformatics Engineering at the Federal University of Ceará, with an emphasis on Biomedical Engineering (2013). He also completed via the Science without Borders program a research internship at the University of Leicester, England, in the Sandwich Doctorate modality (2012). He holds a master's degree in Teleinformatics Engineering (2007) and entered Electrical Engineering (2006), both from the Federal University of Ceará. His current research projects and scientific interests are focused on signals and image digital processing, systems to aid medical diagnosis, computer vision applied in the context of environmental mapping and medical images, and automatic feature extraction within electrocardiogram (ECG) signals.

Preface

Machine learning, a cutting-edge branch of artificial intelligence, has made significant strides in reshaping various industries, and the field of healthcare stands at the forefront of this transformation. In this reprint of "Health and Public Health Applications for Decision Support Using Machine Learning", we delve into the dynamic and ever-evolving landscape where machine learning intersects with health sciences. This compilation brings together a diverse range of research and innovations that demonstrate the potential of data-driven algorithms to revolutionize patient care, disease diagnosis, and public health management.

Throughout this reprint, a wide array of topics and applications that exemplify the transformative power of machine learning in healthcare are explored. Researchers and healthcare professionals will find valuable insights and inspiration within these pages. Topics covered include biomedical relation extraction, blood glucose level forecasting for diabetes management, prediction of walking stability to prevent falls, automated pneumonia-infected volume quantification in CT images, heart sound classification for precision medicine, noninvasive risk assessment for early detection of renal damage, ECG measurement uncertainty analysis, smart-data-driven tools for colony-type distinction, audio-visual stress classification for mental health assessment, early diagnosis of intracranial artery stenosis using non-invasive hemodynamic indices, COVID-19 detection using multiple data modalities, and artificial intelligence models in the diagnosis of adult-onset dementia disorders.

Overall, this "Health and Public Health Applications for Decision Support Using Machine Learning" reprint explores the symbiotic relationship between machine learning and healthcare. The chapters contained herein demonstrate the breadth of possibilities that emerge when data-driven approaches are applied to medical and healthcare challenges. We hope this reprint serves as a catalyst for future research and collaboration, driving us towards a healthier and more technologically advanced future.

Pedro Miguel Rodrigues, João Alexandre Lobo Marques, and João Paulo do Vale Madeiro

Editors

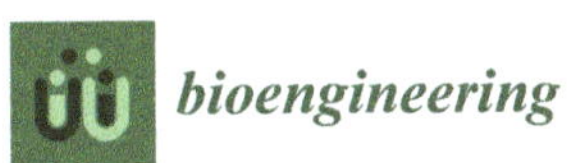 *bioengineering*

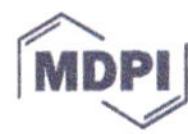

Editorial

Enhancing Health and Public Health through Machine Learning: Decision Support for Smarter Choices

Pedro Miguel Rodrigues [1,*], João Paulo Madeiro [2] and João Alexandre Lobo Marques [3]

[1] CBQF—Centro de Biotecnologia e Química Fina—Laboratório Associado, Escola Superior de Biotecnologia, Universidade Católica Portuguesa, Rua de Diogo Botelho 1327, 4169-005 Porto, Portugal
[2] Department of Computing, Federal University of Ceará, Fortaleza 60440-900, Ceará, Brazil; jpaulo.vale@dc.ufc.br
[3] Laboratory of Applied Neurosciences, University of Saint Joseph, Macao SAR 999078, China; alexandre.lobo@usj.edu.mo
* Correspondence: pmrodrigues@ucp.pt

Citation: Rodrigues, P.M.; Madeiro, J.P.; Marques, J.A.L. Enhancing Health and Public Health through Machine Learning: Decision Support for Smarter Choices. *Bioengineering* **2023**, *10*, 792. https://doi.org/10.3390/bioengineering10070792

Received: 1 June 2023
Accepted: 29 June 2023
Published: 2 July 2023

In recent years, the integration of Machine Learning (ML) techniques in the field of healthcare and public health has emerged as a powerful tool for improving decision-making processes. The ability of ML algorithms to analyze vast amounts of data, identify patterns, and generate actionable insights has opened new avenues for enhancing various aspects of healthcare delivery and public health initiatives. This Special Issue (SI) explores the applications of ML in health and public health decision support systems, highlighting their potential benefits and challenges, mainly in the following areas:

1. Disease Diagnosis and Prognosis—In this area, ML algorithms can analyze patient data, including medical records, lab results, and imaging scans, to aid in the diagnosis and prognosis of various diseases. By training on large datasets, these algorithms can learn to recognize patterns and make accurate predictions, helping healthcare professionals make informed decisions about treatment plans and interventions. ML models have shown promising results in detecting conditions such as cancer [1], cardiovascular diseases [2], neurological diseases [3], and infectious diseases [4], enabling early detection and timely interventions. In this sub-area of study, the SI contributes with the following studies:

- Mirniaharikandehei et al. [5] explore the feasibility of using a modified deep learning (DL) method for automatically segmenting disease-infected regions and predicting disease severity in computed tomography (CT) images. A dataset from 20 COVID-19 patients has been used, incorporating manually annotated lung and infection masks. An ensemble DL model was trained, combining five customized residual attention U-Net models for disease-infected region segmentation and a Feature Pyramid Network model for disease severity stage prediction. The analysis reveals >90% agreement in disease severity classification between the DL model and radiologists for 45 testing cases.

- Chen et al. [6] explore a noninvasive, cost-effective tool to assess the risk of subclinical renal damage (SRD) in asymptomatic individuals. Using ML algorithms, a risk assessment score model was established based on systolic blood pressure, diastolic blood pressure, and body mass index. The model demonstrated excellent classification ability, with an AUC value of 0.778 for SRD estimation and 0.729 for 4-year SRD risk prediction.

- Zhang et al. [7] investigate the effects of atherosclerotic intracranial internal carotid artery stenosis (IICAS) on extracranial internal carotid artery (ICA) flow velocity waveforms to identify sensitive hemodynamic indices for IICAS diagnoses. Hemodynamic indices, including peak systolic velocity (PSV), end-diastolic velocity (EDV), resistive index (RI), and the first harmonic ratio (FHR), were analyzed in simulations with and without IICAS. In a case-control study with patients having mild-to-moderate IICAS, statistical analyses revealed that the average PSV, EDV, and RI were lower in the stenosis group compared to the control group, but without significant differences ($p > 0.05$), except for the PSV of the right ICA ($p = 0.011$). However, the FHR showed a significantly higher value in the stenosis group compared to the control group ($p < 0.001$), indicating its potential as a superior diagnostic index for early IICAS detection using carotid Doppler ultrasound methods.

- Barnawi et al.'s study [8] proposed a simple and efficient approach for recognizing normal and abnormal phonocardiogram (PCG) signals using Physionet data. The method utilizes data selection techniques like kernel density estimation (KDE) for signal duration extraction, signal-to-noise ratio (SNR), and Gaussian mixture model (GMM) clustering. The authors enhance the performance of 17 pre-trained Keras CNN models through these techniques. The results demonstrate excellent classification performance, achieving an overall accuracy of 97%, sensitivity of 94.6%, precision of 94.4%, and specificity of 94.6% by fine-tuning the VGG19 model after selecting the appropriate signal duration using KDE. This approach holds promise for developing accessible and user-friendly Cardiovascular disease recognition solutions, encouraging regular heart screenings for early detection.

- Ribeiro et al. [9] published a literature review paper about the exploration of the infection mechanism, patient symptoms, and laboratory diagnosis regarding COVID-19. They also assess various technologies and computerized models, such as ECG, voice, and X-ray techniques, used for the accurate detection of COVID-19. The state-of-art literature reported high accuracy rates ranging from 85.70% to 100% for the diagnostic models. Based on these findings, they concluded that the existing models for COVID-19 detection have shown promising results, but there is still potential for improvement considering the diverse symptomatology and evolving understanding of the disease in individuals.

- Battineni et al. [10] published a review paper focused on the use of ML models in the diagnosis of adult-onset dementia disorders. The authors explored the combination of ML algorithms with conventional magnetic resonance imaging (MRI) to enhance diagnostic accuracy. The findings indicate that ML techniques combined with MRI improve the diagnostic accuracy, with reported rates ranging from 73.3% to 99%. Alzheimer's disease and vascular dementia were the most common adult-onset dementia disorders identified. The study concludes that ML should be integrated with conventional MRI techniques to achieve precise and early diagnosis of dementia disorders in older adults.

2. Personalized Medicine—ML techniques facilitate personalized medicine by leveraging patient-specific data to develop tailored treatment strategies. By considering individual characteristics, such as genetics, demographics, lifestyle, and medical history, algorithms can assist in predicting treatment outcomes and recommending optimal interventions [11]. This approach enables healthcare providers to deliver targeted therapies, optimize drug prescriptions, and minimize adverse effects, leading to improved patient outcomes and enhanced healthcare efficiency. This sub-area of study benefits from the contributions of the SI through the following research studies:

- Kim et al. [12] used transfer transformers to identify drug–drug and chemical–protein interactions. They utilized the DDI Extraction-2013 Shared Task and BioCreative ChemProt datasets for extracting drug-related interactions. Two models were proposed: BERTGAT, incorporating a graph attention network for sentence structure, and T5slim_dec, adapting T5's generation task for relation classification. T5slim_dec achieved remarkable performance with 91.15% accuracy on the DDI dataset and 94.29% accuracy for the CPR class group in ChemProt. However, BERTGAT did not significantly improve relation extraction. This highlights the language understanding capability of transformer-based approaches, which can comprehend language effectively without relying on additional structural information.

- The study by Khadem et al. [13] addresses the challenge of accurate blood glucose prediction for diabetes management. They highlight the difficulty in determining the appropriate look-back window length, which affects the availability and relevance of information for decision-making. To overcome this challenge, the researchers propose an interconnected lag fusion framework using nested meta-learning analysis. They apply this framework to Ohio type 1 diabetes datasets and rigorously evaluate the models. The study demonstrates the effectiveness of their proposed method in personalized blood glucose level forecasting, providing valuable insights for informed decisions on insulin dosing, diet, and physical activity in diabetes management.

3. Public Health Surveillance and Outbreak Detection–ML plays a crucial role in public health surveillance systems by analyzing diverse data sources, including social media feeds, internet searches, electronic health records, environmental and bacteriological data [14]. By monitoring and detecting patterns, ML algorithms can identify potential disease outbreaks, track the spread of infectious diseases, and forecast disease trends. These insights enable public health authorities to allocate resources effectively, implement timely interventions, and prevent or mitigate the impact of epidemics. The SI makes a significant contribution to this particular sub-area of study through the inclusion of:

- Rodrigues et al. [15] introduced a hybrid method combining pre-trained CNN keras models and classical ML models to visually discriminate different bacterial colonies based on their morphology on culture media. The system achieved high accuracy rates: 92% for Pseudomonas aeruginosa vs. Staphylococcus aureus, 91% for Escherichia coli vs. Staphylococcus aureus, and 84% for Escherichia coli vs. Pseudomonas aeruginosa.

4. Health Behavior Analysis and Intervention—ML algorithms can analyze large-scale health behavior data to identify risk factors, understand population health trends, and develop targeted interventions. By mining data from wearable devices, mobile apps, and social media platforms, ML models can provide insights into individuals' behaviors, habits, and health outcomes [16]. This information can support the design of personalized interventions, health promotion campaigns, and policy recommendations, empowering individuals to make healthier choices and promoting population-level well-being. The SI actively contributes to this sub-area of study by including the following manuscripts:

- Promsri et al. [17] studied the relationship between walking stability and fall risk markers in older adults. Three-dimensional lower-limb kinematic data from 43 healthy individuals were analyzed using principal component analysis (PCA) to extract principal movements (PMs) representing different components of walking. The largest Lyapunov exponent (LyE) was applied to the PMs as a measure of stability. Fall risk was assessed using the Short Physical Performance Battery (SPPB) and the Gait Subscale of Performance-Oriented Mobility Assessment (POMA-G). Results indicated a negative correlation ($p \leq 0.009$) between SPPB and POMA-G scores and LyE in specific PMs, suggesting that increased walking instability is associated with higher fall risk.
- Gupta et al. study [18] aimed to detect and address stress, which is a significant factor affecting mental health and overall well-being. In this study, a novel approach utilizing audio-visual data processing is proposed to detect human mental stress. By employing the cascaded RNN-LSTM strategy, the study achieved a high accuracy of 91% in classifying emotions and distinguishing between stressed and unstressed states using the RAVDESS dataset.

5. Healthcare Resource Optimization—ML can optimize healthcare resource allocation by predicting patient demand, improving scheduling and resource utilization, and optimizing healthcare facility operations. By analyzing historical data and considering factors such as patient demographics, disease prevalence, and resource availability, ML models can assist in optimizing bed occupancy, staff allocation, and healthcare supply chains [19]. This approach enhances operational efficiency, reduces costs, and improves patient access to timely and appropriate care. Within this sub-area of study, the SI offers the following valuable contribution:

- da Silva et al. [20] proposed a methodology to analyze the performance of measurement systems during the design phase using the Monte Carlo method. The methodology was applied to a simulated ECG, estimating a measurement uncertainty of 3.54% with 95% confidence. The analysis revealed that the preamplifier module had a greater impact on the measurement results compared to the final stage module, suggesting that interventions in the preamplifier module would yield more significant improvements.

To conclude, ML has revolutionized health and public health decision support systems by enabling data-driven insights and informed decision-making. By harnessing the power of ML algorithms, healthcare professionals and public health authorities can improve disease diagnosis and prognosis, personalize treatment strategies, detect outbreaks, analyze health behaviors, and optimize resource allocation. As technology continues to advance, the integration of ML in health and public health applications will play an increasingly significant role in transforming healthcare delivery and improving population health outcomes.

Author Contributions: Conceptualization, P.M.R.; methodology, P.M.R.; validation, P.M.R., J.P.M. and J.A.L.M.; investigation, P.M.R.; writing—original draft preparation, P.M.R.; writing—review and editing, P.M.R., J.P.M. and J.A.L.M. All authors have read and agreed to the published version of the manuscript.

Conflicts of Interest: The authors declare no conflict of interest.

References

1. Kourou, K.; Exarchos, T.P.; Exarchos, K.P.; Karamouzis, M.V.; Fotiadis, D.I. Machine learning applications in cancer prognosis and prediction. *Comput. Struct. Biotechnol. J.* **2015**, *13*, 8–17. [CrossRef] [PubMed]
2. Bhatt, C.M.; Patel, P.; Ghetia, T.; Mazzeo, P.L. Effective Heart Disease Prediction Using Machine Learning Techniques. *Algorithms* **2023**, *16*, 88. [CrossRef]
3. Rodrigues, P.M.; Bispo, B.C.; Garrett, C.; Alves, D.; Teixeira, J.P.; Freitas, D. Lacsogram: A New EEG Tool to Diagnose Alzheimer's Disease. *IEEE J. Biomed. Health Inform.* **2021**, *25*, 3384–3395. [CrossRef] [PubMed]
4. Santangelo, O.E.; Gentile, V.; Pizzo, S.; Giordano, D.; Cedrone, F. Machine Learning and Prediction of Infectious Diseases: A Systematic Review. *Mach. Learn. Knowl. Extr.* **2023**, *5*, 175–198. [CrossRef]
5. Mirniaharikandehei, S.; Abdihamzehkolaei, A.; Choquehuanca, A.; Aedo, M.; Pacheco, W.; Estacio, L.; Cahui, V.; Huallpa, L.; Quiñonez, K.; Calderón, V.; et al. Automated Quantification of Pneumonia Infected Volume in Lung CT Images: A Comparison with Subjective Assessment of Radiologists. *Bioengineering* **2023**, *10*, 321. [CrossRef] [PubMed]
6. Chen, C.; Liu, G.; Chu, C.; Zheng, W.; Ma, Q.; Liao, Y.; Yan, Y.; Sun, Y.; Wang, D.; Mu, J. A Novel and Noninvasive Risk Assessment Score and Its Child-to-Adult Trajectories to Screen Subclinical Renal Damage in Middle Age. *Bioengineering* **2023**, *10*, 257. [CrossRef] [PubMed]
7. Zhang, X.; Wu, D.; Li, H.; Fang, Y.; Xiong, H.; Li, Y. Early Diagnosis of Intracranial Internal Carotid Artery Stenosis Using Extracranial Hemodynamic Indices from Carotid Doppler Ultrasound. *Bioengineering* **2022**, *9*, 422. [CrossRef] [PubMed]
8. Barnawi, A.; Boulares, M.; Somai, R. Simple and Powerful PCG Classification Method Based on Selection and Transfer Learning for Precision Medicine Application. *Bioengineering* **2023**, *10*, 294. [CrossRef] [PubMed]
9. Ribeiro, P.; Marques, J.A.L.; Rodrigues, P.M. COVID-19 Detection by Means of ECG, Voice, and X-ray Computerized Systems: A Review. *Bioengineering* **2023**, *10*, 198. [CrossRef] [PubMed]
10. Battineni, G.; Chintalapudi, N.; Hossain, M.A.; Losco, G.; Ruocco, C.; Sagaro, G.G.; Traini, E.; Nittari, G.; Amenta, F. Artificial Intelligence Models in the Diagnosis of Adult-Onset Dementia Disorders: A Review. *Bioengineering* **2022**, *9*, 370. [CrossRef] [PubMed]
11. Sebastiani, M.; Vacchi, C.; Manfredi, A.; Cassone, G. Personalized Medicine and Machine Learning: A Roadmap for the Future. *J. Clin. Med.* **2022**, *11*, 4110. [CrossRef] [PubMed]

12. Kim, S.; Yoon, J.; Kwon, O. Biomedical Relation Extraction Using Dependency Graph and Decoder-Enhanced Transformer Model. *Bioengineering* **2023**, *10*, 586. [CrossRef] [PubMed]
13. Khadem, H.; Nemat, H.; Elliott, J.; Benaissa, M. Blood Glucose Level Time Series Forecasting: Nested Deep Ensemble Learning Lag Fusion. *Bioengineering* **2023**, *10*, 487. [CrossRef] [PubMed]
14. Zeng, D.; Cao, Z.; Neill, D.B. Chapter 22—Artificial intelligence–enabled public health surveillance—From local detection to global epidemic monitoring and control. In *Artificial Intelligence in Medicine*; Xing, L., Giger, M.L., Min, J.K., Eds.; Academic Press: Cambridge, MA, USA , 2021; pp. 437–453. [CrossRef]
15. Rodrigues, P.M.; Ribeiro, P.; Tavaria, F.K. Distinction of Different Colony Types by a Smart-Data-Driven Tool. *Bioengineering* **2022**, *10*, 26. [CrossRef] [PubMed]
16. Goh, Y.S.; Ow Yong, J.Q.Y.; Chee, B.Q.H.; Kuek, J.H.L.; Ho, C.S.H. Machine Learning in Health Promotion and Behavioral Change: Scoping Review. *J. Med. Internet Res.* **2022**, *24*, e35831. [CrossRef] [PubMed]
17. Promsri, A.; Cholamjiak, P.; Federolf, P. Walking Stability and Risk of Falls. *Bioengineering* **2023**, *10*, 471. [CrossRef] [PubMed]
18. Gupta, M.V.; Vaikole, S.; Oza, A.D.; Patel, A.; Burduhos-Nergis, D.P.; Burduhos-Nergis, D.D. Audio-Visual Stress Classification Using Cascaded RNN-LSTM Networks. *Bioengineering* **2022**, *9*, 510. [CrossRef] [PubMed]
19. Tawhid, A.; Teotia, T.; Elmiligi, H. Chapter 13—Machine learning for optimizing healthcare resources. In *Machine Learning, Big Data, and IoT for Medical Informatics*; Kumar, P., Kumar, Y., Tawhid, M.A., Eds.; Intelligent Data-Centric Systems; Academic Press: Cambridge, MA, USA, 2021; pp. 215–239. [CrossRef]
20. da Silva, J.H.B.; Cortez, P.C.; Jagatheesaperumal, S.K.; de Albuquerque, V.H.C. ECG Measurement Uncertainty Based on Monte Carlo Approach: An Effective Analysis for a Successful Cardiac Health Monitoring System. *Bioengineering* **2023**, *10*, 115. [CrossRef] [PubMed]

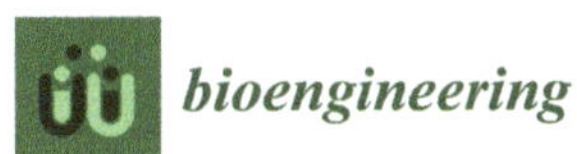 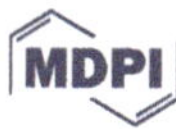

Article

Biomedical Relation Extraction Using Dependency Graph and Decoder-Enhanced Transformer Model

Seonho Kim [1], Juntae Yoon [2,*] and Ohyoung Kwon [3,*]

[1]   Department of Computer Science and Engineering, Sogang University, Seoul 04107, Republic of Korea; shkim.lex@gmail.com

[2]   VAIV Company, Seoul 04107, Republic of Korea

[3]   Department of Future Technology, Korea University of Technology and Education, Cheonan-si 31253, Republic of Korea

*   Correspondence: jtyoon@vaiv.kr (J.Y.); oykwon@koreatech.ac.kr (O.K.)

Abstract: The identification of drug–drug and chemical–protein interactions is essential for understanding unpredictable changes in the pharmacological effects of drugs and mechanisms of diseases and developing therapeutic drugs. In this study, we extract drug-related interactions from the DDI (Drug–Drug Interaction) Extraction-2013 Shared Task dataset and the BioCreative ChemProt (Chemical–Protein) dataset using various transfer transformers. We propose $BERT_{GAT}$ that uses a graph attention network (GAT) to take into account the local structure of sentences and embedding features of nodes under the self-attention scheme and investigate whether incorporating syntactic structure can help relation extraction. In addition, we suggest $T5_{slim\_dec}$, which adapts the autoregressive generation task of the T5 (text-to-text transfer transformer) to the relation classification problem by removing the self-attention layer in the decoder block. Furthermore, we evaluated the potential of biomedical relation extraction of GPT-3 (Generative Pre-trained Transformer) using GPT-3 variant models. As a result, $T5_{slim\_dec}$, which is a model with a tailored decoder designed for classification problems within the T5 architecture, demonstrated very promising performances for both tasks. We achieved an accuracy of 91.15% in the DDI dataset and an accuracy of 94.29% for the CPR (Chemical–Protein Relation) class group in ChemProt dataset. However, $BERT_{GAT}$ did not show a significant performance improvement in the aspect of relation extraction. We demonstrated that transformer-based approaches focused only on relationships between words are implicitly eligible to understand language well without additional knowledge such as structural information.

Keywords: DDI (drug–drug interaction); CPR (chemical–protein relation); transformer; self-attention; GAT (graph-attention network); relation extraction; ChemProt; T5 (text-to-text transfer transformer)

Citation: Kim, S.; Yoon, J.; Kwon, O. Biomedical Relation Extraction Using Dependency Graph and Decoder-Enhanced Transformer Model. *Bioengineering* **2023**, *10*, 586. https://doi.org/10.3390/bioengineering10050586

Academic Editors: Pedro Miguel Rodrigues, João Alexandre Lobo Marques and João Paulo do Vale Madeiro

Received: 1 March 2023
Revised: 6 May 2023
Accepted: 9 May 2023
Published: 12 May 2023

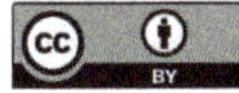

1. Introduction

With the rapid progress in biomedical studies, it is a very challenging issue to extract efficiently useful information described in the biomedical literature. According to LitCOVID [1], over 1000 articles were published in just three months from December 2019, when COVID-19 was first reported, to March 2020. In PubMed [2] which is a biomedical literature retrieval system, more than 35 million biomedical articles are included. Therefore, life science researchers cannot keep up with all journals relevant to their areas of interest and select useful information from the latest research. In order to manage biomedical knowledge, curated databases such as UniProt [3], DrugBank [4], CTD [5], and IUPHAR/BPS [6] are constantly being updated. However, updating or developing a database manually can be time-consuming and labor-intensive work, and the speed is often slow, which makes automatic knowledge extraction and mining from biomedical literature highly demanding. Consequently, many pieces of valuable information with complex relationships between entities still remain unstructured and hidden in raw text.

Recently, AI algorithms have been used to analyze complex forms of medical and life science data to assist human knowledge or to develop protocols for disease prevention and treatment. Moreover, deep learning techniques have been actively applied to various biomedical fields such as drug and personalized medicine development, clinical decision support systems, patient monitoring, and interaction extraction between biomedical entities. For example, protein–protein interaction in biomedical entities are very crucial for understanding various human life phenomena and diseases. Many biochemistry studies go beyond the molecular level of individual genes and focus on the networks and signaling pathways that connect groups or individuals that interact with each other. Similarly, interest in the integration and curation of relationships between biological and drug/chemical entities from text is increasing.

One of valuable information of drugs and chemical compounds is how they interact with certain biomedical entities, in particular genes and proteins. As mentioned in the study [1], metabolic relations are related to construction/curation of metabolic pathways and drug metabolism such as drug–drug interaction and adverse reactions. Inhibitor/activator associations are related to drug design and system biology approaches. Antagonist and agonist interactions helps in drug design, drug discovery, and understanding mechanism of actions. Drug–drug interaction (DDI) can be defined as a change in the effects of one drug by the presence of another drug. Since such information prevents dangers or side-effects caused by drugs, it is also important to extract useful knowledge from pharmaceutical papers.

Compared to other fields, texts of biomedical publications are more easily accessible due to the publicly available database MEDLINE [7] and the search system PubMed [2] However, the complexity and ambiguity in biomedical text are much greater than those of general text. One of characteristics of biomedical text is that multiple biomedical entities appear within a single sentence and one entity may be interacted with multiple entities. In particular, it is very difficult to infer which pairs contain actual relations because all entities in a single sentence share the same context, as shown in Figures 1 and 2. In this work, the relation extraction is simplified as classification task, where the problem is to classify which interaction exists between the given pre-recognized entities at sentence level.

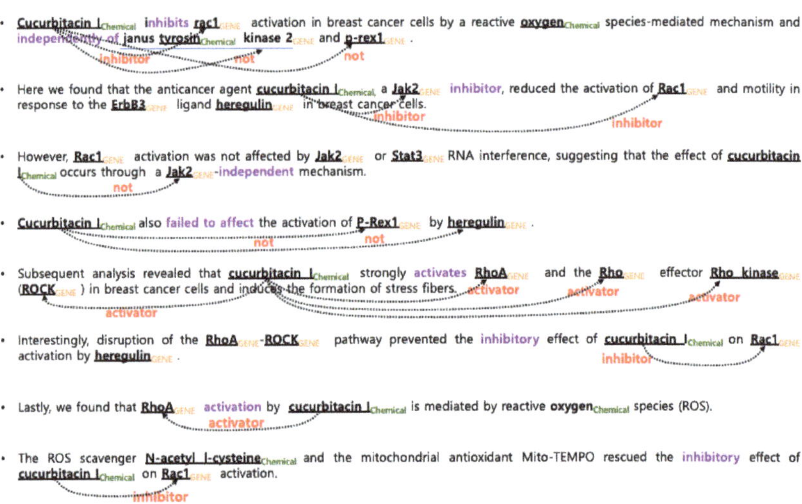

Figure 1. Examples of ChemProt interactions.

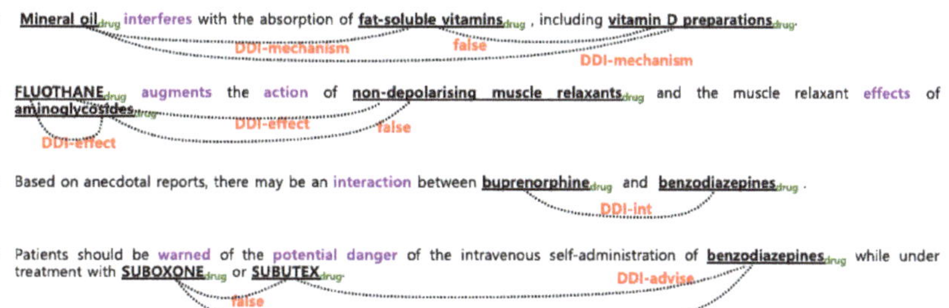

Figure 2. Examples of SemEval13 DDI interactions.

The main objectives of this study are as follows: (1) we apply transfer transformer learning models, which have made impressive performances and progresses in recent years across a wider range of NLP tasks, to the detection of drug-related interactions in biomedical text, and aim to demonstrate which models are effective in biomedical relation extraction. The transformers generate abstract contextual representations of tokens very well by incorporating inter-relations of all tokens in a sequence with the concept of self-attention. As baseline models, three different dominant types of transformers: encoder-only model such as Google's BERT (Bidirectional Encoder Representations from Transformers) [8], decoder-only model such as OpenAI's GPT-3 (Generative Pre-trained Transformer) [9], and encoder–decoder structure of Google's T5 (Text-To-Text Transfer Transformer) [10] are chosen to establish a performance benchmark for our proposed methods. All experiments are conducted using ChemProt corpus [11] and DDI corpus [12] which are a collection of text documents that contains information about chemical/drug–protein/gene interactions and drug–drug interactions, respectively.

(2) The second objective of this study is to investigate the effects of syntactic structure of sentences on biomedical relation extraction by incorporating dependencies between words to enhance self-attention mechanism. According to previous studies, syntactic clues such as grammatical dependencies of a sentence help relation extraction. Some studies [13] have demonstrated that removing tokens outside the subtree rooted at the lowest common ancestor of the two entities or SDP (shortest dependency path) word sequence between two entities from the parse tree can improve relation extraction performance by eliminating irrelevant information from the sentence. However, this simplified representation by considering only the SDP word sequence may fail to capture contextual information, such as the presence of negation, which could be crucial for relation extraction [14].

In this work, we propose BERT$_{GAT}$, a newly developed structure-enhanced encoding model that combines the graph-attention network (GAT) [15] with BERT. We investigate its effectiveness on relation extraction by taking into account not only word token information but also grammatical relevance between words within the attention scheme. To incorporate syntactic information, each dependency tree structure is converted into corresponding adjacency matrix. The GAT model uses an attention mechanism to calculate the importance of words within the input graph. This can allow for the extraction of more relevant information.

(3) Finally, we tailor T5, the encode–decoder transformer which has demonstrated high performances in text generation task, to efficiently handle discriminative, non-autoregressive tasks such as our relation classification problem. Since T5 transformer is designed for text-to-text tasks such as text generation and machine translation, the decoder generates output tokens autoregressively based on previous tokens. This can be less efficient for classification tasks where a single label or output is required. Consequently, decoder's role is not much in classification tasks. We suggest T5$_{slim_dec}$, which determines the interaction category by removing the self-attention block of T5's decoder input.

The rest of the paper is organized as follows. In Section 2, related works in the field of biomedical relation extraction is presented. Section 3 briefly describes the dataset and provides necessary background information about transformers to help readers better understand the rest of the paper. Section 4 introduces the baseline models and proposed approaches in detail. Data statistics, results, and analysis are discussed in Section 5, along with comparisons with state of the art approaches and limitations. Finally, conclusions and outlooks are reported in Section 6.

2. Related Works

In the DDI (drug–drug interaction) extraction task [12], traditional deep-learning systems, such as convolutional neural networks (CNNs) [16] and recurrent neural networks (RNNs) [17] have shown better performances than feature-based approaches. Recently, the transformer-based models including BERT [8], RoBERTa [18], MASS [19], BART [20], MT-DNN [21], GPT-3 [9], and T5 [10] have demonstrated remarkable improvement in performance across various NLP (Natural Language Processing) tasks by obtaining contextualized token representation through a self-supervised learning on a large-scale raw text such as masked language model. The transformer model is originated from the "Attention Is All You Need" paper [22] researched by Google Brain and Google Research. They also attempted the transfer learning which the weights pretrained on a large-scale text dataset for a specific task such as masked language modeling, next sentence prediction or next token prediction were applied to downstream task by fine-tuning the pretrained models on the downstream task. As a result, pretrained language models tend to perform better than learning new knowledge from scratch with no prior knowledge because they utilize previously learned results.

The pretraining on large-scale raw texts has also significantly improved performance in biomedical domain. BERT based on encoder structure and its variants such as SCIBERT [23], BioBERT [24], and PubMedBERT [25] have been successfully applied in biomedical field. Since previous methods consider only the context around entities in the text, some research has encoded various knowledge besides input tokens, resulting in more informative input representations for downstream tasks [26,27].

Asada et al. [26] explored the impact of incorporating drug-related heterogeneous information on DDI extraction, and achieved an F-score of 85.40. They reported it as state-of-the-art performance. They constructed a HKG (heterogeneous knowledge graph) embedding vectors of drugs by performing a link prediction task which predicts an entity, t, that forms triple (h, r, t) for a given entity, h and relation pair, r on the PharmaHKG dataset. The dataset contains graph information: six nodes (entities), i.e., drug, protein, pathway, category, and ATC (Anatomical Therapeutic Chemical) code, molecular structure from different databases/thesauruses and eight edges (relations): category, ATC, pathway, interact, target, enzyme, carrier, and transporter. The input sentence S was tokenized into sub-word tokens by the BERT tokenizer and extended by adding KG vectors of two drugs. Thus, the input sentence is represented with {[CLS], $w_1, \ldots w_{m1}, \ldots, w_{m2}, \ldots$; [SEP], $[KG_{m1}] [KG_{m2}]$}, where w_i corresponds to subword and m_1, to $drug_1$ and m_2, to $drug_2$, and $[KG_{m1}]$ and $[KG_{m2}]$ represent knowledge embeddings for each drug entity.

Similarly, Zhu et al. [28] utilized drug descriptions from Wikipedia and DrugBank to enhance the BERT model with the semantic information of drug entities. They used three kinds of entity-aware attentions to get sentence representation with entity information, mutual drug entity information, and drug entity information. The mutual information vector of two drug entities was obtained by subtracting the BioBERT embeddings of two drugs. For drug description information, all drug description documents were fed into Doc2Vec model and obtained its vector representations for each drug entity appearing in the 2013 DDI corpus. The vectors for entity information were fed into attention layers and retrieve sentence representation vectors integrating entity's multiple information. They reported 80.9 (micro F1-score) on DDI corpus.

LinkBERT [29] used hyperlinks to create better context for learning general-purpose LMs (language model). The hyperlink can offer new, multi-hop knowledge, which is not available in the single article alone. It creates inputs by placing linked documents in the same context window. They joined the segments of two different documents on BERT via special tokens to form an input instance: [CLS] X_A [SEP] X_B [SEP], where X_A segment belongs to document A and X_B segment belongs to document B. They used the Document Relation Prediction (DPR) objective for pretraining, which classifies the relation of two segments X_B to X_A as contiguous (X_B is direct continuation of X_A), random, and linked. They achieved a performance of 83.35 (micro F1-score) on DDI classification task. SciFive [30] and T5-MTFT [31] pretrained on biomedical text using T5 architecture also showed good performance in relation extraction. In particular, SciFive was pretrained on PubMed abstracts and outperformed other encoder-only models.

3. Preliminaries

3.1. Data Sets and Target Relations

The evaluation of transformers is conducted on two datasets, namely ChemProt [11] and DDI [12] which are used for RE (relation extraction) between drug-related entities. This paper is not intended to validate different RE methods across various datasets, but rather than focuses on extraction of drug-related interactions and perform a more in-depth evaluation.

In ChemProt track corpus in BioCreative VI, interactions are annotated to explore recognition of chemical–protein relations from abstracts, as shown in Table 1. The corpus contains directed relations from chemical/drug to gene/protein, indicating how the chemical/drug interacts with the gene/protein. Chemical–protein relations, referred to as 'CPR', are categorized into 10 semantically related classes that share some underlying biological characteristics. For instance, the interactions such as "activator", "indirect upregulator" and "upregulator", which result in an increase in the activity or expression of a target gene or protein, belong to CPR:3 group. The interactions such as "downregulator", "indirect downregulator", and "inhibitor" interactions which all decrease the activity or expression of a target gene or protein, belong to CPR:4. For this task, chemical and protein/gene entity mentions were manually annotated. In the track, only relations belonging to the following five classes were considered for evaluation purposes: CPR:3, CPR:4, CPR:5, CPR:6, and CPR:9.

Table 1. Interaction classes of ChemProt Corpus.

Class Group	ChemProt Relations	Semantic Meaning
CPR:0	UNDEFINED	
CPR:1	PART-OF	Part-of
CPR:2	DIRECT-REGULATOR, INDIRECT-REGULATOR, REGULATOR	Regulator
CPR:3	ACTIVATOR, INDIRECT-UPREGULATOR, UPREGULATOR	Upregulator or activator
CPR:4	DOWNREGULATOR, INDIRECT-DOWNREGULATOR, INHIBITOR	Downregulator or inhibitor
CPR:5	AGONIST, AGONIST-ACTIVATOR, AGONIST-INHIBITOR	Agonist
CPR:6	ANTAGONIST	Antagonist
CPR:7	MODULATOR, MODULATOR-ACTIVATOR, MODULATOR-INHIBITOR	Modulator
CPR:8	COFACTOR	Cofactor
CPR:9	SUBSTRATE, SUBSTRATE_PRODUCT-OF, PRODUCT-OF	Substrate or product-of
CPR:10	NOT	Not

In the DDIExtraction 2013 shared task, five types of interactions are annotated, as shown in Table 2. The false pairs, which are drug pairs that do not interact, were excluded in the evaluation to simplify the evaluation and enable better comparability between systems in the shared task. Tables 3 and 4 display the number of instances for each class.

Figures 1 and 2 illustrate examples of interactions in ChemProt and DDI, respectively. For example, the first sentence in Figure 2 states that 'mineral oil' and 'fat-soluble vitamins' have a DDI-mechanism relationship, while there is no interaction (false) between 'fat-soluble vitamin' and 'vitamin d preparations'. The interaction between 'mineral oil' and 'vitamin d preparation' is a DDI-mechanism. Since three interactions appear in one sentence, when creating instances, separators such as ** (## and ** for ChemProt) are added before and after the target entities to indicate the desired interaction pair.

Table 2. Interaction classes of DDI 2013 Corpus.

Relation Class	Semantic Meaning
DDI-Mechanism	a pharmacokinetic interaction mechanism is described in a sentence
DDI-Effect	the effect of an interaction is described in a sentence
DDI-Advice	a recommendation or advice regarding the concomitant use of two drugs is described in an input sentence
DDI-Int	the sentence mentions that interaction occurs and does not provide any detailed information about the interaction
DDI-False	non-interacting entities

Table 3. The instances of the ChemProt corpus.

Dataset	CPR:0	CPR:1	CPR:2	CPR:3	CPR:4	CPR:5	CPR:6	CPR:7	CPR:8	CPR:9	CPR:10
train	0	550	1656	784	2278	173	235	29	34	727	242
dev	1	328	780	552	1103	116	199	19	2	457	175
test	2	482	1743	667	1667	198	293	25	25	644	267

Table 4. The instances of the DDI extraction 2013 corpus.

Corpus	Advice	Effect	Mechanism	Int	False
train	826	1687	1319	188	15842
test	218	356	302	96	4782

3.2. Transformer and Attention

Before explaining our transformer approaches, we will first introduce the concept of the transformer model and attention. The transformer was designed for sequence-to-sequence tasks. It uses stacked self-attentions to encode contextual information of input sequence. Attention is a mechanism which enables a model to focus on relevant parts of the input sequence to enhance the meaning of the word of interest [32]. The inputs to the transformer model are word embedding vectors. The model weighs these vectors according to their neighboring context within the sentence. For example, in the sentence, "He swam across the river to the other bank", the word, 'bank' has a contextualized vector which is closer to the meaning of 'sloping raised land' rather than 'a financial institution' by focusing on the words "swam" and "river".

The attention provides contextualized representation for each word and captures relatedness between other words occurred in the sequence. BERT processes input tokens through transformer encoder blocks and returns a hidden state vector for each token. These hidden state vectors encapsulate information about each input token and the context of the entire sequence.

The attention score, as represented by Equation (1), is computed after creating a query(Q_i), key(K_i), and value(V_i) embedding vector for each token in a sentence. The calculation involves three parts: (1) computing the attention score between query and key using a dot-product similarity function, (2) normalizing the attention score using softmax, and (3) weighting the original word vectors according to surrounding context using the normalized attention weights.

$$Q_i = QW_i^Q, K_i = KW_i^K, V_i = VW_i^V$$

$$head_i = Attention(Q_i, K_i, V_i) = softmax\left(\frac{Q_i K_i^T}{\sqrt{d_k}}\right) V_i$$

$$softmax(s_i) = \frac{e^{s_j}}{\sum_{j=1}^{n} e^{s_j}}$$

$$Multi_{head(Q,K,V)} = Concat(head_1, head_2, \ldots, head_h) W^O$$

(1)

In Equation (1), d_k is the dimension of query/key/value and n is the sequence length. The matrix multiplication QK^T computes the dot product for every possible pair of queries and keys. If two token vectors are close (similar) to each other, their dot product is going to be big. The shape of each matrix is $n \times n$, where each row represents the attention score between a specific token and all other tokens in the sequence. The softmax and multiplication with value matrices represents a weighted mean and $\sqrt{d_k}$ is a scaling factor. With multi-headed self-attention, multiple sets of $Q/K/V$ weight matrices are used to reflect different representation of the input sequence.

As a result, the attention operation helps focus more on the values associated with keys that have higher similarities and capture important contextual information in the sequence. It produces a contextualized representation of the whole sequence and can be interpreted as connection weights between each word token and all other words in a given sequence. Figure 3 shows how to compute multi-head self-attention for an example sentence: "concomitant administration of other @DRUG$ may potentiate the undesirable effect of @DRUG$." In the case, "concomitant" might be highly associated with "administration" by the self-attention. The outputs of the attention mechanism are concatenated before being further processed and fed to a FFNN (feed-forward neural network). The transformer encoder takes the input sequence and maps it into a representational space. It generates d_{embed}-dimensional vector representation for each position of the input, as shown in Figure 3, which is then sent to the decoder.

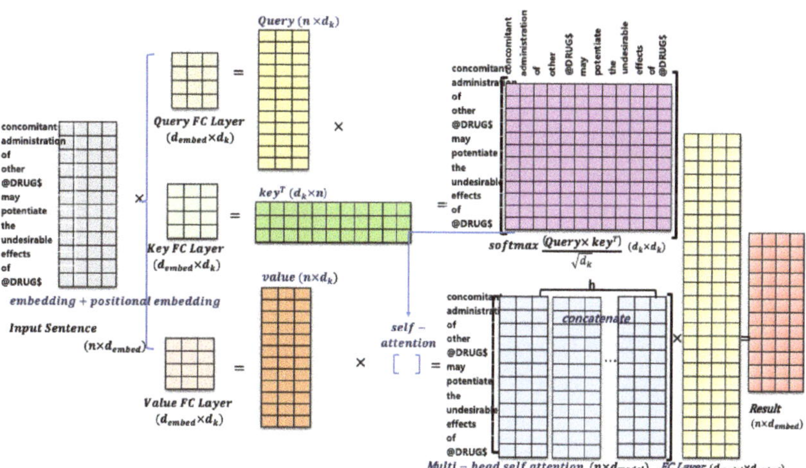

Figure 3. Visualization of multi-head self-attention for an example sentence.

In addition to word embedding, transformer also employs positional embedding to represent a token's positional information. This allows for parallel processing with causal masking, which restricts the use of future information during training by masking future tokens that appears after the current position in the input. The positional embedding vector to each input token can be easily computed using sine and cosine functions with Equation (2), where d_{model} represents the dimension of the input embedding vector.

The transformer consists of a stacked encoder and decoder, both of which are built with two sublayers: multi-head self-attention layers as mentioned earlier and fully connected

FFN (FeedForward Neural Network) layers. The FFN consists of two linear transformations with the ReLU (Rectified Linear Unit) activation as shown in Equation (3). To prevent the model from losing important features of input data during training, residual connections, as shown in Equation (4), are employed around each of the sub-layers, followed by layer normalization:

$$PE_{(pos,2i)} = \sin\left(\frac{pos}{10000^{\frac{2i}{d_{model}}}}\right), PE_{(pos,2i+1)} = \cos\left(\frac{pos}{10000^{\frac{2i}{d_{model}}}}\right) \tag{2}$$

$$FFN(x) = \max(0, xW1 + b1)W2 + b2 \tag{3}$$

$$LayerNorm(x + Sublayer(x)) \tag{4}$$

Besides the two sub-layers, the decoder has an additional sublayer called multi-head cross attentions, which considers the relationship between the output of the encoder and the input of the decoder. The output of the encoder is transformed into a set of K and V vectors and utilized in the cross-attention. The cross attention adopts Q matrix from the self-attention layer of decoder and K and V matrix from the encoder, respectively. Unlike its operation in the encoder, the self-attention layer in the decoder is modified to prevent positions from attending to subsequent positions by masking. This masking ensures that the predictions for position i can depend only on the known outputs at positions less than i.

In practice, the encoder maps an input sequence to a sequence of continuous contextual representation. Given the input representation, the decoder auto-regressively generates an output sequence, one element at a time, using the previously generated elements as additional input when generating the next.

4. Methods

In this section, we first describe three transformers used as baseline models and introduce proposed models, BERT$_{GAT}$ and T5$_{slim_dec}$ for relation extraction.

4.1. Baseline Methods

As baseline models for our research on interaction extraction, we employed three types of transformer: BERT (encoder-only) [8], GPT3 (decoder-only) [9], and T5 (encoder–decoder) [10]. First, BERT is bidirectional transformer which uses only encoder block of the transformer. For a detailed structure and implementation, please refer to the study [22]. BERT is pretrained on two unsupervised tasks: (1) masked language model (MLM), where some of the input tokens are randomly masked and the model is trained to predict the masked tokens and (2) next sentence prediction (NSP), where the model is trained to predict whether one sentence follows another, as shown in Figure 4. It uses WordPiece tokenizer and has a special classification token '[CLS]' in the first token of every sequence which corresponds to the aggregated whole sequence representation.

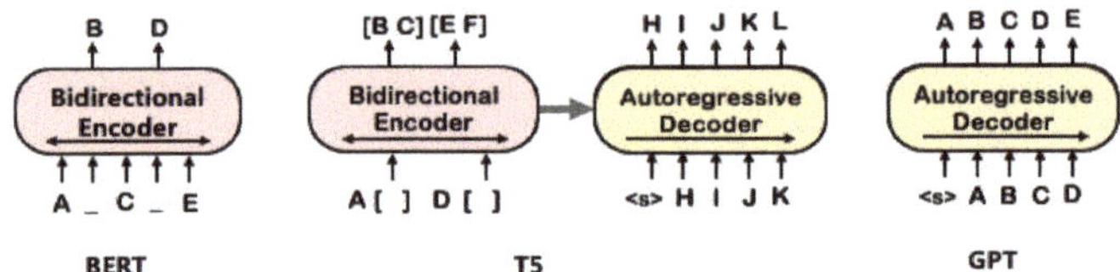

Figure 4. Pretraining methods of transformers.

We initialized the model with SCIBERT [23] for drug-related relationship extraction in order to leverage the domain specific knowledge and then fine-tuned all of the parameters using labeled ChemProt and DDI dataset. SCIBERT has the same architecture as BERT but was pretrained on scientific texts, which consist of 1.14 million papers from the computer science domain (18%) and the broad biomedical domain (82%), sourced from Semantic Scholar [33]. In addition, in-domain WordPiece vocabulary on the scientific corpus was newly constructed. Ultimately, we fed the special '[CLS]' token vector of the final hidden layer into a linear classification layer with softmax output to classify the interaction types.

Secondly, we employed the text-to-text transfer transformer (T5) [10], which is an encoder–decoder model. In the research, the authors experimented with various types of transformers and demonstrated that the encoder–decoder transformer architecture, combined with the denoising (masked language modeling) objective, yielded the best performance for most NLP tasks. T5 was pretrained with self-supervision through a learning objective called span-based language masking, in which a set of consecutive tokens are masked with sentinel tokens and the target sequence is predicted as a concatenation of the real masked spans, as shown in Figure 5. The tokens for pretraining were randomly sampled, and dropped out 15% of tokens in the input sequence. It used SentencePiece tokenizer [34] to encode text.

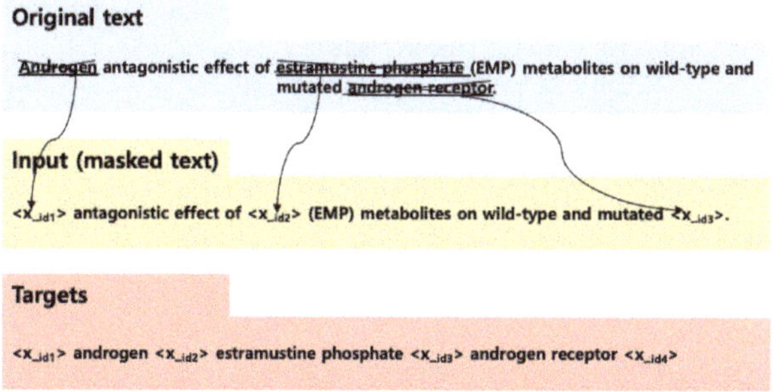

Figure 5. T5's pretraining scheme.

In general, encoder-only model such as BERT are easily applicable to classification or prediction tasks by using the '[CLS]' token, which provides a summary representation of the entire input sentence. On the contrary, T5 treats every text processing problem into a text-to-text generation problem that takes text as input and produce new text as output. Therefore, our relation classification problem is treated as a generation task for interaction types. Initially, we used the pretrained parameters of the SciFive [30] model and then finetuned it on our specific dataset in relation extraction tasks. The SciFive model was retrained on various text combination, which consisted of the C4 corpus [35], PubMed abstracts, and PMC full-text articles, to optimize the pretrained weights from T5 in the context of biomedical literature. Consistent with the original T5 model [10], SciFive learned to generate a target text sequence for a given text input sequence using a learning objective known as span-based mask language modeling. The output sequence is generated during the decoding phase by applying beam search algorithm. This involves maintaining the top n probable output sequences at each timestep and finally generating the output sequence with the highest probability.

Finally, we employed GPT-3 (Generative Pretrained Transformer) [9] which utilizes constrained self-attention where every token can only attend to its left context. As a decoder-only transformer, it was pretrained on a diverse range of web text to predict the next token in an autoregressive manner given the preceding text. It can generate words only conditioned on the left context, so it cannot learn bidirectional interactions.

Previous pretrained models have a limitation in that they need additional large, labeled datasets for a task-specific fine-tuning process to achieve desirable performance. Thus, GPT2 was designed as a general language model for various NLP tasks without the need for extensive fine-tuning. It is capable of performing downstream tasks with little or no fine-tuning, including zero-shot and few-shot learning scenarios, where only a few labeled examples are available for fine-tuning. However, the results were not satisfactory in some tasks. They still need fine-tuning on task-specific labeled data to improve the performance.

In contrast, GPT-3 increased the capacity of transfer language models to 175 billion parameters, thereby allowing the model to utilize its language skills to comprehend tasks with a few examples or natural language instructions. GPT-3 has demonstrated strong performance across a wide range of downstream tasks with a meta-learning technique called 'in-context learning', which allows a language model to develop a broad set of skills and policies for tasks and pattern recognition abilities during unsupervised pretraining. This enables the model to rapidly adapt to a desired task during inference time. Its large-scale, autoregressive language model trained on a massive amount of text data has a deep understanding of the rich context of language and enables the model to generate text, which is similar to human writing.

To achieve this, example sequences for various tasks are used as text input to the pretrained model. For instance, sequences for addition can provide a context for performing arithmetic addition, while error correction sequences can demonstrate how to correct spelling mistakes. Given the context, the model can learn how to perform the intended task and utilize the language skills learned during the pretraining phase.

Recently, OpenAI announced ChatGPT (GPT-3.5) and GPT-4, generative AI models based on reinforcement learning from human feedback (RLHF) and ultra-language models, which have shown very impressive results in generating responses. In this paper, we partially evaluated the potential of GPT-3 on relation extraction using GPT-Neo 125 M and GPT-Neo1.3B models [36] which are dense autoregressive transformer-based language models with 125 M and 1.3 billion parameters trained on 8 million web pages.

4.2. Self-Attention Using Dependency Graph: BERT$_{GAT}$

In this section, we describe BERT$_{GAT}$ to encode the syntactic structure with graph-attention network (GAT) [15]. It leverages the overall graph structure to learn complex relationships between entities, enabling the classification of various types of relationships. In general, dependency trees provide a rich structure to be exploited in relation extraction. Parse trees can have varying structures depending on the input sentences, which may differ in terms of length, complexity, and syntactic construction. Thus, organizing these trees into a fixed-size batch can be difficult. Unlike linear sequences, where tokens can be easily aligned and padded, the hierarchical structure of parse trees complicates this process. In sequence models, padding is used to create equal-length inputs for efficient batch processing. However, for parse trees, padding is not straightforward, as it involves adding artificial tree nodes that might disrupt the tree's structure and introduce noise to the model. Due to these difficulties, it is usually hard to parallelize neural models working on parse trees.

On the contrary, models based on the SDP (shortest dependency path) between two entities are computationally more efficient, but they might exclude crucial information by removing tokens outside the path. In addition, some studies stated that not all tokens in the dependency tree are needed to express the relation of the target entity pair. They have utilized SDP [37] or subtree rooted at the lowest common ancestor (LCA) of the two entities [14] to remove irrelevant information. However, SDP can lead to loss of crucial information and easily hurt robustness. For instance, according to the research by Zhang et al. [14], in the sentence "She was diagnosed with cancer last year, and succumbed this June", the dependency path 'She←diagnosed→cancer' is not sufficient to establish that cancer is the cause of death for the subject unless the conjunction dependency to succumbed is also present. In order to incorporate crucial information off the dependency path, they proposed a path-centric pruning strategy to keep nodes that are directly attached to the dependency path.

To address the issue, we here adapt the graph attention network to consider syntactic dependency tree structure by converting each tree into corresponding adjacency matrix. The graph attention [15] is jointly considered in self-attention sublayer to encode the dependency structure between tokens into vector representations. That helps to capture relevant local structures of dependency edge patterns that are informative for classifying relations by considering the relationships between each node and its neighbors, assigning greater weights to more important neighboring nodes. This approach allows for more effective learning of node representations of graph data, ultimately helping to represent node features more accurately.

For this, the Stanford dependency parser [38] is utilized to retrieve universal dependencies for each sentence. A dependency tree is a type of directed graph where nodes correspond to words and edges indicate the syntactic relations between the head and dependent words. In this work, if there is a dependency between node i and node j, then its opposite direction of dependency, node j and node i is also included. The dependency types of edge such as 'subj' and 'obj' are not considered. A self-loop is also considered for each node in the tree. Since BERT takes as subword units generated by tokenizer instead of word-based linguistic tokens of a parse tree, we introduce additional edges to handle unit differences. Figure 6a shows the architecture of BERT$_{\text{GAT}}$.

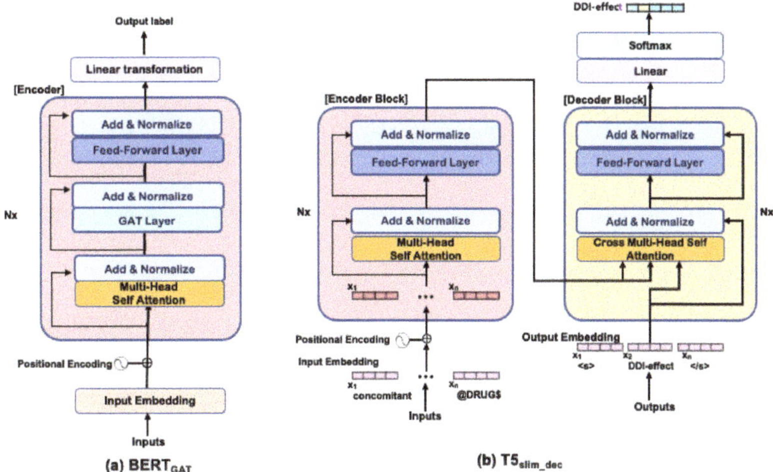

Figure 6. BERT$_{\text{GAT}}$ and T5$_{\text{slim_dec}}$ architecture.

Given a graph with n nodes, we can represent the graph with an $n \times n$ adjacency matrix A, where A_{ij} is 1 if there is a direct edge going from node i to node j. The encoder consists of two sublayers: multi-head self-attention layer and multi-head self-graph attention layer. The final hidden layer of the encoder is fed into a linear classification layer to predict a relation type, which is followed by a softmax operation. That is, the output layer is one-layer task-specific feed-forward network for relation classification.

The output of the BERT model is a contextualized representation for each word in the given text, which is expressed as the hidden state vector of each word. This output vector contains contextual information about the corresponding word. The input to GAT consists of a set of the hidden state vectors obtained from BERT, $\text{h} = \{h_1, h_2, \ldots, h_V\}$, which serve as the initial feature vectors for each token in the text.

The GAT layer in Figure 6a produces a new set of node features, $\text{h}' = \{h'_1, h'_2, \ldots, h'_V\}$, as its output and V is the number of nodes. The Equations (5) and (6) are used to obtain GAT representation. In this study, we follow the formulation of the Graph Attention Network (GAT) as proposed in the original paper by Veličković et al. (2018) [15]. The GAT model is defined by Equations (5) and (6).

In the beginning, a shared linear transformation, parameterized by weight matrix **w** is applied to each node to transform the input features into higher-level features. Here, **w** is a learnable linear projection matrix. Subsequently, a self-attention mechanism a is performed on the nodes and attention coefficients e are computed for every pair of nodes. To calculate the connection importance of node j to node i, the masked attention coefficient $e_{i,j}$ is computed according to Equation (5) only when j is a neighbor of node i in the graph. $\mathcal{N}_i$ represents the set of i's one-hop neighbors, including the i node itself, as a self-loops are permitted.

While the multi-head self-attention layer in Figure 6a uses a scaled dot product function as a similarity function, the GAT layer uses a one-layer feedforward neural network denoted as a after concatenating the key and query. The scoring function e computes a score for every edge (j,i), which indicates the importance of the neighbor j to the node i. It assigns negative value if there is no connection and then the resulting $\alpha_{i,j}$ is normalized with softmax, as shown in Equation (5). It makes the coefficients easily comparable across different nodes. In the equation, the attention mechanism a is a single-layer FFNN, parametrized by a weight vector $\mathbf{a}$ and LeakyReLU nonlinearity activation function is applied where T represents transposition and $||$ is the concatenation operation.

$$
\begin{aligned}
&e_{i,j} = a\left(\mathbf{w}h_i, \mathbf{w}h_j\right), j \in \mathcal{N}_i \\
&a : \text{LeakyReLU}\left(\text{Linear}\left(\text{concat}\left(\mathbf{w}h_i, \mathbf{w}h_j\right)\right)\right) \\
&\alpha_{i,j} = \text{softmax}\left(e_{i,j}\right) = \frac{\exp\left(e_{i,j}\right)}{\sum_{k \in \mathcal{N}_i} \exp\left(e_{i,k}\right)} = \frac{\exp\left(\text{LeakyReLU}\left(\mathbf{a}^{\mathbf{T}}\left[\mathbf{w}h_i || \mathbf{w}h_j\right]\right)\right)}{\sum_{k \in \mathcal{N}_i} \exp\left(\text{LeakyReLU}(\mathbf{a}^{\mathbf{T}}[\mathbf{w}h_i || \mathbf{w}h_k])\right)}
\end{aligned}
\tag{5}
$$

The normalized attention coefficients α are used to compute a weighted sum of the corresponding neighbors and to select its most relevant neighbors, as shown in Equation (6). It utilizes the attention mechanism to aggregate neighborhood representations with different weights. That is, each node gathers and summarizes information from its neighboring nodes in the graph. The aggregated information and value is combined and serves as the final output representation for every node. In this way, a node iteratively aggregates the information from its neighbors and updates the representation. To perform multi-head attention, K heads are used. Here, σ refers to the ReLU activation function and $\alpha_{i,j}^k$ means normalized attention coefficients computed by the k-th attention mechanism. Finally, we use averaging and activation function and then add a linear classifier to predict for the relation type.

$$
\begin{aligned}
&h'_i = \sigma\left(\sum_{j \in \mathcal{N}_i} \alpha_{i,j} \mathbf{W}h_j\right) h'_i = ||_{k=1}^K \sigma\left(\sum_{j \in \mathcal{N}_i} \alpha_{i,j}^k \mathbf{W}^k h_j\right) (mutli\_head) \\
&h'_i = \text{LeakyReLU}\left(\frac{1}{K} \sum_{k=1}^K \sum_{j \in \mathcal{N}_i} \alpha_{i,j}^k \mathbf{W}^k h_j\right)
\end{aligned}
\tag{6}
$$

Figure 7 visualizes an example of graph self-attention for an entity node "Sympathomimetic Agents" in the sentence, "Concomitant administration of other Sympathomimetic Agents may potentiate the undesirable effects of FORADL." The interaction type between the two entities, Sympathomimetic Agents" and "FORDAL" is classified as "DDI-effect". In the Figure, (a) displays the sentence's dependency structure, (b) shows the same dependency structure in the form of a graph, (c) presents the adjacency table reflecting the dependency relationships among words, and (d) illustrates the transformation of the vector representation of node 5, "sympathomimetic agents" through graph attention. In addition, this model can incorporate off-connection but useful information by employing a residual connection around each of the two sub-layers, followed by layer normalization. That is, the output of GAT sublayer is LayerNorm(x + GAT_Sublayer(x)), where x is the output of BERT's self-attention sublayer.

Thus, this model reflects both contextual relatedness and syntactic relatedness between tokens. In addition, the GAT model applies attention to the features of each node's neighbors to combine them and create a new representation of the node. Therefore, by utilizing attention weights that reflect the importance of edge connections, the neighbor information includes not only directly connected nodes but also indirectly connected nodes, effectively capturing local substructures within the graph.

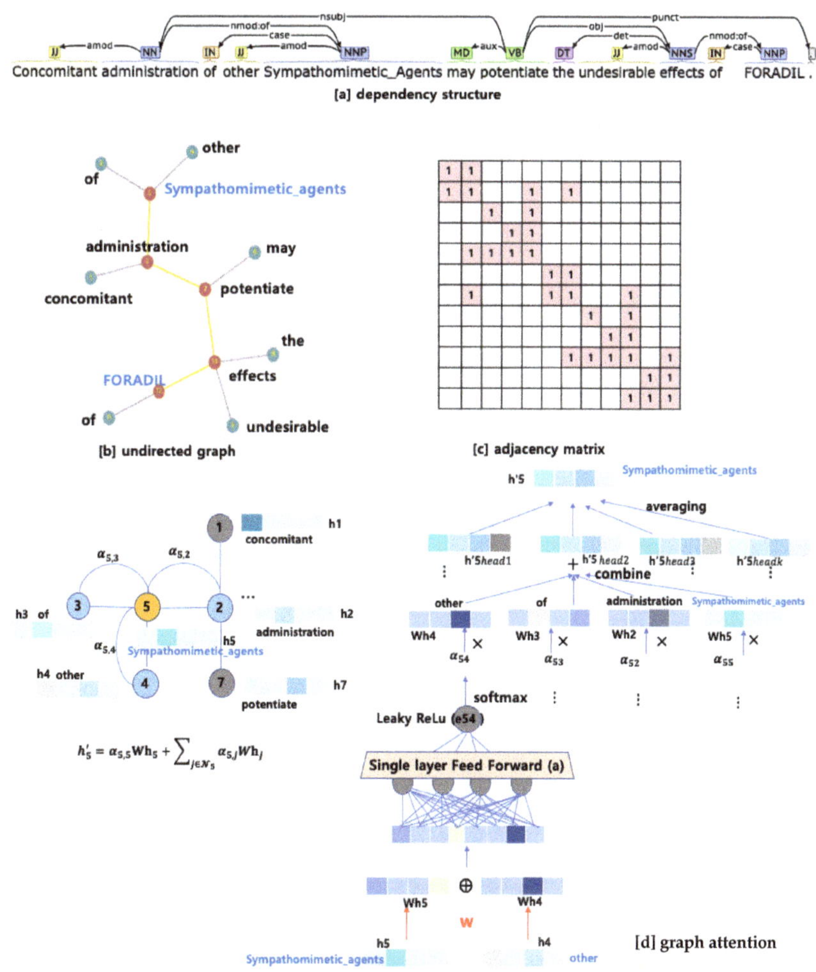

Figure 7. An example of multi-head graph-attention network.

4.3. T5 with Non-Autoregressive Decoder: T5$_{slim_dec}$

As mentioned earlier, T5 [10] converts all text-based language tasks into text-to-text format. As a result, our interaction classification problem is transformed into a relation type generation task, where the model generates a corresponding interaction label between the mentioned entities for a given input sentence. For example, the output label, "DDI-effect" is tokenized as '<s>', '_ DD', 'I',' –', 'effect', '</s>' and "AGONIST" is as '<s>', '_AG', 'ON', 'IST', and '</s>' in T5. These tokens correspond to decoder's inputs. Similar to the encoder, the decoder input of target sequence is also embedded, and its positional encoding is added to indicate the position of each word. The self-attention layer in the decoder only allows earlier position tokens to attend to the output sequence by masking future position tokens. This means that the decoder generates output tokens auto-regressively, predicting one token at a time based on the previous tokens, as shown in Equation (7), until a special end symbol, '</s>', is reached indicating the decoder has completed its output. For a given input sequence X, the target sequence Y with a length m is generated through a chain of conditional probabilities based on the left-to-right sequential dependencies, where $y_{<i}$ denotes the target tokens up to position i.

$$P(Y|X) = \prod_{i=1}^{m} p(y_i|y_{<i}, X) \tag{7}$$

The model learns to predict the next token in a sentence more accurately, as it uses teacher forcing to feed the decoder with the actual target tokens from the ground truth data instead of with its own generated previous tokens, during the training phase. The output sequence is generated by searching for the most likely sequences of tokens. By incorporating beam search, T5 can produce more coherent, accurate, and contextually appropriate text outputs. However, to perform classification task under the text-to-text framework, the target label is treated as output text, which is typically a single word or short string. Thus, the autoregressive task, typically used for generating sequences of output text, is not required for class inference. In our work, the output of T5 corresponds to single interaction string, which represents a label such as "DDI-effect" or "AGONIST". The decoder generates output tokens, each of which represents a specific class from a limited set of class labels. As mentioned in Liu et al.'s study [36], the decoder parameters in T5 model are highly under-utilized for the classification task, in contrast to the typical encoder–decoder models where the decoder layers account for more than half of the total parameters. As a result, when there is only one output token, the decoder has limited previously generated tokens as inputs, which reduces the role of the self-attention mechanism. In such cases, most of the information is passed from the encoder to the decoder and is processed in the cross-attention layer.

Thus, we removed the self-attention block in the decoder, as shown in Figure 6b and tailored the T5 model to fit our interaction-type classification task in a non-autoregressive manner. This approach is inspired by the EncT5 model [39], an encoder-only transformer architecture which reuses T5 encoder layers without code changes. However, we still retained the cross-attention layers to take into account the relationships between the input sentence and output interaction category. The cross-attention plays a role in combining two embedding sequences of the same dimension. It transfers information from an input sequence to the decoder layer to generate output token, which represents the interaction label. The decoder processes the representation of the input sequence through the cross-attention mechanism, yielding a new context-sensitive representation. The embedded vector of the interaction label serves as the query, while the output representation of the encoder is used as both the key and value for the inputs in the cross-attention layer.

For this, we add target labels to vocabulary sets to handle these as whole tokens rather than separated tokens. We also opt for more lexically meaningful labels such as 'ACTIVATOR', 'AGONIST', 'AGONIST-ACTIVATOR', and 'AGONIST-INHIBITOR' instead of generic labels such as "CRP:1" or "CRP2". The model will learn the mapped embedding for this token and the learned embedding will then determine how to optimally pool or aggregate information from the encoder. Finally, the decoder's output is fed into a linear classifier (a fully connected layer), which transforms the high-dimensional context representation into the size of the number of possible labels. The linear classifier generates decoder_output_logits, which represent the raw and unnormalized output values associated with each label in the vocabulary. The decoder_output_logits are passed through softmax function to convert them into a probability distribution over the entire set of possible labels. The label associated with the highest probability is selected as the output text. We will refer to this model as T5$_{\text{slim_dec}}$. Figure 6b presents the overall architecture of T5$_{\text{slim_dec}}$.

Figure 8 visually compares the operational mechanisms of T5 and T5$_{\text{slim_dec}}$, highlighting their differences. As shown in the Figure 8, T5 generates one token at a time based on the input sequence and the previously generated token in the auto-regressive decoding process. For each step of this process, the model calculates decoder_output_logits for all tokens in vocabulary. The token with the highest probability is selected and included in the output sequence and then combines the tokens to form the final readable output text.

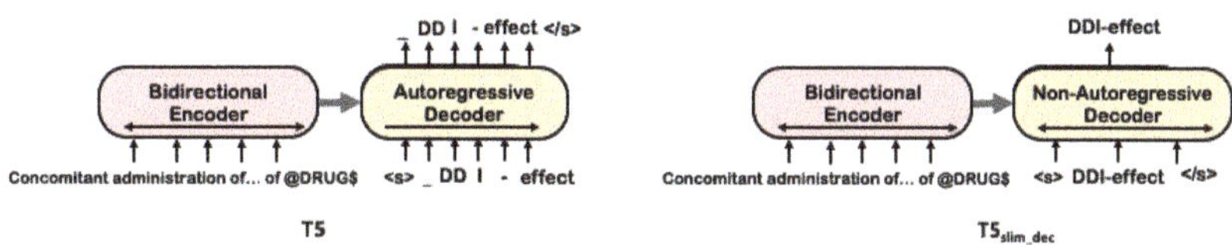

Figure 8. Comparison with T5 and T5$_{slim_dec}$ Models.

5. Results and Discussion

5.1. Experimental Setup

In this section, we discuss the results of transformers we suggested in the previous section and how they can be interpreted in comparison to previous studies. All codes were implemented with HuggingFace's transformers [40] which is a platform that provides APIs and many libraries to access and train state-of-the-art pretrained models. It is available from the HuggingFace hub. We utilized the AdamW optimizer in conjunction with the cross-entropy loss function for training models.

The experimental results were obtained in a GPU-accelerated computing environment using an NVIDIA Tesla V100 32 GB GPU and Google Colab Pro+ with an NVIDIA A100 SXM4 80 GB GPU. To evaluate the model performance, accuracy and F1-score are adopted for evaluation metrics. The accuracy means the proportion of correctly predicted data out of the total data and F1-score is the harmonic mean of precision and recall, designed to balance the two values, as in Equation (8).

$$Accuracy = \frac{TP+TN}{TP+TN+FP+FN}$$
$$Precision = \frac{TP}{TP+FP}, \ Recall(sensitivity) = \frac{TP}{TP+FN} \tag{8}$$
$$F1-score = 2 \times \frac{Precision \times Recall}{Precision + Recall}$$

5.2. Baseline Models

We will begin by presenting the experimental result for the baseline models. In case of encoder–transformer, 'SCIBERT-uncased' pretrained model [23] which has the same structure used in BERT [8] were utilized. The model was trained from scratch using the SCIVOCAB, a new WordPiece vocabulary on scientific corpus using the SentencePiece library. Unlike BERT, the model allows maximum sentence length up to 512 tokens. In our relation classification the final vector of the '[CLS]' token was fed into a linear classification layer with softmax outputs to classify interactions. According to the original SCIBERT study [23], the model achieved a micro F1-score of 0.8364 on the ChemProt dataset. However, in our own experiments, we observed a slightly lower performance with 0.8169. In classification tasks for which every case is guaranteed to be assigned to exactly one class, micro-F1 is equivalent to accuracy.

For T5 [10], our tasks were fine-tuned using 'SciFive-large-Pubmed_PMC' pretrained model [30]. The model was first initialized with pretrained weights from the base T5 model and then re-trained on C4 [35], PubMed abstracts, and PMC full-text articles. It has 24 decoder/encoder layer and 16 heads. The input length, target length and d$_{model}$ are 512, 16, and 1024, respectively. SciFive [30] used the SentencePiece model [34] for the base vocabulary. Its relation extraction performances on ChemProt and DDI sets were reported as 0.8895 and 0.8367 (micro F1-score), respectively. In our experiment, SciFive pretrained model demonstrated performances of 0.9100 and 0.8808 for the same set. The number of beams was set to 2 during the decoding phase.

In case of GPT-3 model, it is one of the largest generative language models with 175 billion parameters, trained on a massive text data set. It is capable of generating high-quality text on a wide range of tasks. However, GPT-3 is not open-source and is only available through OpenAI's API. Therefore, for our experiment, we fine-tuned our tasks using EleutherAI's pretrained models instead. EleutherAI has released several open-source language models called GPT-Neo which perform similarly to GPT-3 but with fewer parameters. Nevertheless, the GPT-NeoX-20B still has 20 billion parameters and requires a large amount of RAM to load the model as well as high-quality computing power to run efficiently. In this experiments, smaller models, such as GPT-Neo1.3b and GPT-Neo125M, were to reduce resource requirements. For future work, the performance of ChatGPT or GPT-4 will be evaluated in the context of biomedical relation extraction to further explore their potential in this domain. Table 5 presents the number of entities in the datasets.

Table 5. The number of entities.

Dataset	Entity Type	Number of Entities
ChemProt	Protein–Chemical	10,031
DDI	Drug–Drug	4920

5.3. Results of the Proposed Models

Table 6 displays the overall performances (accuracy) of the five attempted methods including BERT$_{GAT}$ and T5$_{slim_dec}$. To simplify parsing and reduce the unnecessary complexity caused by multi-word entity terms in a sentence, entities were masked as entity classes with special @CHEM\$ (chemical), @PROT\$ (protein), and @DRUG\$ (drug) tokens. The term "entity masking" in Table 6 indicates those entity replacements. Experiments were conducted on both original datasets as to which entity mentions are kept and datasets with masked entity names. In general, entity masking is known to be beneficial in the generalization capabilities of relation extraction models by encouraging them to focus on context rather than specific entity mentions. This results in better performance when dealing with new and unseen entities and mitigates the risk of overfitting. In Table 6, it is shown that entity masking in DDI interaction extraction proved to be somewhat effective. On the other hand, in the interaction extraction in ChemProt, using the actual tokens of entities rather than their classes resulted in better performance. One possible reason for this is that the training and evaluation datasets are extracted from the same domain and similar entities are likely to appear more frequently, which can contribute to better performance when not masking entities.

Table 6. Experimental results.

Method	ChemProt Accuracy (Micro F1-Score)			DDI Accuracy (Micro F1-Score)		
	Entity Masking	Actual Relation Type	Class Group (CPR)	Entity Masking	4Classes	5Classes -False
SCIBERT		0.8169	0.8844			
SCIBERT	O	0.7852	0.8764	O	0.8703	0.9292
BERT$_{GAT}$	O	0.8089	0.8812			
GPT-Neo125M		0.7647	0.8483			
GPT-Neo1.3b		0.8204	0.9010		0.8950	0.9261
GPT-Neo1.3b	O	0.8282	0.9013	O	0.8978	0.9314
T5$_{sciFive}$		0.8408	0.9100		0.8808	0.9413
T5$_{sciFive}$	O	0.8223	0.9022	O	0.9031	0.9412
T5$_{slim_dec}$		**0.8746**	**0.9429**	O	**0.9193**	**0.9533**

Note that although the ChemProt corpus contains 10 types of relation group classes, only 5 relation types (CPR:3, CPR:4, CPR:5, CPR:6, and CPR:9) were designated to be evaluated in the BioCreative task. In this experiment, two evaluations were conducted: one using the group classes of the CPR-format to which interaction types belong and the other using actual relation types instead of the group classes directly. Consequently, recognizing the interaction class group led to a higher F1-score.

In the case of DDI, the '4classes' in Table 6 indicates that the training and testing were conducted on the four classes (advice, effect, mechanism, int) following the 2013 DDIExtraction shared task evaluation. On the other hand, '5classes' refers to the results of training and testing on the five classes, including 'DDI-false'. In the table, '-false' indicates the accuracy of interaction labels excluding the cases where the gold label is 'DDI-false' during evaluation. In practice, because there were many instances of DDI-false and they were relatively easier to predict, the model achieved a higher F1-score on the 5classes evaluation.

Even though, $BERT_{GAT}$ showed some improvement compared to BERT using entity classes, the performance was still not satisfactory. One reason, the parser is more likely to encounter parsing errors when faced with the complicated biomedical entities and expression. Although the attention mechanism used in GAT allows the model to consider indirectly connected nodes as well as directly connected nodes and BERT's context representation was used as input feature vector for each node, which make it robust to parsing errors, this method partially depends on a correct parse tree to extract crucial information from sentences. Thus, the accurate performance gain of this approach can be accessed on the availability of human-annotated parses for both training and inference. Currently, the effect of incorporating dependency tree information into pretrained transformer remains uncertain. The $BERT_{GAT}$ was experimented only on ChemProt datasets due to the parsing problem.

Another reason could be that the multi-head attention model based on tokens implicitly encodes syntax well enough since it allows the model to learn from input sequence in multiple aspects simultaneously, with each head collecting information from a different subset. This multi-head structure enables the model to analyze the input from various perspectives and make more accurate predictions without restriction of external dependency structure. Thus, implicit syntactic knowledge within sentences might be learned well by transformer models based solely on tokens.

As a result, $T5_{slim\_dec}$ exhibited the best performances on both the ChemProt and DDI datasets and T5 model fine-tuned with SciFive also demonstrated good performances on the datasets. Specially, $T5_{slim\_dec}$ demonstrated noticeable improvements in F1-score, compared to the original T5 model. It showed a 6.36% increase from 0.8223 (F1-score) to 0.8746 on the ChemProt task and a 2.4% increase from 0.89 to 0.9115 on the DDI task. The results indicate that the $T5_{slim\_dec}$ model is performing well on the interaction classification task by tailoring the decoder structure.

Tables 7 and 8 show the F1-scores per interaction type. In addition, macro F1-score, micro F1-score, and weighted F1-score were considered as evaluation metrics as well as standard F1-score. Analyzing these metrics can provide a more comprehensive understanding of the models' performances in multiclass classification by taking into account different aspects of class distribution and the relative importance of each class. In terms of per-class recognition rate, 'DDI-int' had the lowest recognition rate in the DDI dataset while "DOWN-REGULATOR' had lowest recognition rate in the ChemProt dataset. One possible reason for the low performance, the 'DDI-int' relation have relatively fewer instances (5.6%) in the DDI corpus compared to other relations. Similarly, the classes 'AGONIST-ACTIVATOR', and 'AGONIST-INHIBITOR' and 'SUBSTRATE__PRODUCT-OF' appeared infrequently in the training dataset, with only 10, 4, and 14 occurrences, respectively. This limited number of examples in the training data may impact the model's ability to accurately recognize related interactions.

Table 7. F1-score per DDI type.

Relation Type	4Classes				5Classes			
	Precision	Recall	F1-Score	Support	Precision	Recall	F1-Score	Support
DDI-advise	0.9420	0.9548	0.9483	221	0.9019	0.8733	0.8874	221
DDI-effect	0.8706	0.9722	0.9186	360	0.7928	0.8611	0.8256	360
DDI-false					0.9767	0.9820	0.9794	4782
DDI-int	0.9474	0.5625	**0.7059**	96	0.8125	0.4062	**0.5417**	360
DDI-mechanism	0.9628	0.9437	0.9532	302	0.8467	0.8411	0.8439	302
Accuracy			0.9193	979			0.9533	5761
Macro avg.	0.9307	0.8583	0.8815	979	0.8661	0.7927	0.8156	5761
Weighted avg.	0.9227	0.9193	0.9151	979	0.9528	0.9533	0.9518	5761
Micro avg.	0.9193	0.9193	0.9193	979	0.9533	0.9533	0.9533	5761

Table 8. F1-score per ChemProt interaction.

Relation Type	Precision	Recall	F1-Score	Support
ACTIVATOR	0.8571	0.8836	0.8702	292
AGONIST	0.8333	0.9066	0.8684	182
AGONIST-ACTIVATOR	0	0	**0**	4
AGONIST-INHIBITOR	0	0	**0**	12
ANTAGONIST	0.9257	0.9352	0.9304	293
DOWNREGULATOR	0.2381	0.2083	**0.2222**	72
INDIRECT-DOWNREGULATOR	0.7884	0.8765	0.8301	340
INDIRECT-UPREGULATOR	0.8416	0.8114	0.8262	334
INHIBITOR	0.9354	0.9466	0.941	1255
PRODUCT-OF	0.8804	0.8482	0.864	191
SUBSTRATE	0.9505	0.8896	0.919	453
SUBSTRATE_PRODUCT-OF	0.5	1	**0.6667**	1
UPREGULATOR	0	0	**0**	41
Accuracy			0.8746	3470
Macro avg.	0.5961	0.6389	0.6106	3470
Weighted avg.	0.8682	0.8746	0.8709	3470
Micro avg.	0.8746	0.8746	0.8746	3470

Additionally, Figure 9 shows that 'DDI-int' was frequently confused with 'DDI-effect' or 'DDI-false'. The reason may be that this type is assigned when a drug–drug interaction appears in the text without any additional information, which can lead to potential confusion. As shown in Figure 10, 'DOWNREGULATOR' interactions in ChemProt dataset were frequently misclassified as different interaction types belonging to the same class group, such as 'INDIRECT-DOWNREGULATOR' or 'INHIBITOR', as 'AGONIST-ACTIVATOR' was often misclassified as 'AGONIST' with the same CRP group. Since there might be similarities among them related to their interactions. This makes it difficult for the model to distinguish between them. For example, the 'DOWNREGULATOR' represents a chemical that decreases a protein's activity, while the 'INHIBITOR' refers to a chemical that suppresses a specific protein's function. Both classes have a similarity in that they both decrease or inhibit a protein's activity.

5.4. Comparisons with Other Systems

We also compared T5$_{slim_dec}$, which showed the best performance, with other previous studies in terms of per-class F1-score per for DDI extraction. As shown in Table 9, T5$_{slim_dec}$ outperformed other two approaches for DDI interaction extraction across all DDI types on the '4classes' evaluation. Additionally, in the '5classes' evaluation, our model performed well compared to others, except for 'DDI-int'. Since there were limited studies reporting per-class F1-score, few comparisons were presented in Tables 9 and 10. Zhu et al. [28] constructed three different drug entity-aware attentions to get the sentence representations by using external drug description information, mutual drug entity information, and drug entity information, based on BioBERT. Sun et al. [41] proposed a recurrent hybrid convolutional neural network for DDI extraction and introduced an improved focal loss function to handle class imbalance in the multiclass classification task.

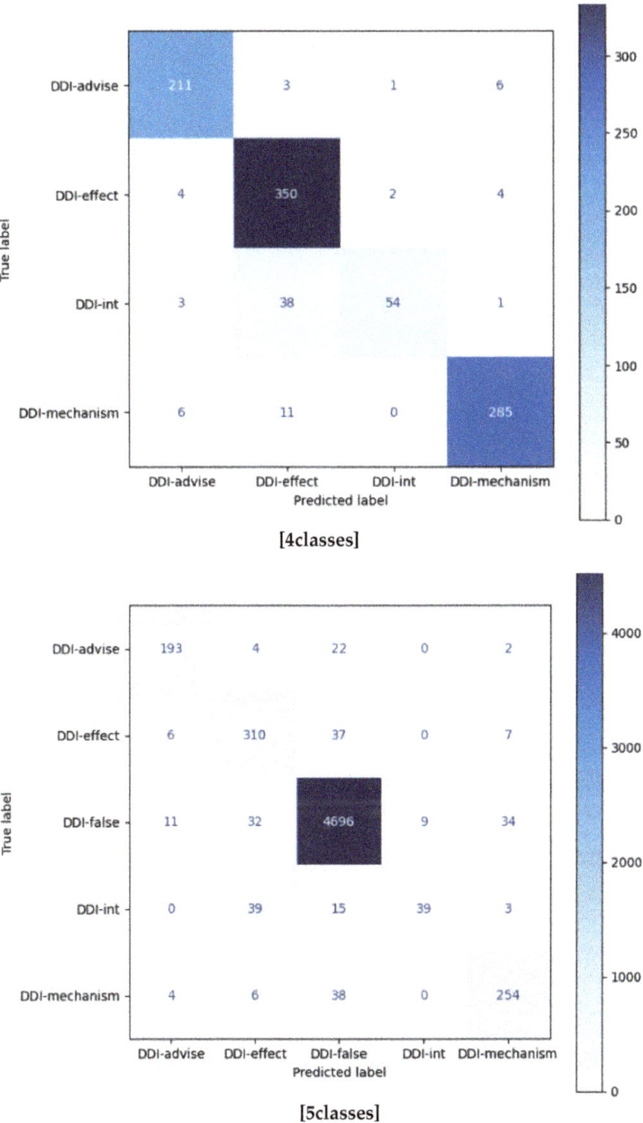

Figure 9. Confusion matrix for T5$_{\text{slim_dec}}$ on DDI test dataset.

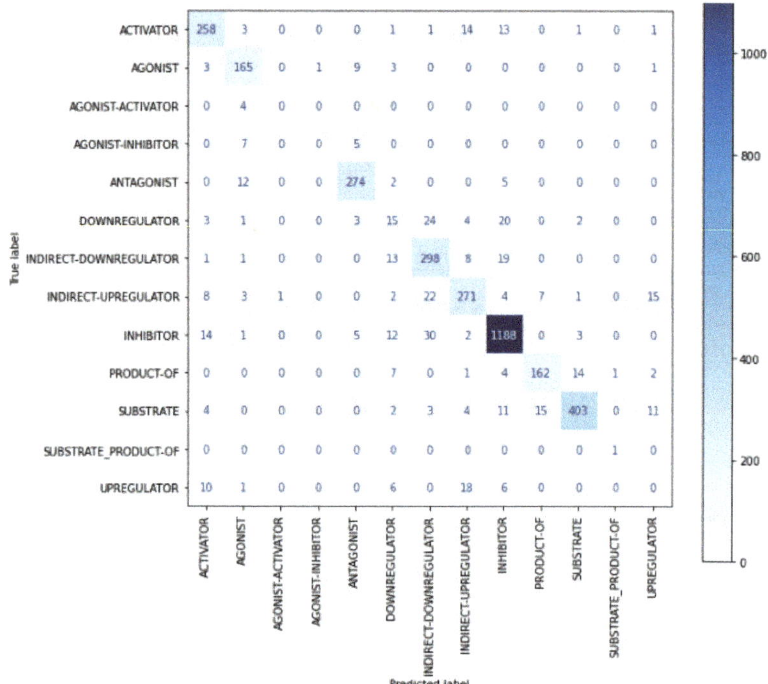

Figure 10. Confusion matrix for T5$_{slim_dec}$ on ChemProt test dataset.

Table 9. Comparisons of per-class F1-scores with other methods (DDI dataset).

Interaction Type	T5$_{slim_dec}$ (4Classes)	T5$_{slim_dec}$ (5Classes)	Zhu et al. [28]	Sun et al. [41]
DDI-advise	0.9483	0.8874	0.860	0.805
DDI-effect	0.9186	0.8256	0.801	0.734
DDI-int	0.7059	0.5417	0.566	0.589
DDI-mechanism	0.9532	0.8439	0.846	0.782

Table 10. Comparisons of per-class F1-scores with other method (ChemProt dataset).

Interaction Type	T5$_{slim_dec}$ F1-Score	Asada et al. F1-Score [26]
ACTIVATOR	0.8702	0.771
AGONIST	0.8684	0.790
AGONIST-ACTIVATOR	0	0
AGONIST-INHIBITOR	0	0
ANTAGONIST	0.9304	0.919
DOWNREGULATOR	0.2222	?
INDIRECT-DOWNREGULATOR	0.8301	0.779
INDIRECT-UPREGULATOR	0.8262	0.752
INHIBITOR	0.941	0.853
PRODUCT-OF	0.864	0.669
SUBSTRATE	0.919	0.708
SUBSTRATE_PRODUCT-OF	0.6667	0
UPREGULATOR	0	?

Table 10 shows the comparison of per class F1-score in the ChemProt dataset. Asada et al. [26] encoded sentence representation vectors by concatenating the drug knowledge graph embedding with word token embedding. The knowledge graph embedding took into account various external information, such as hierarchical categorical information, interacting protein information, related pathway information, textual drug information, and drug molecular structural information. Our $T5_{slim\_dec}$ model achieved better classification results for all ChemProt interaction types compared to the current state-of-the-art (SOTA) system [26]. $T5_{slim\_dec}$ model with previous systems on DDI and ChemProt relation extraction. Based on the evaluation metric F1-score, our system showed very promising performance in both interaction extraction tasks.

Consequently, $T5_{slim\_dec}$ effectively extracted drug-related interactions compared to previous state-of-the-art systems without utilizing external information for entities, simply by tailoring the encoder–decoder transformer architecture to suit the classification task and by not tokenizing the decoder input.

Finally, Table 11 shows an overall performance comparison of our $T5_{slim\_dec}$ model with previous systems on DDI and ChemProt relation extraction. The notation 'CPR' indicates that the model determines an interaction type by CPR class group, as mentioned earlier. Our experiments showed that SciFive [30], a T5 model trained on large biomedical corpora for domain-specific tasks, performed competitively on both DDI and ChemProt datasets, achieving an accuracy of 0.90 for the 4classes of DDI and 0.91 for the CPR class group of ChemProt. According to our knowledge, SciFive is a state-of-the-art system for drug-related interaction extraction.

Table 11. Comparisons with previous SOTA systems.

Method	Accuracy (Micro F1-Score) DDI	Our Experiment	Accuracy (Micro F1-Score) ChemProt	Our Experiment
CNN (Liu et al., 2016) [16]	0.6701			
BiLSTM (Sahu and Anand, 2018) [17]	0.6939			
BioBERT (Lee et al., 2019) [24]			0.7646	
SCIBERT (Beltagy et al., 2019) [23]			0.8364	0.8169
BioMegatron (Shin et al., 2020) [42]			0.77	
KeBioLM (Yuan et al., 2021) [27]	0.8190		0.775	
PubMedBERT(Gu et al., 2021) [25]	0.8236		0.7724	
SciFive (Phan et al., 2021) [30]	0.8367	$0.9031_{4classes}$	**0.8895**	0.9100_{CPR}
BioM-BERT (Alrowili et al., 2021) [43]			0.80	
BioLinkBERT (Yasunaga et al., 2022) [29]	0.8335		0.7998	
PubMedBERT+HKG (Asada et al., 2022) [26]	**0.8540**			
BioBERT+multi entity-aware attention (Zhu et al.) [28]	0.8090			
Our Method ($T5_{slim\_dec}$)	$0.9533_{5classes}$ $0.9115_{4classes}$		0.8746 0.9429_{CPR}	

As a result, our $T5_{slim\_dec}$ model outperformed SciFive with an accuracy of 0.91 for the 4class classification and 0.95 for the 5class classification in the DDI dataset. Additionally, our model achieved an accuracy of 0.94 for the CPR-based class group and 0.87 for 13 interaction types. As shown in the table, encoder-only transformers such as BioBERT, SCIBERT, PubMedBERT, BioM-BERT, and BioLinkBERT exhibited lower performance than encoder–decoder transformer models such as T5 and $T5_{slim\_dec}$. Moreover, the PubMedBERT + HKG model, which leverages external knowledge, also showed strong classification accuracy.

5.5. Limitations

In this section, we will address several limitations that need to be considered for future improvements. The $BERT_{GAT}$ model encoded dependencies between tokens by converting each tree into a corresponding adjacency matrix. Although the model utilized an attention mechanism to calculate the importance of words within the input graph structure and incorporated BERT's contextualized representation as embedding feature vectors for input graph nodes, it still requires more sophisticated techniques for incorporating syntactic and semantic information to enhance biomedical relation extraction performance. This is further complicated by errors in the dependency tree which can potentially introduce confusion in relation classification, emphasizing the need for a method that is robust to such issues. Even though the attention mechanism used in GAT allows the model to consider indirectly connected nodes and capture complex relationships in the graph, it is necessary to develop strategies that effectively address these challenges.

In addition, as shown in Figure 10, the $T5_{slim\_dec}$ occasionally misclassifies terms with opposite meanings, such as confusing ACTIVATOR with INHIBITOR and AGONIST with ANTAGONIST. This indicates a need for further in-depth research and investigation regarding negation handling to improve the model's performance in such cases.

Furthermore, due to computing limitations, we were unable to fully validate the performance of GPT-3 in this study, and GPT-Neo1.3b did not outperform the T5 model. Recently, ultra-large language models such as ChatGPT (GPT-3.5) and GPT-4 have demonstrated remarkable performances in text generation. Therefore, further research to explore the potential of ChatGPT or GPT-4 APIs on biomedical interaction extraction is needed.

Finally, the transformer models we proposed were currently designed to perform sentence-level relation extraction, even though transformers can handle multiple sentences simultaneously by using [SEP] to separate them. Thus, they have limitations in handling n-ary relation or cross-sentence n-ary relation extraction tasks, as there could be more than two entities across multiple sentences.

6. Conclusions

In this work, we demonstrated the effectiveness of transfer learning that utilizes transformer models pretrained on a large-scale language dataset and fine-tuned the parameters on relation extraction task dataset.

Although we did not compare the performance of high-capacity parameter models such as GPT-3 or GPT-3.5 (Instruct GPT, ChatGPT) on the relation extraction task, the encoder–decoder transformer T5 consistently demonstrated strong performance in drug-related interaction classification.

We proposed $T5_{slim\_dec}$, a modified version of T5 for interaction classification tasks by removing the self-attention layer from the decoder and adding the target labels to the vocabulary. As a result, $T5_{slim\_dec}$ can handle the target labels as whole tokens rather than requiring them to be predicted sequentially in an autoregressive manner. The model demonstrates the effectiveness for DDI and ChemProt interaction extraction tasks and achieved improved classification performance compared to state-of-the-art models.

The relation extraction can be a challenging task for transformer models when dealing with complex sentence structures. This difficulty arises from several factors, including long or nested sentences, entities spanning multiple sentences, and domain-specific language structure. To address this difficulty, we incorporated explicit syntactic information to enhance context vector representation of a sentence using structural information of the sentence. We presented $BERT_{GAT}$ to augment the transformer with dependency parsing results. However, that model did not demonstrate a significant performance improvement and additional research is required.

The proposed DDI extraction method can be applied to pharmacovigilance and drug safety surveillance by identifying potential adverse drug interactions. The ChemProt extraction can be utilized in drug discovery and development by facilitating the identification of potential protein targets for new drugs.

Author Contributions: Conceptualization, S.K., J.Y. and O.K.; methodology, S.K., J.Y. and O.K.; software, S.K. and J.Y.; validation, S.K., J.Y. and O.K.; formal analysis, S.K. and J.Y.; investigation, S.K.; resources, S.K., J.Y. and O.K.; data curation, S.K.; writing—original draft preparation, S.K.; writing—review and editing, S.K., J.Y. and O.K.; visualization, S.K. and J.Y.; supervision, S.K.; project administration, S.K.; funding acquisition, S.K. All authors have read and agreed to the published version of the manuscript.

Funding: This research was supported by Basic Science Research Program through the National Research Foundation of Korea (NRF) funded by the Ministry of Education (NRF-2020R1I1A1A01073125).

Institutional Review Board Statement: Not applicable.

Informed Consent Statement: Not applicable.

Data Availability Statement: Not applicable.

Conflicts of Interest: The authors declare no conflict of interest.

References

1. Chen, Q.; Allot, A.; Lu, Z. Keep up with the latest coronavirus research. *Nature* **2020**, *579*, 193. [CrossRef] [PubMed]
2. PubMed. Available online: https://pubmed.ncbi.nlm.nih.gov (accessed on 28 February 2023).
3. Bairoch, A.; Apweiler, R. The SWISS-PROT protein sequence data bank and its supplement TrEMBL in 2000. *Nucleic Acids Res.* **1997**, *25*, 31–36. [CrossRef] [PubMed]
4. Wishart, D.S.; Knox, C.; Guo, A.; Shrivastava, S.; Hassanali, M.; Stothard, P.; Chang, Z.; Woolsey, J. DrugBank. A comprehensive resource for in silico drug discovery and exploration. *Nucleic Acids Res.* **2006**, *34*, D668–D672. [CrossRef] [PubMed]
5. Davis, A.P.; Wiegers, T.C.; Johnson, R.J.; Sciaky, D.; Wiegers, J.; Mattingly, C.J. Comparative Toxicogenomics Database (CTD): Update 2023. *Nucleic Acids Res.* **2023**, *51*, D1257–D1262. [CrossRef] [PubMed]
6. Harmar, A.J.; Hills, R.A.; Rosser, E.M.; Jones, M.; Buneman, O.P.; Dunbar, D.R.; Greenhill, S.D.; Hale, V.A.; Sharman, J.L.; Bonner, T.I.; et al. IUPHAR-DB: The IUPHAR database of G protein-coupled receptors and ion channels. *Nucleic Acids Res.* **2008**, *37*, D680–D685. [CrossRef] [PubMed]
7. MEDLINE. Available online: https://www.nlm.nih.gov/medline/index.html (accessed on 28 February 2023).
8. Devlin, J.; Chang, M.W.; Lee, K.; Toutanova, K. BERT: Pre-training of deep bidirectional transformers for language understanding. In Proceedings of the NAACL-HLT 2019, Minneapolis, MN, USA, 2–7 June 2019; pp. 4171–4186.
9. Brown, T.B.; Mann, B.; Ryder, N.; Subbiah, M.; Kaplan, J.; Dhariwal, P.; Neelakantan, A.; Shyam, P.; Sastry, G.; Askell, A.; et al. Language Models are Few-Shot Learners. In Proceedings of the 34th Conference on Neural Information Processing Systems (NeurIPS 2020), Vancouver, Canada, 6–12 December 2020.
10. Raffel, C.; Shazeer, N.; Roberts, A.; Lee, K.; Narang, S.; Matena, M.; Zhou, Y.; Li, W.; Liu, P.J. Exploring the Limits of Transfer Learning with a Unified Text-to-Text Transformer. *J. Mach. Learn. Res.* **2020**, *21*, 5485–5551.
11. Krallinger, M. Overview of the Chemical-Protein relation extraction track. In Proceedings of the BioCreative VI Workshop, Bethesda, MD, USA, 20 October 2017.
12. Segura-Bedmar, I.; Martínez, P.; Herrero-Zazo, M. SemEval-2013 Task 9: Extraction of Drug-Drug Interactions from Biomedical Texts (DDIExtraction 2013). In Proceedings of the Second Joint Conference on Lexical and Computational Semantics (*SEM), Volume 2: Seventh International Workshop on Semantic Evaluation (SemEval 2013), Atlanta, GA, USA, 14–15 June 2013; pp. 341–350.
13. Kanjirangat, V.; Rinaldi, F. Enhancing Biomedical Relation Extraction with Transformer Models using Shortest Dependency Path Features and Triplet Information. *J. Biomed. Inform.* **2021**, *122*, 103893. [CrossRef] [PubMed]
14. Zhang, Y.; Qi, P.; Manning, C.D. Graph Convolution over Pruned Dependency Trees Improves Relation Extraction. In Proceedings of the 2018 Conference on Empirical Methods in Natural Language Processing, Brussels, Belgium, 31 October–4 November 2018; pp. 2205–2215.
15. Veličković, P.; Casanova, A.; Liò, P.; Cucurull, G.; Romero, A.; Bengio, Y. Graph attention networks. In Proceedings of the 6th International Conference on Learning Representations, Vancouver, Canada, 30 April 2018.
16. Liu, S.; Tang, B.; Chen, Q.; Wang, X. Drug-Drug Interaction Extraction via Convolutional Neural Networks. *Comput. Math. Methods Med.* **2016**, *2016*, 6918381. [CrossRef] [PubMed]
17. Sahu, S.K.; Anand, A. Drug-drug interaction extraction from biomedical texts using long short-term memory network. *J. Biomed. Inform.* **2018**, *86*, 15–24. [CrossRef] [PubMed]
18. Liu, Y.; Ott, M.; Goyal, N.; Du, J.; Joshi, M.; Chen, D.; Levy, O.; Lewis, M.; Zettlemoyer, L.; Stoyanov, V. RoBERTa: A Robustly Optimized BERT Pretraining Approach. In Proceedings of the 20th China National Conference on Computational Linguistics, Hohhot, China, 13–15 August 2021; pp. 1218–1227.
19. Song, K.; Tan, X.; Qin, T.; Lu, J.; Liu, T. MASS: Masked Sequence to Sequence Pre-training for Language Generation. In Proceedings of the 36th International Conference on Machine Learning, Long Beach, CA, USA, 9–15 June 2019; pp. 5926–5936.

20. Lewis, M.; Liu, Y.; Goyal, N.; Ghazvininejad, M.; Mohamed, A.; Levy, O.; Stoyanov, V.; Zet-tlemoyer, L. BART: Denoising Sequence-to-Sequence Pre-training for Natural Language Generation, Translation, and Comprehension. In Proceedings of the 58th Annual Meeting of the Association for Computational Linguistics, Online, 6–8 July 2020; pp. 7871–7880.
21. Liu, X.; He, P.; Chen, W.; Gao, J. Multi-Task Deep Neural Networks for Natural Language Understanding. In Proceedings of the 57th Annual Meeting of the Association for Computational Linguistics, Florence, Italy, July 2019; pp. 4487–4496.
22. Vaswani, A.; Shazeer, N.; Parmar, N.; Uszkoreit, J.; Jones, L.; Gomez, A.N.; Kaiser, L.; Polosukhin, I. Attention Is All You Need. In Proceedings of the Advances in Neural Information Processing Systems (NIPS 2017), Long Beach, CA, USA, 4–9 December 2017.
23. Beltagy, I.; Lo, K.; Cohan, A. SCIBERT: A Pretrained Language Model for Scientific Text. In Proceedings of the 2019 Conference on Empirical Methods in Natural Language Processing and the 9th International Joint Conference on Natural Language Processing (EMNLP-IJCNLP), Hong Kong, China, 3–7 November 2019; pp. 3615–3620.
24. Lee, J.; Yoon, W.; Kim, S.; Kim, D.; Kim, S.; So, C.H.; Kang, J. BioBERT: A pre-trained biomedical language representation model for biomedical text mining. *Bioinformatics* **2019**, *36*, 1234–1240. [CrossRef] [PubMed]
25. Yuxian, G.; Robert Tinn, R.; Hao Cheng, H.; Lucas, M.; Usuyama, N.; Liu, X.; Naumann, T.; Gao, J.; Poon, H. Domain-Specific Language Model Pretraining for Biomedical Natural Language Processing. *ACM Trans. Comput. Health* **2021**, *3*, 1–23.
26. Asada, M.; Miwa, M.; Sasaki, Y. Integrating heterogeneous knowledge graphs into drug–drug interaction extraction from the literature. *Bioinformatics* **2022**, *39*, btac754. [CrossRef] [PubMed]
27. Yuan, Z.; Liu, Y.; Tan, C.; Huang, S.; Huang, F. Improving Biomedical Pretrained Language Models with Knowledge. In Proceedings of the BioNLP 2021 Workshop, Online, 11 June 2021; pp. 180–190. [CrossRef]
28. Zhu, Y.; Li, L.; Lu, H.; Zhou, A.; Qin, X. Extracting drug-drug interactions from texts with BioBERT and multiple entity-aware attentions. *J. Biomed. Inform.* **2020**, *106*, 103451. [CrossRef] [PubMed]
29. Yasunaga, M.; Jure Leskovec, J.; Liang, P. LinkBERT: Pretraining Language Models with Document Links. In Proceedings of the 60th Annual Meeting of the Association for Computational Linguistics, Dublin, Ireland, 22–27 May 2022; pp. 8003–8016.
30. Phan, L.N.; Anibal, J.T.; Tran, H.; Chanana, S.; Bahadıro, E.; Peltekian, A.; Altan-Bonnet, G. SciFive: A text-to-text transformer model for biomedical literature. *arXiv* **2021**, arXiv:2106.03598.
31. Sarrouti, M.; Tao, C.; Randriamihaja, Y.M. Comparing Encoder-Only and Encoder-Decoder Transformers for Relation Extraction from Biomedical Texts: An Empirical Study on Ten Benchmark Datasets. In Proceedings of the BioNLP 2022 Workshop, Dublin, Ireland, 26 May 2022; pp. 376–382. [CrossRef]
32. Bahdanau, D.; Cho, K.; Bengio, Y. Neural Machine Translation by Jointly Learning to Align and Translate. In Proceedings of the 3rd International Conference on Learning Representations (ICLR 2015), San Diego, CA, USA, 7–9 May 2015.
33. Fricke, S. Semantic Scholar. *J. Med. Libr. Assoc.* **2018**, *106*, 145–147. [CrossRef]
34. Kudo, T.; Richardson, J. SentencePiece: A simple and language independent subword tokenizer and detokenizer for Neural Text Processing. In Proceedings of the 2018 Conference on Empirical Methods in Natural Language Processing: System Demonstrations, Brussels, Belgium, 2–4 November 2018; pp. 66–77.
35. Dodge, J.; Sap, M.; Marasović, A.; Agnew, W.; Ilharco, G.; Groeneveld, D.; Mitchell, M.; Gardner, M. Documenting Large Webtext Corpora: A Case Study on the Colossal Clean Crawled Corpus. In Proceedings of the 2021 Conference on Empirical Methods in Natural Language Processing, Online, 7–11 November 2021; pp. 1286–1305.
36. Black, S.; Biderman, S.; Hallahan, E.; Anthony, Q.; Leo Gao, L.; Golding, L.; He, H.; Leahy, C.; McDonell, K.; Phang, J.; et al. GPT-NeoX-20B: An Open-Source Autoregressive Language Model. In Proceedings of the ACL Workshop on Challenges & Perspectives in Creating Large Language Models, Dublin, Ireland, 27 May 2022.
37. Xu, Y.; GeLi, L.; Chen, Y.; Peng, H.; Jin, Z. Classifying relations via long short term memory networks along shortest dependency paths. In Proceedings of the EMNLP, Lisbon, Portugal, 17–21 September 2015.
38. Marneffe, M.; Manning, C.D. Stanford Typed Dependencies Manual. 2016. Available online: https://downloads.cs.stanford.edu/nlp/software/dependencies_manual.pdf (accessed on 28 February 2023).
39. Liu, F.; Huang, T.; Lyu, S.; Shakeri, S.; Yu, H.; Li, J. EncT5: A Framework for Fine-tuning T5 as Non-autoregressive Models. *arXiv* **2021**, arXiv:2110.08426.
40. Wolf, T.; Debut, L.; Sanh, V.; Chaumond, J.; Delangue, C.; Moi, A.; Cistac, P.; Rault, T.; Louf, R.; Funtowicz, M.; et al. HuggingFace's Transformers: State-of-the-Art Natural Language Processing. In Proceedings of the 2020 Conference on Empirical Methods in Natural Language Processing: System Demonstrations, Online, October 2020; pp. 38–45.
41. Sun, X.; Dong, K.; Ma, L.; Sutcliffe, R.; He, F.; Chen, S.; Feng, J. Drug-Drug Interaction Extraction via Recurrent Hybrid Convolutional Neural Networks with an Improved Focal Loss. *Entropy* **2019**, *21*, 37. [CrossRef] [PubMed]
42. Shin, H.C.; Zhang, Y.; Bakhturina, E.; Puri, R.; Patwary, M.; Shoeybi, M.; Mani, R. BioMegatron: Larger Biomedical Domain Language Model. In Proceedings of the EMNLP, Online, 16–20 November 2020.
43. Alrowili, S.; Vijay-Shanker, K. BioM-Transformers: Building Large Biomedical Language Models with BERT, ALBERT and ELECTRA. In Proceedings of the BioNLP 2021 Workshop, Online, 11 June 2021; pp. 221–227.

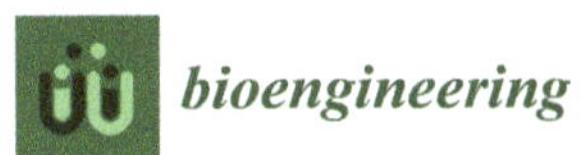 *bioengineering*

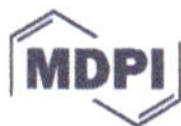

Article

Blood Glucose Level Time Series Forecasting: Nested Deep Ensemble Learning Lag Fusion

Heydar Khadem [1,*]**, Hoda Nemat** [1]**, Jackie Elliott** [2,3] **and Mohammed Benaissa** [1]

[1] Department of Electronic and Electrical Engineering, University of Sheffield, Sheffield S10 2TN, UK
[2] Department of Oncology and Metabolism, University of Sheffield, Sheffield S10 2TN, UK
[3] Department of Diabetes and Endocrinology, Sheffield Teaching Hospitals, Sheffield S5 7AU, UK
[*] Correspondence: h.khadem@sheffield.ac.uk

Abstract: Blood glucose level prediction is a critical aspect of diabetes management. It enables individuals to make informed decisions about their insulin dosing, diet, and physical activity. This, in turn, improves their quality of life and reduces the risk of chronic and acute complications. One conundrum in developing time-series forecasting models for blood glucose level prediction is to determine an appropriate length for look-back windows. On the one hand, studying short histories foists the risk of information incompletion. On the other hand, analysing long histories might induce information redundancy due to the data shift phenomenon. Additionally, optimal lag lengths are inconsistent across individuals because of the domain shift occurrence. Therefore, in bespoke analysis, either optimal lag values should be found for each individual separately or a globally suboptimal lag value should be used for all. The former approach degenerates the analysis's congruency and imposes extra perplexity. With the latter, the fine-tunned lag is not necessarily the optimum option for all individuals. To cope with this challenge, this work suggests an interconnected lag fusion framework based on nested meta-learning analysis that improves the accuracy and precision of predictions for personalised blood glucose level forecasting. The proposed framework is leveraged to generate blood glucose prediction models for patients with type 1 diabetes by scrutinising two well-established publicly available Ohio type 1 diabetes datasets. The models developed undergo vigorous evaluation and statistical analysis from mathematical and clinical perspectives. The results achieved underpin the efficacy of the proposed method in blood glucose level time-series prediction analysis.

Keywords: deep learning; time-series forecasting; blood glucose; diabetes; ensemble learning; artificial neural network

Citation: Khadem, H.; Nemat, H.; Elliott, J.; Benaissa, M. Blood Glucose Level Time Series Forecasting: Nested Deep Ensemble Learning Lag Fusion. *Bioengineering* **2023**, *10*, 487. https://doi.org/10.3390/bioengineering10040487

Academic Editors: Pedro Miguel Rodrigues, João Alexandre Lobo Marques and João Paulo do Vale Madeiro

Received: 21 March 2023
Revised: 12 April 2023
Accepted: 17 April 2023
Published: 19 April 2023

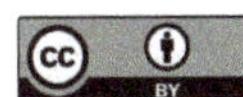

1. Introduction

Type 1 diabetes is a chronic metabolic disorder [1]. The disease is currently incurable [2,3]. Nevertheless, its effective management can dramatically mitigate the symptoms and the risk of associated short-term and long-term complications [4,5]. Accordingly, people with type 1 diabetes and their potential carers are normally educated on the standard practices to control the illness [6–8].

Self-management of type 1 diabetes is, however, burdensome and prone to human errors [9–11]. Hence, automating the management tasks would be highly beneficial [12,13]. Some developments have already been made related to this concern [14–16]. For example, technological breakthroughs, such as continuous glucose monitoring biosensors [17,18] and insulin pumps [19,20], nowadays, serve myriads of type 1 diabetes patients. The former, in a minimally invasive fashion, takes regular snapshots of blood glucose levels in alignment with the general advice on a frequent review of glycaemic state [21,22]. The latter semiautomates insulin administration, requiring minimum user interference [23–25]. Moreover, there are ongoing efforts to develop fully noninvasive continuous blood glucose level monitoring sensors to help more effective diabetes management [26–29].

Despite the advancements achieved so far, continued progress in the automation process is still demanded to further facilitate and effectuate the management of type 1 diabetes [30,31]. In this respect, engineering accurate blood glucose predictor devices would be game changing [32,33]. Such instruments can provide early warning about possible adverse glycaemic events so that automated or nonautomated pre-emptive measures can be taken [34,35]. Additionally, these devices are a prerequisite for the advent of a closed-loop artificial pancreas as the current vision for the ultimate automated management of type 1 diabetes [36,37].

For predicting blood glucose levels, physiological, data-driven, and hybrid modelling approaches can be pursued [38,39]. In the data-driven approach, also used in this research, current and past values of diabetes-management-related variables are studied to project future blood glucose excursion [38,40].

For constructing data-driven blood glucose level predictors, one of the three main categories of time-series forecasting approaches is typically used: classical time-series forecasting, traditional machine learning, or deep learning analysis. Among these, deep learning, as a member of the modern artificial intelligence family, has proven potency in solving complicated computational tasks, including complex time-series forecasting [41–46].

Predicting the blood glucose levels of individuals with type 1 diabetes is a convoluted forecasting mission due to the highly erratic behaviour of the phenomenon [47]. Thus, in line with many other time-series forecasting areas, deep learning has gained enormous popularity in the blood glucose level prediction realm [48,49]. Subsequently, extensive research has been underway to advance the analysis. Notwithstanding all the enhancements in this field so far, there still exist challenges to be addressed adequately [50]. This work contributes to addressing one such challenge.

When applying deep learning algorithms for data-driven time-series blood glucose level forecasting, lag observations of data are studied to predict specific future values. Here, a quandary is to select the appropriate length of history to be investigated. This issue is even more pronounced when considering the fact that due to the significant discrepancy in the blood glucose profile across type 1 diabetes patients, the common practice is to generate personalised models. In this circumstance, finding an optimal length of history separately for each individual entails further disparity and complexity in the analysis. To address this difficulty, the present work suggests a compound lag fusion approach by exploiting the potential of nested ensemble learning over typical ensemble learning analysis. This is the first paper, to the best of our knowledge, that incorporates nested meta-learning analysis in the field of blood glucose level prediction.

The rest of the article is outlined as follows. Section 2 reviews some recent studies on type 1 diabetes blood glucose level prediction. Section 3 concisely describes the datasets used in this research. Section 4 explains model development and assessment analysis. Section 5 presents the results of the model assessment analysis along with the relevant discussions. Finally, Section 6 summarises and concludes the work.

2. Literature Survey

In the following, a number of recent articles on data-driven blood glucose level prediction are succinctly overviewed. For further alignment with the contents of this study, the focus of this overview is on the application of state-of-the-art machine learning techniques and the use of Ohio type 1 diabetes datasets for model development and evaluation. A more comprehensive review of the latest revolutions in the blood glucose level prediction area can be studied at these references [51–54].

A recent article offered a multitask approach for blood glucose level prediction by experimenting on the Ohio datasets [55]. The methods are based on the concept of transfer learning. The study explicitly targets addressing the challenge of the need for extensively large amounts of data for personalised blood glucose level prediction. For this purpose, it suggests pre-training a model on a source domain and a multitask model on the whole dataset and then using these learning experiences in constructing personalised models.

The authors showcase the efficacy of their propositions by comparing the performance of their approach with sequential transfer learning and subject-isolated learning.

An autonomous channel setup was recently presented for deep learning blood glucose level prediction using the Ohio datasets [56]. The proposed method chose the history lengths for different variables adaptively by affecting the time-dependency scale. The crux is to avoid dismissing useful information from variables with enduring influence and engaging uninformative data from variables with transient impact at the same time. The models generated in the study undergo comparison analysis with standard non-autonomous channel structures deploying mathematical and clinical assessments.

A deep learning approach based on dilated recurrent neural networks accompanied by transfer learning concepts is introduced for blood glucose level prediction [57]. In the study, personalised models are created for individuals with type 1 diabetes using an Ohio dataset. The method is examined for short-term forecasting tasks. Its supremacy over standard methods, including autoregressive models, support vector regression, and conventional neural networks, is shown.

Another study suggests an efficient method for univariate blood glucose level prediction [58]. In the analysis, recurrent neural networks were used as learners. The learners are trained in an end-to-end approach to predict future blood glucose levels 30 and 60 min in advance using only histories of blood glucose data. The models are developed and assessed using an Ohio dataset. The results achieved are comparable with the state-of-the-art research on the dataset. In addition to accuracy analysis, the study investigates the certainty in the predictions. To do so, a parameterised univariate Gaussian is tasked with calculating the standard deviation of the predictions as a representative of uncertainty.

Employing the concepts of the Internet of things, a study compares four broadly used models of glycaemia, including support vector machine, Bayesian regularised neural network, multilayer perceptron, and Gaussian approach [59]. These models are used to investigate the possibility of completing the data collected from 25 individuals with type 1 diabetes by mapping intricate patterns of data. The findings highlight the potential of such analysis in contributing to improved diabetes management. Further, among the approaches examined, Bayesian regularised neural networks outperform others by delivering the best root mean square error and coefficient of determination.

3. Material

For generating blood glucose level prediction models, this study uses two well-established, publicly accessible Ohio type 1 diabetes datasets [60]. The first dataset includes data for six individuals with type 1 diabetes. The participants' age at the time of data collection was in a range of 40 to 60 years. The sample comprised four females and two males. This dataset was initially released for the first blood glucose challenge in Knowledge Discovery at the Healthcare Data conference in 2018. This dataset is referred to as the Ohio 2018 dataset hereafter. The second dataset also contains six people with type 1 diabetes, different from those in the first dataset. The data contributors in this dataset were in an age range of 20 to 80 years at the point of data acquisition. Five of them were male and one female. This dataset was originally distributed for the second blood glucose level prediction challenge in Knowledge Discovery at the Healthcare Data conference in 2020. Hereafter, we refer to this dataset as the Ohio 2020 dataset.

Both datasets contain diabetes-related modalities, including blood glucose, physical activity, carbohydrate intake, and bolus insulin injection. Blood glucose and bolus insulin data were collected automatically using physiological sensors. For the former, a Medtronic Enlite continuous glucose monitoring device was used. For the latter, patients in the Ohio 2018 dataset wore a Basis Peak fitness band that collected heart rate data as a representative of physical activity. Alternatively, subjects in the Ohio 2020 dataset wore an Empatica Embrace fitness band that tracked the magnitude of acceleration as a representative of physical activity data. On the other hand, carbohydrate and bolus insulin data were self-reported by individuals in both datasets.

In both datasets, data were collected for eight weeks. The data come with the training and testing set already separated by the data collection and distribution team. The last ten days of data are allocated as a testing set and the remaining former data points as the training set. In the present study, using training sets only, bespoke predictive models are created for future values of blood glucose levels from historical values of blood glucose itself as the indigenous variable, along with exogenous variables of physical activity, carbohydrate intake, and bolus insulin injection. The testing sets are then used to evaluate the generated models. Table 1 displays individuals' identification number, sex, and age information together with a short representation of the statistical properties of blood glucose as the intrinsic variable in the dataset. A more comprehensive description of the Ohio datasets and the data collection process can be found in the original documentation [60].

Table 1. Demographic information of contributors and summary of statistical properties of blood glucose data (the focal modality) in the Ohio datasets.

Dataset	PID	Sex	Age	Set	Blood Glucose Data							
					Count	Range (mg/dL)	Mean (mg/dL)	SD (mg/dL)	MR (%)	HOR (%)	ER (%)	HRR (%)
2018	559	female	40–60	Train	10,655	40–400	167.53	70.44	12.06	3.65	55.98	40.37
				Test	2444	45–400	168.93	67.78	14.81	3.03	59.86	37.11
	563	male	40–60	Train	11,013	40–400	146.94	50.51	8.80	2.82	72.81	24.36
				Test	2569	62–313	167.38	46.15	4.71	0.70	60.45	38.85
	570	male	40–60	Train	10,981	46–377	187.5	62.33	5.73	1.97	42.97	55.07
				Test	2672	60–388	215.71	66.99	5.05	0.41	29.04	70.55
	575	female	40–60	Train	11,865	40–400	141.77	60.27	10.43	8.71	68.62	22.66
				Test	2589	40–342	150.49	60.53	4.94	5.37	63.50	31.13
	588	female	40–60	Train	12,639	40–400	164.99	50.51	3.69	1.04	63.56	35.40
				Test	2606	66–354	175.98	48.66	3.42	0.15	53.26	46.58
	591	female	40–60	Train	10,846	40–397	156.01	58.03	17.59	3.94	63.97	32.09
				Test	2759	43–291	144.83	51.42	3.15	5.18	67.27	27.55
2020	540	male	20–40	Train	11,914	40–369	136.78	54.75	9.76	7.08	72.66	20.25
				Test	2360	52–400	149.94	66.46	6.74	5.64	68.18	26.19
	544	male	40–60	Train	10,533	48–400	165.12	60.08	19.11	1.47	63.78	34.75
				Test	2715	62–335	156.48	54.14	15.47	1.22	68.29	30.50
	552	male	20–40	Train	8661	45–345	146.88	54.63	22.30	3.89	72.05	24.06
				Test	1792	47–305	138.11	50.23	85.71	3.57	80.02	16.41
	567	female	20–40	Train	10,750	40–400	154.43	60.88	24.91	6.75	63.40	29.84
				Test	2388	40–351	146.25	55.00	20.18	8.33	67.38	24.29
	584	male	40–60	Train	12,027	40–400	192.34	65.29	9.13	0.80	47.69	51.51
				Test	2661	41–400	170.48	60.76	12.40	1.01	61.86	37.13
	596	male	60–80	Train	10,858	40–367	147.17	49.34	25.35	2.08	73.99	23.93
				Test	2663	49–305	146.98	50.79	9.76	2.78	75.07	22.16

Note. PID: patient identification; SD: standard deviation; MR: missingness rate; HOR: hypoglycaemic rate; ER: euglycaemic rate; HRR: hyperglycaemic rate. Hypoglycaemia, euglycaemia, and hyperglycaemia refer to when the blood glucose level is, respectively, less than 70 mg/dL, between 70 and 180 mg/dL, and more than 180 mg/dL. Both hypoglycaemia and hyperglycaemia are adverse glycaemic events.

4. Methods

This section explicates the methodological implementations for blood glucose level prediction model generation and evaluation. First, some curation steps performed to prepare the data for formal prediction modelling analysis are explained. Next, time-series forecasting models constructed for blood glucose level prediction are described. After that, the criteria considered for evaluating the generated predictive models are presented. Finally, statistical analysis operated on the model outputs is outlined.

4.1. Data Curation

The following pre-modelling curation steps are operated on the raw data to render the ensuing formal deep learning prediction modelling analysis more effective.

4.1.1. Missingness Treatment

The first data curation stage deals with the missing values presented in the automatically collected blood glucose and physical activity data. At the beginning and end of the blood glucose and physical activity series, there are some timespans where data are absent. This unavailability occurred because the subject did not start and finish wearing the sensing devices exactly at the same time. As an initial missing value treatment step, the head and tail of all series are trimmed by removing the void timestamps so that variables start and end from the same point. Afterwards, the linear interpolation technique is used to fill in missing values in the training sets of blood glucose and physical activity. Alternatively, for the testing sets of these modalities, the linear extrapolation technique is used to fill in missing values. This technique precludes future value observation in the evaluation stage, so the models created possess applicability for real-time monitoring.

4.1.2. Sparsity Handling

The sparsity of the self-reported carbohydrate and bolus insulin data is the next pre-modelling issue to be addressed. A reasonable assumption as to the unavailable values of these modalities in the majority of timestamps is that there has been no occurrence to be reported in those points. Therefore, for these two modalities, as a simple yet acceptable practice, zero values are assigned to non-reported timestamps.

4.1.3. Data Alignment

Another data curation step is to unify the frequency of exogenous modalities and align their timestamps with the blood glucose level as the indigenous variable. Initially, acceleration data are downsampled from a one-minute frequency to a five-minute frequency. For this purpose, the entries in the nearest neighbourhood to blood glucose timestamps are kept, and the remaining data points are removed. Following that, timestamps of all extrinsic variables are aligned with those of blood glucose levels with the minimum possible shifts.

4.1.4. Data Transformation

As the next data curation step, as a common practice, feature values are converted into a standardised form that machine learning models can analyse more effectively. For each variable, first, the average of training set values is subtracted from all values in both the training and testing sets. Then, all obtained values are divided by the standard deviation of the training set to make unit variance variables.

4.1.5. Stationarity Inspection

Stationary time-series data have statistical characteristics, including variance and mean, that do not change over time. In this data treatment step, the stationarity condition in the time-series data is satisfied. By conducting the feature transformation step explained in Section 4.1.4, the variances in the series are stabilised. To stabilise the mean of the series, the first-order differencing method is applied. Subsequently, the outcomes are examined using two prevalent statistical tests of Kwiatkowski–Phillips–Schmidt–Shin [61] and Augmented Dickey–Fuller [62], where both confirm the stationary of the series.

4.1.6. Problem Reframing

The final data curation phase translates the time-series blood glucose level prediction question to the supervised machine learning language. Hence, pairs of independent and dependent variables need to be constructed from the time-series data. To this end, a rolling window approach is used to appoint sequences of lag observations for blood glucose, physical activity, carbohydrate, and bolus insulin as the independent variables and sequences of blood glucose in the prediction horizon as the dependent variable.

4.2. Modelling

This subsection describes time-series forecasting models created for blood glucose level prediction 30 and 60 min into the future. This work undertakes a sequence-to-sequence fashion for multi-step-ahead time-series prediction. Prior to explaining the formal modelling process, it is useful to provide a brief explanation of stacking as an ensemble learning variation used in this work.

4.2.1. Preliminary

Ensemble learning is an advanced machine learning method that attempts to improve analysis performance by combining the decisions of multiple models [63]. Stacking is a type of ensemble learning in which a meta-learner intakes predictions of a number of base learners as an input feature to make final decisions [64].

4.2.2. Model Development

The diagram in Figure 1 displays the procedure contrived in this work for model creation. According to the diagram, the models are constructed by training three categories of learners: non-stacking, stacking, and nested stacking. The models generated based on the block diagram in Figure 1 are described below.

A non-stacking model takes a specific length of historical blood glucose, physical activity, carbohydrate, and bolus insulin data as multivariate input and returns a sequence of forecasted future blood glucose levels over a predefined prediction horizon of 30 or 60 min. According to the diagram in Figure 1, for each prediction horizon of 30 and 60 min, eight non-stacking models are created in aggregate. For this purpose, a multilayer perceptron network and a long short-term memory network are trained separately on four different lag lengths of 30, 60, 90, and 120 min.

A stacking model is a meta-model that takes sequence predictions from four non-stacking models with a homogenous learner (multilayer perceptron network or long short-term memory network) as multivariate input and fuses them to generate new prediction outputs. According to v, for each prediction horizon of 30 and 60 min, two stacking models are created, one with multilayer perceptron networks and the other with long short-term memory networks as the underlying embedded learners.

A nested stacking model is a nested meta-model. It receives the outcomes of the two stacking models described above as multivariate inputs and returns new predictions. As can be seen in Figure 1, two nested stacking models are generated for each prediction horizon of 30 and 60 min; one employs a multilayer perceptron network and the other a long short-term memory network as the nested stacking learner.

According to Figure 1, in all model creation scenarios, the learners recruited are either multilayer perceptron or long short-term memory networks. For simplicity and coherency, all multilayer perceptron networks have similar architectures consisting of an input layer, a hidden dense layer with 100 nodes, followed by another dense layer as output. Additionally, all long short-term memory networks are the vanilla type with an input layer, a hidden 100-node LSTM layer, and a dense output layer. Given the five-minute resolution of time-series data investigated, the number of nodes in the output layer is 6 and 12 for

30 min and 60 min prediction horizons, respectively. In all networks, He uniform is set as the initialiser, Adam as the optimiser, ReLU as the activation function, and mean square error as the loss function. Moreover, in all training scenarios, epoch size and batch size are set to 100 and 32, respectively. In addition, the learning rate is initiated from 0.01, and then using the ReduceLROnPlateau callback, it is reduced by a factor of 0.1 once the validation loss reduction stagnates with patience of ten iterations.

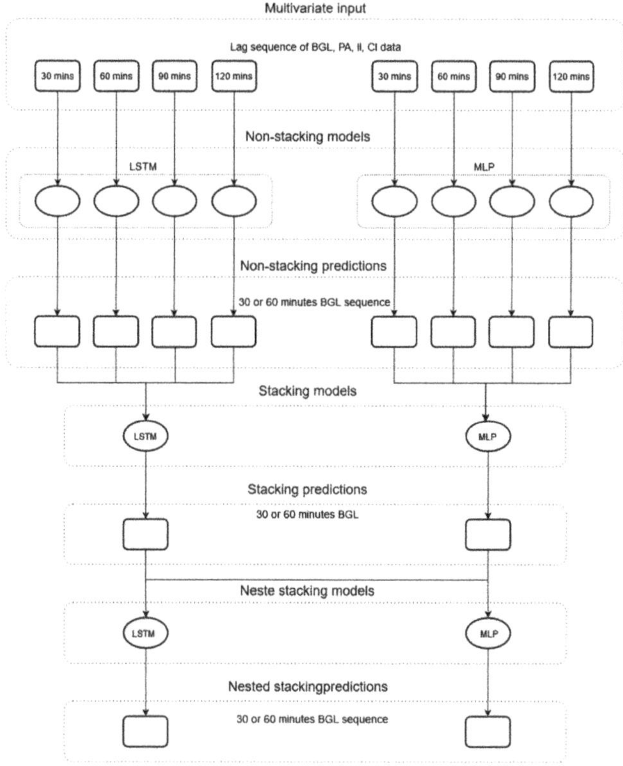

Figure 1. Blueprint for generating non-stacking, stacking, and nested stacking blood glucose level prediction models. Rectangular and oval blocks represent sequences of lag or future data and regression learners, respectively. Note. BGL: blood glucose level; PA: physical activity; II: insulin injection; CI: carbohydrate intake; LSTM: long short-term memory; MLP: multilayer perceptron.

4.3. Model Assessment

This section describes the analyses performed to validate the functionality of the developed blood glucose level prediction models. The generated models are assessed from regression, clinical, and statistical perspectives, as discussed below.

4.3.1. Regression Evaluation

Four broadly applied regression metrics are determined to verify the performance of the constructed models from a mathematical viewpoint. Mean absolute error (Equation (1)), root mean square error (Equation (2)), and mean absolute percentage error (Equation (3)) rate the accuracy of predictions. Further, the coefficient of determination (Equation (4)) measures the correlation between the reference and predicted blood glucose levels.

$$\text{MAE} = \left(\sum_{i=1}^{N} \left| \text{BGL}_i - \hat{\text{BGL}}_i \right| \right) / N \tag{1}$$

$$\text{RMSE} = \sqrt{\left(\sum_{i=1}^{N} (\text{BGL}_i - \hat{\text{BGL}}_i)^2\right)/N} \tag{2}$$

$$\text{MAPE} = \left(\left(\sum_{i=1}^{N} \left|(\text{BGL}_i - \hat{\text{BGL}}_i)/\text{BGL}_i\right|\right)/N\right) \times 100 \tag{3}$$

$$r^2 = 1 - \left(\left(\sum_{i=1}^{N} (\text{BGL}_i - \hat{\text{BGL}}_i)^2\right)\left(\sum_{i=1}^{N} (\text{BGL}_i - \overline{\text{BGL}})^2\right)\right) \tag{4}$$

where MAE: mean absolute error; BGL: blood glucose level; N: the size of the testing set; RMSE: root mean square error; MAPE: mean absolute prediction error; r^2: coefficient of determination.

4.3.2. Clinical Evaluation

Two criteria are employed to evaluate the developed models from a clinical standpoint. One criterion is the Matthew's correlation coefficient [65]. It is a factor fundamentally used for assessing the effectuality of binary classifications. In this work, this metric, calculated as Equation (5), is exploited to investigate the potency of the blood glucose prediction models in discriminating adverse glycaemic events from euglycaemic events. Hereby, an adverse glycaemic event is defined as a blood glucose level lower than 70 mg/dL (hypoglycaemia) or more than 180 mg/dL (hyperglycaemia), and a euglycaemia event as a blood glucose level between 70 mg/dL and 180 mg/dL.

$$\text{MCC} = (\text{TP} \times \text{TN} - \text{FP} \times \text{FN})/\sqrt{(\text{TP}+\text{FP})(\text{TP}+\text{FN})(\text{TN}+\text{FP})(\text{TN}+\text{FN})} \tag{5}$$

where TP: true positive (the count of correctly predicted adverse glycaemic events); TN: true negative (the count of correctly predicted euglycaemic events); FP: false positive (the count of falsely predicted adverse glycaemic events); FN: false negative (the count of falsely predicted euglycaemic events).

The other considered clinical evaluation criterion is surveillance error [66]. It is based on error grid analysis to identify the clinical risk of inaccuracies in blood glucose level predictions. Detailed calculations of surveillance error can be found in the original article [66]. However, a concise elucidation of the outcome of the calculations is as follows. A unitless error value is measured for each predicted blood glucose level. Errors smaller than 0.5 indicate clinically risk-free predictions. Errors between 0.5 and 1.5 indicate clinically slight-risk predictions. Errors between 1.5 and 2.5 indicate clinically moderate-risk predictions. Errors between 2.5 and 3.5 indicate clinically high-risk predictions. Finally, errors bigger than 3.5 indicate clinically critical-risk predictions. We adopt two evaluation metrics based on surveillance error calculation outcomes. One is the average of surveillance errors across the entire testing set, and the other is the proportion of obtained surveillance errors less than 0.5 (clinically riskless predictions) across the entire testing set.

4.3.3. Statistical Analysis

Statistical analysis is conducted for further side-by-side performance assessment for different models. In this sense, the non-parametric Friedman test is exercised to compare the outcomes of different models [67]. This test is privileged for inter-model comparative analysis across multiple datasets with no normality assumption requirement as opposed to the counterpart ANOVA test [68]. In this study, the test is assigned to compare the performance of different types of models considering individuals as independent data sources. To do so, a significant level of five percent is considered to examine the consistency of results achieved for evaluation metrics. The null hypothesis for the test is that the results of the non-stacking, stacking, and nested stacking models have identical distributions. In the next step, for cases where the global Friedman test detects the existence of a statistically significant difference amongst the models' performance, the local Nemenyi test [69], as a post hoc procedure, compares the models in a pairwise manner. In this multi-comparison analysis, the Holm–Bonferroni method is used to adjust the significance level [70]. Finally, the heuristic critical difference approach is employed to visualise the outcomes of the post hoc analysis [71]. The statistical tests are operated on all evaluation metrics in both prediction horizons of 30 and 60 min. Both multilayer perceptron and long short-term memory networks are examined as learners separately.

5. Results and Discussion

This section presents the outcomes of model assessment analyses and the relevant discussion. Initially, the results of regression-wise and clinical-wise evaluation investigations are given for the non-stacking, stacking, and nested stacking models. Therein, for each metric, mean and standard deviation values achieved over five model runs are reported, a common practice in deep learning to counteract the stochastic nature of the analysis. After presenting the evaluation results, the results of the statistical analysis performed for more detailed comparison inspections between different types of models are exhibited.

The full evaluation results of the non-stacking models are compartmentalised in four tables given in Appendix A. Table A1 is dedicated to models with multilayer perceptron learners created on the Ohio 2018 dataset, Table A2 to models with multilayer perceptron learners created on the Ohio 2020 dataset, Table A3 to models with long short-term memory learners created on the Ohio 2018 dataset, and Table A4 to models with long short-term memory learners created on the Ohio 2020.

In the non-stacking analysis, there are four modelling scenarios for each patient: blood glucose level prediction 30 and 60 min in advance, once assigning multilayer perceptron and once long short-term memory as the learner. As can be seen in the Appendix A tables, for each scenario, four models are created by training the learner on 30, 60, 90, or 120 min of historical data separately. Additionally, there are four parallel modelling scenarios for stacking and nested stacking analysis: blood glucose level prediction 30 and 60 min in advance, once employing multilayer perceptron and once long short-term memory as the last-level learner. On the other hand, one model is created for each scenario in stacking and nested stacking analysis because different lags are not separately studied.

To compare the stacking and nested stacking analyses with the non-stacking analyses, initially, for each patient, one of the four non-stacking models created for each modelling scenario is selected as the representative. Then, the representative non-stacking models are studied in parallel with the counterpart stacking and nested stacking models. To select the representative non-stacking models, first, the best evaluation metrics achieved in each modelling scenario are marked in bold font in the Appendix A tables. Subsequently, the model delivering the highest number of best-obtained evaluation metrics, highlighted in grey in the tables, is deemed as the representative. For eligibility, the results for these models are given in Table 2. Moreover, the complete evaluation results for the stacking and nested stacking models are recorded in Tables 3 and 4 respectively.

After picking the representative non-stacking models, the overall performance of these models is compared with the stacking and nested stacking counterparts. To this end, first, the Friedman test is conducted on these models' outcomes. p-values less than a significance level of 5% reveal scenarios in which there is a statistically meaningful distinction in the outputs of the three types of models for a specific evaluation metric. To elicit the performance difference for these cases, critical difference analysis integrated with post hoc Nemenyi test is used. The results of the critical difference analysis are shown in Figure 2. These diagrams show the average ranking of the modelling approaches in generating superior outcomes for a given evaluation metric. In each figure, models with statistically different average rankings are linked via a thick horizontal line. From Figure 2, the nested stacking models yielded superior evaluation outcomes overall. These findings substantiate the effectiveness of the propositions in addressing the challenge of lag optimisation while conducting enhanced outcomes.

Table 2. The evaluation results for the best non-stacking models created using Ohio datasets.

Dataset	PID	Learner	PH	Evaluation Metric						
				RMSE ± SD (mg/dL)	MAE ± SD (mg/dL)	MAPE ± SD (%)	r^2 ± SD (%)	MCC ± SD (%)	SE < 0.5 ± SD (%)	ASE ± SD
2018	559	MLP	30	19.65 ± 0.06	13.56 ± 0.03	8.78 ± 0.03	90.75 ± 0.05	0.77 ± 0.00	0.90 ± 0.00	0.19 ± 0.00
			60	31.36 ± 0.06	22.78 ± 0.06	15.18 ± 0.07	76.30 ± 0.08	0.63 ± 0.00	0.79 ± 0.00	0.31 ± 0.00
		LSTM	30	23.12 ± 0.43	16.60 ± 0.66	11.10 ± 0.63	87.19 ± 0.47	0.74 ± 0.01	0.86 ± 0.01	0.24 ± 0.01
			60	36.08 ± 1.47	25.38 ± 0.84	16.62 ± 0.25	68.60 ± 2.56	0.59 ± 0.02	0.75 ± 0.01	0.34 ± 0.01
	563	MLP	30	18.71 ± 0.05	13.46 ± 0.06	8.47 ± 0.04	82.97 ± 0.09	0.74 ± 0.00	0.91 ± 0.00	0.19 ± 0.00
			60	30.65 ± 0.01	21.69 ± 0.04	13.46 ± 0.04	54.36 ± 0.04	0.57 ± 0.01	0.81 ± 0.00	0.30 ± 0.00
		LSTM	30	21.59 ± 0.64	15.33 ± 0.45	9.69 ± 0.19	77.31 ± 1.34	0.72 ± 0.01	0.89 ± 0.00	0.22 ± 0.00
			60	33.02 ± 0.62	24.13 ± 0.61	15.07 ± 0.18	47.03 ± 2.01	0.51 ± 0.01	0.75 ± 0.02	0.33 ± 0.01
	570	MLP	30	17.44 ± 0.03	12.47 ± 0.03	6.38 ± 0.03	93.34 ± 0.03	0.86 ± 0.00	0.96 ± 0.00	0.12 ± 0.00
			60	29.00 ± 0.14	20.97 ± 0.13	10.73 ± 0.04	81.62 ± 0.18	0.79 ± 0.00	0.91 ± 0.00	0.20 ± 0.00
		LSTM	30	22.92 ± 1.49	16.16 ± 1.15	8.04 ± 0.65	88.47 ± 1.52	0.81 ± 0.02	0.94 ± 0.01	0.15 ± 0.01
			60	35.80 ± 1.50	26.75 ± 1.85	12.68 ± 0.43	71.95 ± 2.31	0.75 ± 0.00	0.88 ± 0.01	0.23 ± 0.01
	575	MLP	30	24.12 ± 0.06	16.05 ± 0.10	11.43 ± 0.09	84.48 ± 0.07	0.73 ± 0.00	0.86 ± 0.00	0.24 ± 0.00
			60	35.63 ± 0.17	25.66 ± 0.20	18.91 ± 0.17	66.19 ± 0.32	0.57 ± 0.01	0.71 ± 0.00	0.38 ± 0.00
		LSTM	30	27.20 ± 0.57	18.25 ± 0.45	13.14 ± 0.71	80.24 ± 0.82	0.69 ± 0.00	0.82 ± 0.02	0.28 ± 0.01
			60	38.09 ± 0.03	27.47 ± 0.52	20.48 ± 1.20	61.36 ± 0.07	0.54 ± 0.02	0.70 ± 0.00	0.41 ± 0.01
	588	MLP	30	18.07 ± 0.35	13.50 ± 0.15	8.29 ± 0.01	85.66 ± 0.56	0.76 ± 0.01	0.93 ± 0.00	0.18 ± 0.00
			60	30.36 ± 0.11	22.68 ± 0.13	14.16 ± 0.12	59.60 ± 0.28	0.58 ± 0.00	0.77 ± 0.00	0.31 ± 0.00
		LSTM	30	19.23 ± 0.11	14.16 ± 0.11	8.53 ± 0.12	83.77 ± 0.19	0.74 ± 0.00	0.92 ± 0.00	0.19 ± 0.00
			60	30.46 ± 0.60	22.48 ± 0.39	14.04 ± 0.23	59.33 ± 1.61	0.60 ± 0.01	0.79 ± 0.01	0.30 ± 0.01
	591	MLP	30	22.98 ± 0.11	16.61 ± 0.05	12.99 ± 0.03	80.32 ± 0.18	0.65 ± 0.01	0.80 ± 0.00	0.29 ± 0.00
			60	34.98 ± 0.05	26.93 ± 0.08	21.91 ± 0.13	54.41 ± 0.12	0.39 ± 0.00	0.65 ± 0.00	0.45 ± 0.00
		LSTM	30	26.33 ± 0.42	19.55 ± 0.24	15.65 ± 0.40	74.16 ± 0.83	0.60 ± 0.00	0.75 ± 0.01	0.34 ± 0.01
			60	36.51 ± 0.20	28.36 ± 0.26	23.32 ± 0.27	50.32 ± 0.54	0.37 ± 0.02	0.63 ± 0.00	0.47 ± 0.00
2020	540	MLP	30	22.88 ± 0.13	17.45 ± 0.10	12.71 ± 0.04	87.60 ± 0.14	0.68 ± 0.00	0.81 ± 0.00	0.27 ± 0.00
			60	39.84 ± 0.14	30.49 ± 0.12	22.96 ± 0.13	62.48 ± 0.27	0.52 ± 0.00	0.66 ± 0.00	0.44 ± 0.00
		LSTM	30	24.84 ± 0.42	18.48 ± 0.70	13.81 ± 1.24	85.37 ± 0.49	0.67 ± 0.02	0.80 ± 0.01	0.29 ± 0.02
			60	41.36 ± 0.58	30.69 ± 0.37	22.40 ± 0.20	59.56 ± 1.12	0.50 ± 0.02	0.66 ± 0.00	0.44 ± 0.00
	544	MLP	30	17.37 ± 0.03	12.14 ± 0.03	8.21 ± 0.03	88.26 ± 0.04	0.78 ± 0.00	0.92 ± 0.00	0.18 ± 0.00
			60	28.49 ± 0.03	20.74 ± 0.04	14.16 ± 0.05	68.32 ± 0.07	0.63 ± 0.00	0.78 ± 0.00	0.30 ± 0.00
		LSTM	30	21.23 ± 0.53	15.00 ± 0.49	9.93 ± 0.35	82.45 ± 0.87	0.76 ± 0.01	0.89 ± 0.00	0.21 ± 0.01
			60	30.45 ± 0.12	22.09 ± 0.45	14.81 ± 0.52	63.83 ± 0.29	0.59 ± 0.02	0.78 ± 0.01	0.31 ± 0.01
	552	MLP	30	14.06 ± 0.03	8.25 ± 0.11	6.48 ± 0.09	86.18 ± 0.05	0.75 ± 0.00	0.92 ± 0.00	0.14 ± 0.00
			60	23.83 ± 0.03	14.57 ± 0.10	11.75 ± 0.12	60.36 ± 0.09	0.64 ± 0.00	0.84 ± 0.00	0.22 ± 0.00
		LSTM	30	16.72 ± 0.44	10.31 ± 0.24	8.04 ± 0.22	80.45 ± 1.01	0.71 ± 0.02	0.90 ± 0.01	0.16 ± 0.01
			60	25.47 ± 0.30	16.27 ± 0.24	13.02 ± 0.27	54.73 ± 1.05	0.61 ± 0.01	0.83 ± 0.01	0.24 ± 0.01
	567	MLP	30	22.72 ± 0.04	16.47 ± 0.04	12.48 ± 0.03	84.80 ± 0.05	0.64 ± 0.00	0.80 ± 0.00	0.28 ± 0.00
			60	38.38 ± 0.02	29.51 ± 0.04	23.24 ± 0.06	56.68 ± 0.04	0.46 ± 0.00	0.64 ± 0.00	0.47 ± 0.00
		LSTM	30	24.64 ± 0.97	17.85 ± 0.81	13.48 ± 0.66	82.10 ± 1.41	0.60 ± 0.01	0.78 ± 0.01	0.31 ± 0.01
			60	40.13 ± 1.22	30.57 ± 1.14	25.05 ± 1.96	52.61 ± 2.86	0.45 ± 0.01	0.62 ± 0.02	0.50 ± 0.03
	584	MLP	30	22.78 ± 0.04	16.92 ± 0.04	11.34 ± 0.03	85.49 ± 0.05	0.77 ± 0.00	0.87 ± 0.00	0.23 ± 0.00
			60	35.99 ± 0.05	27.29 ± 0.02	18.40 ± 0.03	63.67 ± 0.11	0.60 ± 0.00	0.72 ± 0.00	0.37 ± 0.00
		LSTM	30	25.31 ± 1.32	18.27 ± 0.95	11.49 ± 0.52	82.05 ± 1.89	0.75 ± 0.01	0.86 ± 0.01	0.23 ± 0.01
			60	41.45 ± 1.58	31.50 ± 1.91	21.43 ± 2.17	51.75 ± 3.64	0.55 ± 0.03	0.67 ± 0.04	0.42 ± 0.04
	596	MLP	30	17.87 ± 0.08	12.89 ± 0.06	9.67 ± 0.03	86.99 ± 0.12	0.74 ± 0.00	0.89 ± 0.00	0.20 ± 0.00
			60	35.99 ± 0.05	27.29 ± 0.02	18.40 ± 0.03	63.67 ± 0.11	0.60 ± 0.00	0.72 ± 0.00	0.37 ± 0.00
		LSTM	30	19.96 ± 0.28	14.31 ± 0.03	10.83 ± 0.18	83.78 ± 0.45	0.70 ± 0.01	0.87 ± 0.00	0.23 ± 0.00
			60	30.28 ± 0.72	22.17 ± 0.71	16.97 ± 0.45	62.72 ± 1.77	0.56 ± 0.02	0.79 ± 0.00	0.32 ± 0.01

Note. PID: patient identification; PH: prediction horizon; LL: lag length; RMSE: root mean square error; SD: standard deviation; MAE: mean absolute error; MAPE: mean absolute percentage error; r^2: coefficient of determination; MCC: Matthew's correlation coefficient; SE: surveillance error; ASE: average surveillance error.

Table 3. The evaluation results for the stacking models created using Ohio datasets.

Dataset	PID	Learner	PH	RMSE ± SD (mg/dL)	MAE ± SD (mg/dL)	MAPE ± SD (%)	r^2 ± SD (%)	MCC ± SD (%)	SE < 0.5 ± SD (%)	ASE ± SD
2018	559	MLP	30	19.00 ± 0.11	13.19 ± 0.08	8.79 ± 0.05	91.35 ± 0.10	0.78 ± 0.00	0.90 ± 0.00	0.19 ± 0.00
			60	31.25 ± 0.41	22.67 ± 0.22	15.22 ± 0.24	76.46 ± 0.61	0.64 ± 0.00	0.79 ± 0.00	0.31 ± 0.00
		LSTM	30	22.90 ± 0.49	15.77 ± 0.17	9.97 ± 0.09	87.43 ± 0.54	0.76 ± 0.01	0.89 ± 0.00	0.21 ± 0.00
			60	34.95 ± 0.17	24.99 ± 0.11	16.61 ± 0.05	70.56 ± 0.29	0.61 ± 0.01	0.76 ± 0.00	0.33 ± 0.00
	563	MLP	30	18.54 ± 0.05	13.03 ± 0.03	8.10 ± 0.00	83.28 ± 0.08	0.74 ± 0.01	0.92 ± 0.00	0.18 ± 0.00
			60	29.87 ± 0.18	21.22 ± 0.14	13.36 ± 0.04	56.67 ± 0.51	0.58 ± 0.01	0.81 ± 0.00	0.30 ± 0.00
		LSTM	30	21.25 ± 0.05	14.97 ± 0.06	9.38 ± 0.02	78.05 ± 0.11	0.73 ± 0.00	0.89 ± 0.00	0.21 ± 0.00
			60	33.20 ± 0.16	23.55 ± 0.07	14.44 ± 0.02	46.46 ± 0.53	0.52 ± 0.00	0.78 ± 0.00	0.32 ± 0.00
	570	MLP	30	17.49 ± 0.11	12.43 ± 0.10	6.36 ± 0.03	93.30 ± 0.09	0.86 ± 0.01	0.96 ± 0.00	0.12 ± 0.00
			60	28.65 ± 0.08	20.90 ± 0.07	10.91 ± 0.04	82.06 ± 0.10	0.78 ± 0.00	0.91 ± 0.00	0.20 ± 0.00
		LSTM	30	21.58 ± 1.50	15.59 ± 1.55	7.70 ± 0.49	89.77 ± 1.44	0.84 ± 0.01	0.94 ± 0.00	0.14 ± 0.01
			60	32.48 ± 0.69	23.55 ± 0.62	11.82 ± 0.06	76.93 ± 0.98	0.76 ± 0.00	0.89 ± 0.00	0.22 ± 0.00
	575	MLP	30	24.21 ± 0.04	15.70 ± 0.09	11.25 ± 0.19	84.36 ± 0.05	0.74 ± 0.00	0.86 ± 0.00	0.24 ± 0.00
			60	36.42 ± 0.41	26.35 ± 0.77	19.85 ± 1.57	64.68 ± 0.79	0.57 ± 0.02	0.71 ± 0.00	0.40 ± 0.02
		LSTM	30	27.73 ± 0.12	18.09 ± 0.09	12.67 ± 0.09	79.48 ± 0.18	0.66 ± 0.00	0.82 ± 0.00	0.27 ± 0.00
			60	38.34 ± 0.09	27.48 ± 0.06	19.59 ± 0.12	60.86 ± 0.18	0.54 ± 0.00	0.68 ± 0.00	0.41 ± 0.00
	588	MLP	30	18.24 ± 0.19	13.51 ± 0.12	8.17 ± 0.02	85.39 ± 0.30	0.75 ± 0.01	0.93 ± 0.00	0.18 ± 0.00
			60	29.65 ± 0.21	21.84 ± 0.18	13.14 ± 0.08	61.46 ± 0.55	0.57 ± 0.01	0.80 ± 0.00	0.29 ± 0.00
		LSTM	30	18.91 ± 0.08	14.03 ± 0.14	8.43 ± 0.25	84.30 ± 0.13	0.75 ± 0.00	0.92 ± 0.00	0.18 ± 0.01
			60	30.67 ± 0.20	22.29 ± 0.25	13.54 ± 0.49	58.76 ± 0.54	0.60 ± 0.01	0.81 ± 0.01	0.29 ± 0.01
	591	MLP	30	22.88 ± 0.07	16.60 ± 0.04	13.03 ± 0.06	80.49 ± 0.12	0.65 ± 0.00	0.80 ± 0.00	0.29 ± 0.00
			60	34.43 ± 0.06	26.80 ± 0.05	22.09 ± 0.09	55.84 ± 0.14	0.41 ± 0.00	0.65 ± 0.00	0.45 ± 0.00
		LSTM	30	25.51 ± 0.01	18.80 ± 0.05	14.79 ± 0.08	75.73 ± 0.03	0.59 ± 0.00	0.76 ± 0.00	0.33 ± 0.00
			60	36.68 ± 0.16	28.44 ± 0.05	23.78 ± 0.03	49.87 ± 0.44	0.42 ± 0.00	0.64 ± 0.00	0.47 ± 0.00
2020	540	MLP	30	22.34 ± 0.02	17.13 ± 0.03	12.58 ± 0.03	88.18 ± 0.02	0.68 ± 0.00	0.82 ± 0.00	0.27 ± 0.00
			60	39.40 ± 0.09	30.32 ± 0.13	22.95 ± 0.10	63.29 ± 0.17	0.52 ± 0.00	0.66 ± 0.00	0.44 ± 0.00
		LSTM	30	24.13 ± 0.14	18.24 ± 0.06	13.57 ± 0.03	86.20 ± 0.17	0.66 ± 0.00	0.80 ± 0.00	0.29 ± 0.00
			60	40.86 ± 0.05	30.62 ± 0.11	23.06 ± 0.18	60.53 ± 0.09	0.51 ± 0.00	0.66 ± 0.00	0.44 ± 0.00
	544	MLP	30	16.96 ± 0.02	12.01 ± 0.05	8.14 ± 0.08	88.81 ± 0.03	0.79 ± 0.00	0.92 ± 0.00	0.18 ± 0.00
			60	28.36 ± 0.17	20.72 ± 0.04	14.21 ± 0.08	68.62 ± 0.37	0.64 ± 0.00	0.78 ± 0.00	0.30 ± 0.00
		LSTM	30	20.85 ± 0.25	14.84 ± 0.20	10.01 ± 0.14	83.08 ± 0.40	0.73 ± 0.00	0.88 ± 0.00	0.22 ± 0.00
			60	31.30 ± 0.23	22.55 ± 0.10	15.44 ± 0.07	61.77 ± 0.57	0.59 ± 0.00	0.76 ± 0.00	0.33 ± 0.00
	552	MLP	30	14.19 ± 0.03	9.00 ± 0.06	7.10 ± 0.03	85.92 ± 0.05	0.72 ± 0.00	0.91 ± 0.00	0.15 ± 0.00
			60	23.78 ± 0.04	15.52 ± 0.20	12.62 ± 0.18	60.53 ± 0.14	0.61 ± 0.01	0.84 ± 0.00	0.23 ± 0.00
		LSTM	30	17.65 ± 0.22	11.92 ± 0.20	9.79 ± 0.21	78.23 ± 0.53	0.69 ± 0.00	0.88 ± 0.01	0.19 ± 0.01
			60	26.93 ± 0.23	17.97 ± 0.17	15.04 ± 0.14	49.39 ± 0.85	0.58 ± 0.01	0.78 ± 0.00	0.28 ± 0.00
	567	MLP	30	22.67 ± 0.22	16.17 ± 0.22	12.39 ± 0.21	84.86 ± 0.29	0.64 ± 0.01	0.81 ± 0.00	0.28 ± 0.00
			60	37.82 ± 0.24	28.14 ± 0.18	22.42 ± 0.23	57.94 ± 0.52	0.48 ± 0.00	0.66 ± 0.00	0.46 ± 0.00
		LSTM	30	23.74 ± 0.09	16.86 ± 0.14	12.96 ± 0.14	83.41 ± 0.13	0.62 ± 0.00	0.79 ± 0.00	0.30 ± 0.00
			60	38.75 ± 0.41	29.24 ± 0.31	23.40 ± 0.46	55.84 ± 0.92	0.47 ± 0.01	0.64 ± 0.01	0.48 ± 0.01
	584	MLP	30	21.89 ± 0.09	15.96 ± 0.14	10.64 ± 0.13	86.60 ± 0.11	0.77 ± 0.00	0.89 ± 0.00	0.22 ± 0.00
			60	35.42 ± 0.42	26.73 ± 0.52	17.97 ± 0.53	64.79 ± 0.83	0.60 ± 0.01	0.73 ± 0.01	0.36 ± 0.01
		LSTM	30	24.79 ± 0.06	18.21 ± 0.08	12.51 ± 0.13	82.82 ± 0.08	0.76 ± 0.00	0.86 ± 0.00	0.25 ± 0.00
			60	38.65 ± 0.29	29.33 ± 0.12	20.14 ± 0.01	58.09 ± 0.63	0.60 ± 0.00	0.70 ± 0.00	0.39 ± 0.00
	596	MLP	30	17.76 ± 0.09	12.85 ± 0.09	9.71 ± 0.11	87.16 ± 0.13	0.75 ± 0.00	0.90 ± 0.00	0.20 ± 0.00
			60	28.80 ± 0.19	21.37 ± 0.13	16.53 ± 0.11	66.29 ± 0.44	0.59 ± 0.01	0.80 ± 0.00	0.31 ± 0.00
		LSTM	30	19.06 ± 0.16	13.55 ± 0.08	10.27 ± 0.06	85.21 ± 0.24	0.72 ± 0.00	0.88 ± 0.00	0.22 ± 0.00
			60	30.01 ± 0.10	22.25 ± 0.10	17.31 ± 0.16	63.39 ± 0.25	0.56 ± 0.00	0.80 ± 0.00	0.32 ± 0.00

Note. PID: patient identification; PH: prediction horizon; LL: lag length; RMSE: root mean square error; SD: standard deviation; MAE: mean absolute error; MAPE: mean absolute percentage error; r^2: coefficient of determination; MCC: Matthew's correlation coefficient; SE: surveillance error; ASE: average surveillance error.

Table 4. The evaluation results for the nested stacking models created using Ohio datasets.

Dataset	PID	Learner	PH	Evaluation Metric						
				RMSE ± SD (mg/dL)	MAE ± SD (mg/dL)	MAPE ± SD (%)	r^2 ± SD (%)	MCC ± SD (%)	SE < 0.5 ± SD (%)	ASE ± SD
2018	559	MLP	30	19.67 ± 0.05	13.54 ± 0.05	8.89 ± 0.03	90.72 ± 0.05	0.79 ± 0.00	0.90 ± 0.00	0.19 ± 0.00
			60	33.44 ± 0.28	23.54 ± 0.16	15.27 ± 0.04	73.05 ± 0.46	0.63 ± 0.00	0.78 ± 0.00	0.31 ± 0.00
		LSTM	30	19.69 ± 0.19	13.51 ± 0.18	8.83 ± 0.17	90.71 ± 0.18	0.79 ± 0.00	0.90 ± 0.00	0.19 ± 0.00
			60	33.93 ± 0.48	23.82 ± 0.28	15.31 ± 0.05	72.25 ± 0.79	0.63 ± 0.01	0.78 ± 0.00	0.31 ± 0.00
	563	MLP	30	18.85 ± 0.10	13.15 ± 0.08	8.27 ± 0.02	82.72 ± 0.19	0.76 ± 0.01	0.91 ± 0.00	0.18 ± 0.00
			60	31.82 ± 0.54	22.38 ± 0.38	13.84 ± 0.11	50.81 ± 1.66	0.55 ± 0.01	0.80 ± 0.01	0.30 ± 0.00
		LSTM	30	19.00 ± 0.07	13.24 ± 0.06	8.31 ± 0.03	82.44 ± 0.13	0.76 ± 0.01	0.91 ± 0.00	0.19 ± 0.00
			60	31.65 ± 0.51	22.37 ± 0.61	13.79 ± 0.10	51.35 ± 1.59	0.55 ± 0.03	0.80 ± 0.01	0.31 ± 0.01
	570	MLP	30	18.34 ± 0.11	12.85 ± 0.08	6.58 ± 0.05	92.64 ± 0.09	0.86 ± 0.00	0.96 ± 0.00	0.12 ± 0.00
			60	31.09 ± 0.28	22.21 ± 0.14	11.54 ± 0.03	78.88 ± 0.38	0.77 ± 0.00	0.89 ± 0.00	0.21 ± 0.00
		LSTM	30	18.57 ± 0.22	13.11 ± 0.12	6.65 ± 0.08	92.45 ± 0.18	0.86 ± 0.00	0.96 ± 0.00	0.12 ± 0.00
			60	31.61 ± 0.60	22.60 ± 0.54	11.53 ± 0.02	78.16 ± 0.84	0.77 ± 0.00	0.90 ± 0.00	0.21 ± 0.00
	575	MLP	30	26.18 ± 0.09	16.60 ± 0.19	12.40 ± 0.27	81.71 ± 0.12	0.73 ± 0.00	0.84 ± 0.00	0.26 ± 0.01
			60	36.98 ± 0.33	26.43 ± 0.50	19.46 ± 1.39	63.57 ± 0.65	0.54 ± 0.01	0.70 ± 0.01	0.40 ± 0.02
		LSTM	30	26.01 ± 0.91	16.47 ± 0.32	12.02 ± 0.66	81.93 ± 1.25	0.73 ± 0.00	0.84 ± 0.01	0.25 ± 0.01
			60	37.05 ± 0.62	26.29 ± 0.28	18.96 ± 0.13	63.44 ± 1.22	0.54 ± 0.00	0.70 ± 0.00	0.39 ± 0.00
	588	MLP	30	18.50 ± 0.11	13.63 ± 0.08	8.11 ± 0.05	84.98 ± 0.17	0.74 ± 0.00	0.93 ± 0.00	0.18 ± 0.00
			60	29.43 ± 0.07	21.42 ± 0.17	13.01 ± 0.42	62.05 ± 0.17	0.62 ± 0.00	0.82 ± 0.01	0.28 ± 0.01
		LSTM	30	18.26 ± 0.14	13.56 ± 0.27	8.23 ± 0.32	85.37 ± 0.22	0.76 ± 0.01	0.93 ± 0.00	0.18 ± 0.01
			60	29.54 ± 0.28	21.33 ± 0.21	12.84 ± 0.09	61.77 ± 0.74	0.62 ± 0.01	0.82 ± 0.00	0.27 ± 0.00
	591	MLP	30	23.07 ± 0.09	16.48 ± 0.04	12.89 ± 0.06	80.16 ± 0.15	0.64 ± 0.01	0.80 ± 0.00	0.29 ± 0.00
			60	35.68 ± 0.11	27.65 ± 0.08	23.12 ± 0.07	52.56 ± 0.29	0.42 ± 0.00	0.65 ± 0.00	0.46 ± 0.00
		LSTM	30	23.08 ± 0.10	16.52 ± 0.07	12.98 ± 0.08	80.14 ± 0.17	0.63 ± 0.00	0.80 ± 0.00	0.29 ± 0.00
			60	35.68 ± 0.21	27.69 ± 0.12	23.16 ± 0.08	52.57 ± 0.55	0.42 ± 0.00	0.65 ± 0.01	0.46 ± 0.00
2020	540	MLP	30	22.36 ± 0.03	16.96 ± 0.05	12.59 ± 0.03	88.15 ± 0.03	0.67 ± 0.00	0.82 ± 0.00	0.27 ± 0.00
			60	38.81 ± 0.26	29.34 ± 0.14	22.04 ± 0.10	64.38 ± 0.47	0.53 ± 0.01	0.68 ± 0.00	0.43 ± 0.00
		LSTM	30	22.39 ± 0.11	16.99 ± 0.09	12.61 ± 0.08	88.12 ± 0.12	0.67 ± 0.01	0.81 ± 0.00	0.27 ± 0.00
			60	38.74 ± 0.18	29.32 ± 0.18	22.05 ± 0.15	64.52 ± 0.33	0.53 ± 0.01	0.68 ± 0.00	0.43 ± 0.00
	544	MLP	30	16.86 ± 0.11	11.89 ± 0.06	8.02 ± 0.06	88.94 ± 0.14	0.78 ± 0.00	0.92 ± 0.00	0.17 ± 0.00
			60	28.92 ± 0.14	20.88 ± 0.05	14.33 ± 0.02	67.36 ± 0.31	0.63 ± 0.00	0.77 ± 0.00	0.30 ± 0.00
		LSTM	30	16.96 ± 0.15	11.95 ± 0.11	8.07 ± 0.09	88.80 ± 0.19	0.78 ± 0.01	0.92 ± 0.00	0.18 ± 0.00
			60	28.84 ± 0.19	20.81 ± 0.10	14.34 ± 0.13	67.54 ± 0.42	0.63 ± 0.00	0.77 ± 0.00	0.30 ± 0.00
	552	MLP	30	13.87 ± 0.16	8.88 ± 0.32	7.07 ± 0.24	86.56 ± 0.32	0.72 ± 0.01	0.92 ± 0.00	0.15 ± 0.01
			60	24.61 ± 0.11	16.04 ± 0.36	13.43 ± 0.30	57.73 ± 0.38	0.60 ± 0.00	0.82 ± 0.00	0.25 ± 0.00
		LSTM	30	13.86 ± 0.02	9.00 ± 0.06	7.13 ± 0.06	86.58 ± 0.03	0.72 ± 0.00	0.92 ± 0.00	0.15 ± 0.00
			60	23.97 ± 0.44	15.47 ± 0.32	12.76 ± 0.38	59.91 ± 1.47	0.61 ± 0.00	0.83 ± 0.01	0.24 ± 0.01
	567	MLP	30	21.81 ± 0.28	15.58 ± 0.14	11.71 ± 0.30	86.00 ± 0.35	0.65 ± 0.01	0.82 ± 0.01	0.27 ± 0.01
			60	37.50 ± 0.18	27.95 ± 0.13	21.97 ± 0.18	58.65 ± 0.39	0.49 ± 0.00	0.66 ± 0.00	0.46 ± 0.00
		LSTM	30	22.02 ± 0.07	15.70 ± 0.05	11.96 ± 0.07	85.72 ± 0.08	0.64 ± 0.00	0.82 ± 0.00	0.27 ± 0.00
			60	37.77 ± 0.25	28.19 ± 0.22	22.38 ± 0.36	58.05 ± 0.55	0.48 ± 0.00	0.66 ± 0.00	0.46 ± 0.00
	584	MLP	30	22.35 ± 0.58	16.74 ± 0.67	11.54 ± 0.54	86.03 ± 0.73	0.77 ± 0.01	0.88 ± 0.01	0.24 ± 0.01
			60	35.77 ± 0.49	27.25 ± 0.49	18.79 ± 0.44	64.11 ± 0.99	0.61 ± 0.01	0.73 ± 0.01	0.37 ± 0.01
		LSTM	30	22.19 ± 0.11	16.54 ± 0.17	11.38 ± 0.17	86.24 ± 0.13	0.77 ± 0.00	0.88 ± 0.00	0.23 ± 0.00
			60	36.02 ± 0.06	27.37 ± 0.12	18.91 ± 0.14	63.60 ± 0.12	0.61 ± 0.00	0.72 ± 0.00	0.37 ± 0.00
	596	MLP	30	17.78 ± 0.24	12.67 ± 0.13	9.52 ± 0.10	87.13 ± 0.35	0.74 ± 0.00	0.89 ± 0.00	0.20 ± 0.00
			60	28.54 ± 0.24	20.79 ± 0.09	15.74 ± 0.27	66.89 ± 0.55	0.58 ± 0.02	0.81 ± 0.00	0.30 ± 0.00
		LSTM	30	17.57 ± 0.25	12.49 ± 0.14	9.35 ± 0.09	87.43 ± 0.36	0.75 ± 0.01	0.89 ± 0.00	0.20 ± 0.00
			60	28.68 ± 0.37	20.97 ± 0.07	15.96 ± 0.31	66.55 ± 0.87	0.58 ± 0.02	0.81 ± 0.00	0.31 ± 0.00

Note. PID: patient identification; PH: prediction horizon; LL: lag length; RMSE: root mean square error; SD: standard deviation; MAE: mean absolute error; MAPE: mean absolute percentage error; r^2: coefficient of determination; MCC: Matthew's correlation coefficient; SE: surveillance error; ASE: average surveillance error.

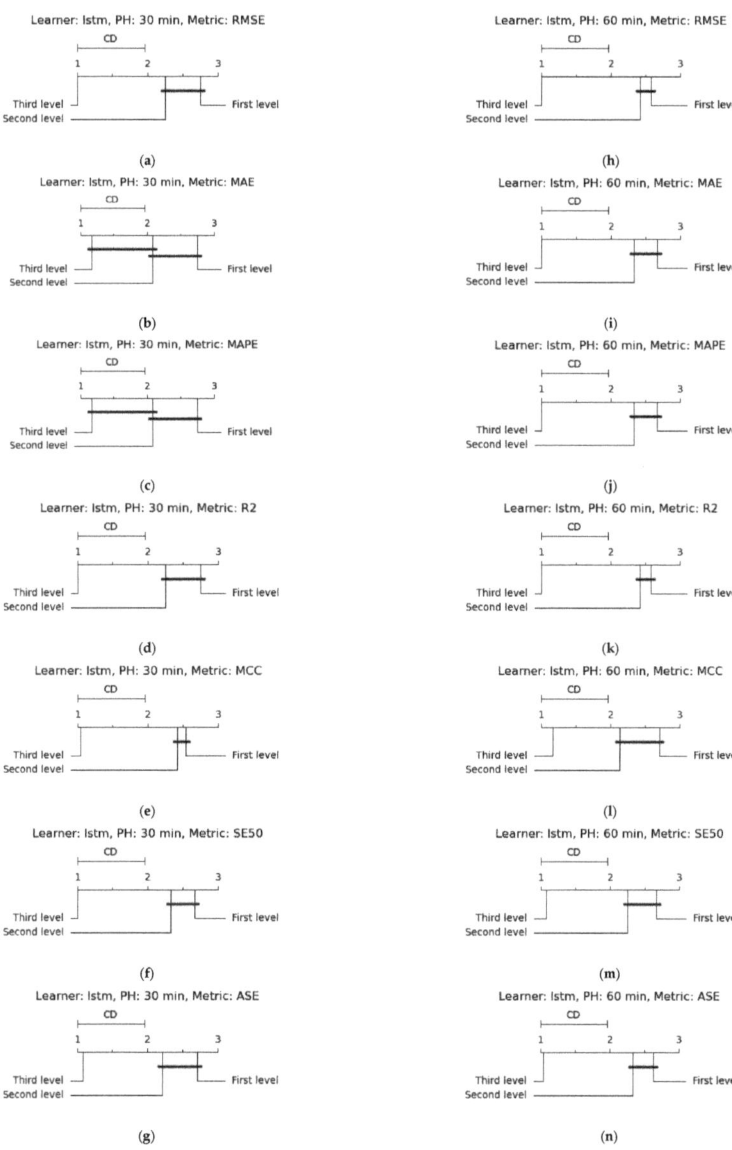

Figure 2. Critical difference diagrams based on Nemenyi test for pairwise comparison of the non-stacking, stacking, and nested stacking modelling approaches: (**a**) LSTM learner, 30 min PH, and RMSE metric, (**b**) LSTM learner, 30 min PH, and MAE metric, (**c**) LSTM learner, 30 min PH, and MAPE metric, (**d**) LSTM learner, 30 min PH, and r^2 metric, (**e**) LSTM learner, 30 min PH, and MCC metric, (**f**) LSTM learner, 30 min PH, and SE50 metric, (**g**) LSTM learner, 30 min PH, and ASE metric, (**h**) LSTM learner, 60 min PH, and RMSE metric, (**i**) LSTM learner, 60 min PH, and MAE metric, (**j**) LSTM learner, 60 min PH, and MAPE metric, (**k**) LSTM learner, 60 min PH, and r^2 metric, (**l**) LSTM learner, 60 min PH, and MCC metric, (**m**) LSTM learner, 60 min PH, and SE50 metric, (**n**) LSTM learner, 60 min PH, and ASE metric. Note. LSTM: long short-term memory; PH: prediction horizon; RMSE: root mean square error; MAE: mean absolute error; MAPE: mean absolute percentage error; r^2: coefficient of determination; MCC: Matthew's correlation coefficient; SE: surveillance error; ASE: average surveillance error.

It is noteworthy that, according to the highlighted models in the Appendix A tables, an inconsistency in the efficient lag to be investigated for different patients, prediction horizons, and learners can be observed. In detail, the optimal lag is 30 min in 19 cases, 60 min in 19 cases, 90 min in 5 cases, and 120 min in 5 cases. Such disparity further accentuates the utility of the nested stacking analyses that efficaciously circumvent the lag optimisation process.

6. Summary and Conclusions

This work offers a nested meta-learning lag fusion approach to address the challenge of history length optimisation in personalised blood glucose level prediction. For this purpose, in lieu of examining different lengths of history from a search space and picking a local optimum for each subject or a global suboptimum for all subjects, all the lags in the search space are studied autonomously, and the results are amalgamated. A multilayer perceptron and long short-term memory network are initially trained on four different lags separately, resulting in four non-stacking models from each network. The outcomes of the four non-stacking multilayer perceptron models are then combined into new outcomes using a stacking multilayer perceptron model. Similarly, a stacking long short-term memory model fuses the results of the four non-stacking long short-term memory models. Finally, the decisions of the two stacking prediction models are ensembled once using a multilayer perceptron and once using a long short-term memory network as a nested stacking model. These investigations are performed for two commonly studied prediction horizons of 30 and 60 min in blood glucose level prediction research. The generated models undergo in-depth regression-wise, clinical-wise, and statistic-wise assessments. The results obtained substantiate the effectiveness of the proposed stacking and nested stacking methods in addressing the challenge of lag optimisation in blood glucose level prediction analysis.

7. Software and Code

For developing and evaluating blood glucose level prediction models, this research used Python 3.6 [72] programming. The libraries and packages employed include Tensor-Flow [73], Keras [73], Pandas [74], NumPy [75], Sklearn [76], SciPy [77], statsmodels [78], scikit-post hocs [79], and cd-diagram [80]. The source code for implementations is available on this Gitlab repository.

Author Contributions: H.K.: conceptualisation, methodology, software, validation, formal analysis, investigation, data curation, writing the original draft, review and editing, visualisation. H.N.: conceptualisation, methodology, software, validation, formal analysis, investigation, data curation, review and editing. J.E.: conceptualisation, validation, review and editing, supervision. M.B.: conceptualisation, methodology, validation, investigation, resources, review and editing. All authors have read and agreed to the published version of the manuscript.

Funding: University of Sheffield Institutional Open Access Fund.

Institutional Review Board Statement: Not applicable.

Informed Consent Statement: Not applicable.

Data Availability Statement: The Ohio datasets used in this research are publicly accessible upon request by following the instructions provided in this link.

Appendix A

In this section, the complete outcomes of evaluation analysis on the non-stacking models are provided in four tables, as below.

Table A1. The evaluation results for non-stacking models created by multilayer perceptron learners using Ohio 2018 dataset.

PID	PH	LL	RMSE ± SD (mg/dL)	MAE ± SD (mg/dL)	MAPE ± SD (%)	r^2 ± SD (%)	MCC ± SD (%)	SE < 0.5 ± SD (%)	ASE ± SD
559	30	30	19.96 ± 0.09	13.78 ± 0.11	8.83 ± 0.11	90.45 ± 0.08	**0.77 ± 0.00**	**0.90 ± 0.00**	**0.19 ± 0.00**
		60	**19.65 ± 0.06**	**13.56 ± 0.03**	**8.78 ± 0.03**	**90.75 ± 0.05**	**0.77 ± 0.00**	**0.90 ± 0.00**	**0.19 ± 0.00**
		90	19.85 ± 0.01	13.73 ± 0.02	8.81 ± 0.04	90.56 ± 0.01	**0.77 ± 0.00**	**0.90 ± 0.00**	**0.19 ± 0.00**
		120	19.88 ± 0.07	13.83 ± 0.05	8.81 ± 0.04	90.53 ± 0.07	**0.77 ± 0.00**	**0.90 ± 0.00**	**0.19 ± 0.00**
	60	30	33.73 ± 0.04	24.46 ± 0.04	16.49 ± 0.05	72.59 ± 0.06	0.58 ± 0.00	0.77 ± 0.00	0.33 ± 0.00
		60	32.04 ± 0.05	23.12 ± 0.09	15.43 ± 0.11	75.26 ± 0.08	0.62 ± 0.01	**0.79 ± 0.00**	**0.31 ± 0.00**
		90	31.67 ± 0.05	22.84 ± 0.06	15.23 ± 0.04	75.82 ± 0.08	**0.64 ± 0.00**	**0.79 ± 0.00**	**0.31 ± 0.00**
		120	**31.36 ± 0.06**	**22.78 ± 0.06**	15.18 ± 0.07	**76.30 ± 0.08**	0.63 ± 0.00	**0.79 ± 0.00**	**0.31 ± 0.00**
563	30	30	**18.71 ± 0.05**	13.46 ± 0.06	8.47 ± 0.04	**82.97 ± 0.09**	0.74 ± 0.00	**0.91 ± 0.00**	**0.19 ± 0.00**
		60	18.89 ± 0.03	**13.33 ± 0.03**	**8.30 ± 0.02**	82.65 ± 0.05	0.74 ± 0.00	**0.91 ± 0.00**	**0.19 ± 0.00**
		90	19.09 ± 0.03	13.42 ± 0.03	8.34 ± 0.02	82.27 ± 0.06	**0.74 ± 0.01**	**0.91 ± 0.00**	**0.19 ± 0.00**
		120	19.29 ± 0.01	13.61 ± 0.00	8.45 ± 0.00	81.91 ± 0.02	0.73 ± 0.01	**0.91 ± 0.00**	**0.19 ± 0.00**
	60	30	30.44 ± 0.08	22.46 ± 0.08	14.40 ± 0.06	55.00 ± 0.23	0.49 ± 0.00	0.78 ± 0.00	0.33 ± 0.00
		60	**30.43 ± 0.05**	21.75 ± 0.02	13.57 ± 0.02	**55.02 ± 0.14**	0.56 ± 0.01	0.80 ± 0.00	0.30 ± 0.00
		90	30.65 ± 0.01	**21.69 ± 0.04**	**13.46 ± 0.04**	54.36 ± 0.04	**0.57 ± 0.01**	**0.81 ± 0.00**	0.30 ± 0.00
		120	30.68 ± 0.15	21.72 ± 0.09	13.47 ± 0.05	54.28 ± 0.44	0.57 ± 0.00	**0.81 ± 0.00**	0.30 ± 0.00
570	30	30	18.24 ± 0.19	13.27 ± 0.15	6.74 ± 0.08	92.71 ± 0.15	0.84 ± 0.00	0.95 ± 0.00	0.13 ± 0.00
		60	**17.44 ± 0.03**	**12.47 ± 0.03**	**6.38 ± 0.03**	**93.34 ± 0.03**	**0.86 ± 0.00**	**0.96 ± 0.00**	**0.12 ± 0.00**
		90	17.58 ± 0.03	12.54 ± 0.03	6.45 ± 0.01	**93.24 ± 0.03**	**0.86 ± 0.00**	**0.96 ± 0.00**	**0.12 ± 0.00**
		120	17.71 ± 0.13	12.53 ± 0.11	6.41 ± 0.06	93.13 ± 0.10	**0.86 ± 0.00**	**0.96 ± 0.00**	**0.12 ± 0.00**
	60	30	30.36 ± 0.08	23.08 ± 0.07	11.89 ± 0.03	79.85 ± 0.10	0.74 ± 0.00	0.89 ± 0.00	0.22 ± 0.00
		60	**28.89 ± 0.03**	21.33 ± 0.04	10.92 ± 0.01	**81.76 ± 0.04**	0.78 ± 0.00	**0.91 ± 0.00**	**0.20 ± 0.00**
		90	28.95 ± 0.10	**21.07 ± 0.09**	10.82 ± 0.02	81.68 ± 0.13	**0.79 ± 0.00**	**0.91 ± 0.00**	**0.20 ± 0.00**
		120	29.00 ± 0.14	20.97 ± 0.13	**10.73 ± 0.04**	81.62 ± 0.18	**0.79 ± 0.00**	**0.91 ± 0.00**	**0.20 ± 0.00**
575	30	30	**24.12 ± 0.06**	16.05 ± 0.10	11.43 ± 0.09	**84.48 ± 0.07**	0.73 ± 0.00	**0.86 ± 0.00**	0.24 ± 0.00
		60	24.49 ± 0.04	**15.93 ± 0.02**	**11.39 ± 0.02**	84.00 ± 0.06	0.73 ± 0.00	0.85 ± 0.00	0.25 ± 0.00
		90	24.38 ± 0.09	15.97 ± 0.13	11.56 ± 0.11	84.13 ± 0.12	0.74 ± 0.00	0.85 ± 0.00	0.25 ± 0.00
		120	24.35 ± 0.09	16.07 ± 0.12	11.72 ± 0.16	84.17 ± 0.12	**0.75 ± 0.00**	0.85 ± 0.01	0.25 ± 0.00
	60	30	36.22 ± 0.10	26.77 ± 0.12	19.49 ± 0.10	65.08 ± 0.19	0.51 ± 0.00	0.69 ± 0.00	0.40 ± 0.00
		60	36.27 ± 0.20	26.24 ± 0.25	18.96 ± 0.17	64.96 ± 0.39	0.54 ± 0.01	0.70 ± 0.00	0.39 ± 0.00
		90	35.90 ± 0.23	25.73 ± 0.11	**18.79 ± 0.09**	65.68 ± 0.44	0.55 ± 0.00	0.70 ± 0.00	0.39 ± 0.00
		120	**35.63 ± 0.17**	**25.66 ± 0.20**	18.91 ± 0.17	**66.19 ± 0.32**	0.57 ± 0.01	0.71 ± 0.00	0.38 ± 0.00
588	30	30	18.80 ± 0.09	13.99 ± 0.09	8.63 ± 0.07	84.49 ± 0.15	**0.75 ± 0.00**	0.92 ± 0.00	0.19 ± 0.00
		60	18.27 ± 0.42	13.61 ± 0.20	8.36 ± 0.06	85.35 ± 0.68	0.75 ± 0.02	**0.93 ± 0.00**	**0.18 ± 0.00**
		90	**18.07 ± 0.35**	**13.50 ± 0.15**	8.29 ± 0.01	85.66 ± 0.56	0.76 ± 0.01	**0.93 ± 0.00**	**0.18 ± 0.00**
		120	18.44 ± 0.67	13.64 ± 0.37	**8.26 ± 0.13**	85.06 ± 1.09	0.75 ± 0.02	**0.93 ± 0.01**	**0.18 ± 0.00**
	60	30	**30.36 ± 0.11**	22.68 ± 0.13	14.16 ± 0.12	**59.60 ± 0.28**	**0.58 ± 0.00**	0.77 ± 0.00	0.31 ± 0.00
		60	30.72 ± 0.26	22.76 ± 0.25	13.62 ± 0.16	58.65 ± 0.69	0.56 ± 0.01	0.79 ± 0.00	0.30 ± 0.00
		90	30.58 ± 0.05	**22.47 ± 0.10**	13.41 ± 0.08	59.01 ± 0.13	0.56 ± 0.00	**0.80 ± 0.00**	**0.29 ± 0.00**
		120	30.48 ± 0.25	22.39 ± 0.26	**13.33 ± 0.19**	59.29 ± 0.67	0.57 ± 0.01	**0.80 ± 0.00**	**0.29 ± 0.00**
591	30	30	**22.89 ± 0.02**	16.68 ± 0.02	**12.98 ± 0.02**	**80.47 ± 0.04**	0.62 ± 0.00	0.79 ± 0.00	0.29 ± 0.00
		60	22.98 ± 0.11	**16.61 ± 0.05**	12.99 ± 0.03	80.32 ± 0.18	**0.65 ± 0.01**	**0.80 ± 0.00**	**0.29 ± 0.00**
		90	23.01 ± 0.06	16.71 ± 0.01	13.12 ± 0.02	80.26 ± 0.09	0.64 ± 0.01	**0.80 ± 0.00**	**0.29 ± 0.00**
		120	22.97 ± 0.07	16.78 ± 0.05	13.21 ± 0.11	80.32 ± 0.12	0.64 ± 0.01	**0.80 ± 0.00**	**0.29 ± 0.00**
	60	30	35.00 ± 0.05	27.27 ± 0.06	22.01 ± 0.07	54.35 ± 0.14	0.36 ± 0.00	0.64 ± 0.00	**0.45 ± 0.00**
		60	35.93 ± 0.07	27.77 ± 0.02	22.37 ± 0.07	51.89 ± 0.19	0.35 ± 0.00	0.63 ± 0.00	0.46 ± 0.00
		90	34.98 ± 0.05	**26.93 ± 0.08**	**21.91 ± 0.13**	54.41 ± 0.12	**0.39 ± 0.00**	**0.65 ± 0.00**	**0.45 ± 0.00**
		120	**34.91 ± 0.07**	27.12 ± 0.16	22.19 ± 0.25	**54.60 ± 0.19**	**0.39 ± 0.00**	**0.65 ± 0.00**	**0.45 ± 0.00**

Note. Values in bold indicate the best evaluation outcome for each metric in each learning scenario, and grey highlights denote the best model in each scenario based on the best-achieved evaluation metrics. Note. PID: patient identification; PH: prediction horizon; LL: lag length; RMSE: root mean square error; SD: standard deviation; MAE: mean absolute error; MAPE: mean absolute percentage error; r^2: coefficient of determination; MCC: Matthew's correlation coefficient; SE: surveillance error; ASE: average surveillance error.

Table A2. The evaluation results for non-stacking models created by multilayer perceptron learners using Ohio 2020 dataset.

PID	PH	LL	RMSE ± SD (mg/dL)	MAE ± SD (mg/dL)	MAPE ± SD (%)	r^2 ± SD (%)	MCC ± SD (%)	SE < 0.5 ± SD (%)	ASE ± SD
540	30	30	23.48 ± 0.04	17.73 ± 0.03	12.88 ± 0.00	86.93 ± 0.04	0.67 ± 0.00	**0.81 ± 0.00**	**0.28 ± 0.00**
		60	**22.88 ± 0.13**	**17.45 ± 0.10**	**12.71 ± 0.04**	87.60 ± 0.14	**0.68 ± 0.00**	0.81 ± 0.00	0.27 ± 0.00
		90	23.41 ± 0.08	17.79 ± 0.04	12.84 ± 0.04	87.02 ± 0.09	**0.68 ± 0.00**	0.81 ± 0.00	0.28 ± 0.00
		120	23.61 ± 0.13	17.92 ± 0.07	12.86 ± 0.02	**86.79 ± 0.15**	0.67 ± 0.00	0.81 ± 0.00	0.28 ± 0.00
	60	30	40.74 ± 0.16	31.20 ± 0.15	23.55 ± 0.12	60.76 ± 0.32	0.49 ± 0.00	0.65 ± 0.00	0.45 ± 0.00
		60	**39.84 ± 0.14**	**30.49 ± 0.12**	**22.96 ± 0.13**	**62.48 ± 0.27**	**0.52 ± 0.00**	**0.66 ± 0.00**	**0.44 ± 0.00**
		90	40.15 ± 0.16	30.68 ± 0.15	23.09 ± 0.14	61.90 ± 0.30	0.52 ± 0.01	0.66 ± 0.00	0.44 ± 0.00
		120	40.38 ± 0.16	30.88 ± 0.14	23.16 ± 0.07	61.45 ± 0.31	0.52 ± 0.00	0.66 ± 0.00	0.44 ± 0.00
544	30	30	17.76 ± 0.06	12.45 ± 0.07	8.47 ± 0.07	87.73 ± 0.09	0.78 ± 0.00	0.91 ± 0.00	0.18 ± 0.00
		60	**17.37 ± 0.03**	**12.14 ± 0.03**	**8.21 ± 0.03**	**88.26 ± 0.04**	0.78 ± 0.00	0.92 ± 0.00	0.18 ± 0.00
		90	17.61 ± 0.03	12.42 ± 0.04	8.35 ± 0.03	87.94 ± 0.05	0.77 ± 0.00	0.91 ± 0.00	0.18 ± 0.00
		120	17.78 ± 0.10	12.49 ± 0.04	8.39 ± 0.03	87.71 ± 0.13	0.77 ± 0.00	0.91 ± 0.00	0.19 ± 0.00
	60	30	29.25 ± 0.08	21.79 ± 0.08	15.29 ± 0.08	66.61 ± 0.19	0.59 ± 0.00	0.75 ± 0.00	0.32 ± 0.00
		60	**28.49 ± 0.03**	**20.74 ± 0.04**	**14.16 ± 0.05**	**68.32 ± 0.07**	**0.63 ± 0.00**	**0.78 ± 0.00**	**0.30 ± 0.00**
		90	28.92 ± 0.09	21.03 ± 0.02	14.29 ± 0.04	67.35 ± 0.20	0.63 ± 0.00	0.77 ± 0.00	0.30 ± 0.00
		120	29.14 ± 0.12	21.12 ± 0.09	14.32 ± 0.04	66.86 ± 0.27	0.62 ± 0.00	0.77 ± 0.00	0.31 ± 0.00
552	30	30	**14.06 ± 0.03**	**8.25 ± 0.11**	**6.48 ± 0.09**	**86.18 ± 0.05**	**0.75 ± 0.00**	**0.92 ± 0.00**	**0.14 ± 0.00**
		60	14.32 ± 0.08	8.91 ± 0.08	7.03 ± 0.06	85.67 ± 0.16	0.73 ± 0.00	0.91 ± 0.00	0.15 ± 0.00
		90	14.47 ± 0.10	9.25 ± 0.09	7.30 ± 0.09	85.36 ± 0.20	0.72 ± 0.00	0.91 ± 0.00	0.15 ± 0.00
		120	14.60 ± 0.08	9.42 ± 0.03	7.44 ± 0.03	85.09 ± 0.16	0.72 ± 0.00	0.91 ± 0.00	0.15 ± 0.00
	60	30	23.83 ± 0.03	**14.57 ± 0.10**	**11.75 ± 0.12**	60.36 ± 0.09	**0.64 ± 0.00**	**0.84 ± 0.00**	**0.22 ± 0.00**
		60	**23.71 ± 0.06**	14.94 ± 0.06	12.07 ± 0.06	**60.78 ± 0.18**	0.63 ± 0.00	**0.84 ± 0.00**	**0.22 ± 0.00**
		90	23.75 ± 0.08	15.44 ± 0.09	12.42 ± 0.06	60.66 ± 0.26	**0.64 ± 0.00**	**0.84 ± 0.00**	0.23 ± 0.00
		120	23.87 ± 0.07	15.50 ± 0.09	12.47 ± 0.08	60.25 ± 0.22	**0.64 ± 0.00**	**0.84 ± 0.00**	0.23 ± 0.00
567	30	30	**22.72 ± 0.04**	**16.47 ± 0.04**	**12.48 ± 0.03**	**84.80 ± 0.05**	**0.64 ± 0.00**	**0.80 ± 0.00**	**0.28 ± 0.00**
		60	22.98 ± 0.07	16.63 ± 0.07	12.93 ± 0.07	84.44 ± 0.10	**0.64 ± 0.00**	**0.80 ± 0.00**	0.29 ± 0.00
		90	23.48 ± 0.18	17.24 ± 0.15	13.48 ± 0.12	83.77 ± 0.25	0.62 ± 0.00	0.79 ± 0.00	0.31 ± 0.00
		120	24.18 ± 0.20	17.98 ± 0.15	14.18 ± 0.12	82.78 ± 0.29	0.61 ± 0.00	0.78 ± 0.00	0.32 ± 0.00
	60	30	**38.38 ± 0.02**	29.51 ± 0.04	**23.24 ± 0.06**	**56.68 ± 0.04**	0.46 ± 0.00	**0.64 ± 0.00**	**0.47 ± 0.00**
		60	39.00 ± 0.07	**29.36 ± 0.01**	23.95 ± 0.01	55.27 ± 0.15	**0.48 ± 0.00**	**0.64 ± 0.00**	0.48 ± 0.00
		90	39.46 ± 0.07	29.96 ± 0.01	24.71 ± 0.03	54.22 ± 0.17	0.46 ± 0.00	0.63 ± 0.00	0.49 ± 0.00
		120	40.39 ± 0.15	30.91 ± 0.08	25.66 ± 0.09	52.01 ± 0.35	0.44 ± 0.00	0.62 ± 0.00	0.51 ± 0.00
584	30	30	23.25 ± 0.08	**16.72 ± 0.06**	**11.00 ± 0.07**	84.88 ± 0.10	0.76 ± 0.00	0.87 ± 0.00	**0.23 ± 0.00**
		60	**22.78 ± 0.04**	16.92 ± 0.04	11.34 ± 0.03	**85.49 ± 0.05**	**0.77 ± 0.00**	0.87 ± 0.00	**0.23 ± 0.00**
		90	22.80 ± 0.02	17.17 ± 0.03	11.51 ± 0.02	85.47 ± 0.03	0.76 ± 0.00	**0.88 ± 0.00**	0.24 ± 0.00
		120	23.30 ± 0.10	17.59 ± 0.10	11.79 ± 0.08	84.82 ± 0.13	0.75 ± 0.00	0.87 ± 0.00	0.25 ± 0.00
	60	30	37.53 ± 0.03	27.65 ± 0.22	**18.33 ± 0.27**	60.48 ± 0.07	0.59 ± 0.00	0.71 ± 0.01	**0.37 ± 0.00**
		60	**35.99 ± 0.05**	**27.29 ± 0.02**	18.40 ± 0.03	**63.67 ± 0.11**	**0.60 ± 0.00**	**0.72 ± 0.00**	**0.37 ± 0.00**
		90	36.04 ± 0.06	27.64 ± 0.06	18.72 ± 0.07	63.56 ± 0.12	0.59 ± 0.00	**0.72 ± 0.00**	0.38 ± 0.00
		120	36.39 ± 0.04	27.83 ± 0.09	18.84 ± 0.12	62.85 ± 0.08	0.58 ± 0.00	0.71 ± 0.00	0.38 ± 0.00
596	30	30	18.66 ± 0.09	13.47 ± 0.11	10.09 ± 0.10	85.82 ± 0.14	0.71 ± 0.00	0.89 ± 0.00	0.21 ± 0.00
		60	**17.87 ± 0.08**	**12.89 ± 0.06**	**9.67 ± 0.03**	**86.99 ± 0.12**	0.74 ± 0.00	0.89 ± 0.00	**0.20 ± 0.00**
		90	17.87 ± 0.09	12.93 ± 0.06	9.71 ± 0.03	86.99 ± 0.13	**0.75 ± 0.00**	0.89 ± 0.00	**0.20 ± 0.00**
		120	17.95 ± 0.05	12.98 ± 0.03	9.76 ± 0.02	86.89 ± 0.07	0.74 ± 0.00	**0.90 ± 0.00**	**0.20 ± 0.00**
	60	30	30.46 ± 0.10	22.78 ± 0.08	17.57 ± 0.08	62.29 ± 0.25	0.52 ± 0.00	0.78 ± 0.00	0.33 ± 0.00
		60	29.00 ± 0.13	21.43 ± 0.14	16.36 ± 0.13	65.83 ± 0.30	0.56 ± 0.00	0.80 ± 0.00	**0.31 ± 0.00**
		90	**28.79 ± 0.05**	**21.35 ± 0.07**	**16.28 ± 0.07**	**66.32 ± 0.13**	0.57 ± 0.01	0.80 ± 0.00	**0.31 ± 0.00**
		120	28.83 ± 0.16	21.37 ± 0.16	16.34 ± 0.16	66.22 ± 0.37	0.57 ± 0.01	**0.81 ± 0.00**	**0.31 ± 0.00**

Note. Values in bold indicate the best evaluation outcome for each metric in each learning scenario, and grey highlights denote the best model in each scenario based on the best-achieved evaluation metrics. Note. PID: patient identification; PH: prediction horizon; LL: lag length; RMSE: root mean square error; SD: standard deviation; MAE: mean absolute error; MAPE: mean absolute percentage error; r^2: coefficient of determination; MCC: Matthew's correlation coefficient; SE: surveillance error; ASE: average surveillance error.

Table A3. The evaluation results for non-stacking models created by long short-term memory learners using Ohio 2018 dataset.

PID	PH	LL	Evaluation Metric						
			RMSE ± SD (mg/dL)	MAE ± SD (mg/dL)	MAPE ± SD (%)	r^2 ± SD (%)	MCC ± SD (%)	SE < 0.5 ± SD (%)	ASE ± SD
559	30	30	**23.12 ± 0.43**	**16.60 ± 0.66**	11.10 ± 0.63	**87.19 ± 0.47**	**0.74 ± 0.01**	0.86 ± 0.01	0.24 ± 0.01
		60	23.51 ± 0.36	16.79 ± 0.54	11.02 ± 0.64	86.76 ± 0.40	**0.74 ± 0.01**	**0.87 ± 0.01**	0.23 ± 0.01
		90	25.50 ± 1.19	17.44 ± 0.64	**10.71 ± 0.13**	84.39 ± 1.44	0.72 ± 0.03	**0.87 ± 0.01**	**0.23 ± 0.00**
		120	32.86 ± 13.20	23.72 ± 10.60	15.55 ± 8.01	71.35 ± 23.13	0.63 ± 0.19	0.78 ± 0.16	0.31 ± 0.15
	60	30	38.39 ± 0.82	27.05 ± 0.53	16.65 ± 0.21	64.46 ± 1.52	0.57 ± 0.01	**0.75 ± 0.00**	0.35 ± 0.00
		60	38.73 ± 4.41	27.75 ± 3.58	17.37 ± 1.50	63.53 ± 8.42	0.54 ± 0.07	0.73 ± 0.05	0.37 ± 0.05
		90	37.77 ± 3.27	26.72 ± 2.04	16.92 ± 0.47	65.46 ± 6.01	0.58 ± 0.02	0.75 ± 0.01	0.35 ± 0.02
		120	**36.08 ± 1.47**	**25.38 ± 0.84**	**16.62 ± 0.25**	**68.60 ± 2.56**	**0.59 ± 0.02**	0.75 ± 0.01	**0.34 ± 0.01**
563	30	30	**21.59 ± 0.64**	**15.33 ± 0.45**	**9.69 ± 0.19**	77.31 ± 1.34	0.72 ± 0.01	**0.89 ± 0.00**	**0.22 ± 0.00**
		60	21.73 ± 0.46	15.52 ± 0.33	9.82 ± 0.32	**77.03 ± 0.96**	**0.73 ± 0.00**	**0.89 ± 0.00**	0.22 ± 0.01
		90	24.91 ± 1.84	17.49 ± 1.38	10.96 ± 1.02	69.71 ± 4.55	0.69 ± 0.03	0.87 ± 0.02	0.24 ± 0.02
		120	24.04 ± 1.89	16.94 ± 1.15	10.65 ± 0.72	71.79 ± 4.43	0.69 ± 0.01	0.87 ± 0.01	0.24 ± 0.01
	60	30	**33.02 ± 0.62**	**24.13 ± 0.61**	**15.07 ± 0.18**	**47.03 ± 2.01**	0.51 ± 0.01	0.75 ± 0.02	**0.33 ± 0.01**
		60	34.44 ± 2.48	25.05 ± 2.24	15.80 ± 1.37	42.17 ± 8.46	0.48 ± 0.09	0.74 ± 0.06	0.35 ± 0.03
		90	34.32 ± 1.23	24.45 ± 1.04	15.16 ± 0.63	42.73 ± 4.13	**0.52 ± 0.01**	**0.77 ± 0.02**	0.34 ± 0.01
		120	34.13 ± 1.59	24.66 ± 1.10	15.27 ± 0.62	43.33 ± 5.27	0.50 ± 0.02	0.76 ± 0.02	0.34 ± 0.01
570	30	30	24.78 ± 3.96	18.97 ± 3.76	8.84 ± 1.30	86.33 ± 4.12	**0.82 ± 0.01**	0.94 ± 0.01	0.16 ± 0.02
		60	25.83 ± 5.11	19.99 ± 4.76	9.28 ± 1.87	85.02 ± 5.59	0.81 ± 0.03	0.93 ± 0.02	0.17 ± 0.03
		90	23.09 ± 2.28	17.15 ± 2.09	8.26 ± 0.74	88.25 ± 2.30	**0.82 ± 0.01**	**0.94 ± 0.00**	**0.15 ± 0.01**
		120	**22.92 ± 1.49**	**16.16 ± 1.15**	**8.04 ± 0.65**	**88.47 ± 1.52**	0.81 ± 0.02	0.94 ± 0.01	**0.15 ± 0.01**
	60	30	38.34 ± 2.65	29.98 ± 2.52	13.56 ± 0.95	67.77 ± 4.48	0.75 ± 0.01	**0.88 ± 0.01**	0.25 ± 0.02
		60	**35.80 ± 1.50**	**26.75 ± 1.85**	**12.68 ± 0.43**	**71.95 ± 2.31**	**0.75 ± 0.00**	**0.88 ± 0.01**	**0.23 ± 0.01**
		90	37.00 ± 2.48	27.94 ± 1.86	13.17 ± 0.99	69.98 ± 4.09	0.75 ± 0.03	0.87 ± 0.02	0.24 ± 0.02
		120	35.80 ± 2.62	25.82 ± 2.70	12.58 ± 0.95	71.89 ± 4.09	0.75 ± 0.02	0.88 ± 0.01	0.23 ± 0.02
575	30	30	**27.20 ± 0.57**	**18.25 ± 0.45**	13.14 ± 0.71	**80.24 ± 0.82**	**0.69 ± 0.00**	0.82 ± 0.02	**0.28 ± 0.01**
		60	27.52 ± 0.76	18.26 ± 0.37	**13.07 ± 0.32**	79.77 ± 1.13	0.69 ± 0.01	**0.82 ± 0.00**	**0.28 ± 0.01**
		90	28.37 ± 0.99	18.89 ± 0.88	13.78 ± 0.69	78.51 ± 1.51	0.68 ± 0.01	0.80 ± 0.01	0.30 ± 0.01
		120	29.33 ± 1.12	19.83 ± 1.63	13.69 ± 0.60	77.03 ± 1.74	0.65 ± 0.05	0.80 ± 0.02	0.29 ± 0.01
	60	30	**38.09 ± 0.03**	**27.47 ± 0.52**	**20.48 ± 1.20**	**61.36 ± 0.07**	**0.54 ± 0.02**	**0.70 ± 0.00**	**0.41 ± 0.01**
		60	39.96 ± 0.84	28.84 ± 0.27	21.39 ± 1.07	57.46 ± 1.78	0.55 ± 0.03	0.68 ± 0.01	0.44 ± 0.01
		90	38.15 ± 0.52	27.58 ± 0.22	20.56 ± 0.49	61.24 ± 1.06	0.52 ± 0.01	0.68 ± 0.01	0.42 ± 0.01
		120	39.47 ± 1.28	28.64 ± 0.43	21.35 ± 0.44	58.48 ± 2.69	0.54 ± 0.01	0.67 ± 0.01	0.43 ± 0.01
588	30	30	**19.23 ± 0.11**	**14.16 ± 0.11**	**8.53 ± 0.12**	**83.77 ± 0.19**	**0.74 ± 0.00**	**0.92 ± 0.00**	**0.19 ± 0.00**
		60	19.60 ± 0.23	14.57 ± 0.15	8.83 ± 0.07	83.13 ± 0.39	0.74 ± 0.01	**0.92 ± 0.00**	**0.19 ± 0.00**
		90	20.33 ± 0.86	15.00 ± 0.73	8.87 ± 0.36	81.84 ± 1.54	0.73 ± 0.01	0.92 ± 0.00	0.19 ± 0.01
		120	21.99 ± 1.74	16.39 ± 1.07	9.64 ± 0.77	78.69 ± 3.39	0.69 ± 0.02	0.91 ± 0.02	0.20 ± 0.02
	60	30	31.32 ± 0.53	23.12 ± 0.56	14.05 ± 0.68	57.00 ± 1.48	0.57 ± 0.01	0.79 ± 0.02	0.30 ± 0.02
		60	**30.46 ± 0.60**	**22.48 ± 0.39**	**14.04 ± 0.23**	**59.33 ± 1.61**	**0.60 ± 0.01**	**0.79 ± 0.01**	**0.30 ± 0.01**
		90	32.01 ± 0.53	23.06 ± 0.33	14.11 ± 0.47	55.07 ± 1.48	0.58 ± 0.02	0.80 ± 0.01	**0.30 ± 0.01**
		120	35.57 ± 4.21	25.60 ± 2.74	15.65 ± 1.69	44.02 ± 13.55	0.50 ± 0.08	0.76 ± 0.03	0.33 ± 0.03
591	30	30	**26.00 ± 0.54**	19.63 ± 0.54	15.81 ± 0.75	**74.78 ± 1.04**	0.58 ± 0.01	0.74 ± 0.00	0.35 ± 0.01
		60	26.33 ± 0.42	**19.55 ± 0.24**	15.65 ± 0.40	74.16 ± 0.83	**0.60 ± 0.00**	**0.75 ± 0.01**	**0.34 ± 0.01**
		90	27.44 ± 1.02	20.46 ± 0.58	**15.63 ± 0.98**	71.90 ± 2.10	0.55 ± 0.05	0.74 ± 0.01	**0.34 ± 0.01**
		120	27.16 ± 0.88	20.13 ± 0.63	15.75 ± 0.85	72.48 ± 1.78	0.57 ± 0.03	0.74 ± 0.02	**0.34 ± 0.01**
	60	30	**36.51 ± 0.20**	**28.36 ± 0.26**	23.32 ± 0.27	**50.32 ± 0.54**	0.37 ± 0.02	**0.63 ± 0.00**	**0.47 ± 0.00**
		60	37.52 ± 0.93	28.36 ± 0.32	**22.47 ± 0.57**	47.52 ± 2.58	0.36 ± 0.04	0.63 ± 0.01	**0.47 ± 0.00**
		90	37.92 ± 1.44	29.32 ± 1.16	24.31 ± 1.51	46.38 ± 4.10	**0.39 ± 0.04**	0.63 ± 0.01	0.48 ± 0.01
		120	37.07 ± 1.67	28.38 ± 1.14	22.37 ± 0.89	48.73 ± 4.57	0.37 ± 0.02	0.63 ± 0.02	0.47 ± 0.02

Note. Values in bold indicate the best evaluation outcome for each metric in each learning scenario, and grey highlights denote the best model in each scenario based on the best-achieved evaluation metrics. Note. PID: patient identification; PH: prediction horizon; LL: lag length; RMSE: root mean square error; SD: standard deviation; MAE: mean absolute error; MAPE: mean absolute percentage error; r^2: coefficient of determination; MCC: Matthew's correlation coefficient; SE: surveillance error; ASE: average surveillance error.

Table A4. The evaluation results for non-stacking models created by long short-term memory learners using Ohio 2020 dataset.

PID	PH	LL	RMSE ± SD (mg/dL)	MAE ± SD (mg/dL)	MAPE ± SD (%)	r² ± SD (%)	MCC ± SD (%)	SE < 0.5 ± SD (%)	ASE ± SD
540	30	30	25.76 ± 1.26	19.38 ± 0.62	14.84 ± 0.24	84.25 ± 1.55	**0.67 ± 0.01**	0.79 ± 0.00	0.31 ± 0.00
		60	**24.84 ± 0.42**	**18.48 ± 0.70**	**13.81 ± 1.24**	**85.37 ± 0.49**	0.67 ± 0.02	**0.80 ± 0.01**	**0.29 ± 0.02**
		90	28.02 ± 3.64	21.40 ± 2.68	15.98 ± 2.30	81.18 ± 4.68	0.63 ± 0.03	0.76 ± 0.03	0.33 ± 0.04
		120	27.92 ± 1.82	21.00 ± 1.99	15.38 ± 2.29	81.48 ± 2.40	0.63 ± 0.02	0.76 ± 0.02	0.32 ± 0.04
	60	30	42.60 ± 1.15	31.84 ± 0.41	23.25 ± 0.53	57.07 ± 2.32	0.48 ± 0.02	0.64 ± 0.01	0.45 ± 0.00
		60	**41.36 ± 0.58**	**30.69 ± 0.37**	**22.40 ± 0.20**	**59.56 ± 1.12**	**0.50 ± 0.02**	**0.66 ± 0.00**	**0.44 ± 0.00**
		90	43.78 ± 2.80	32.44 ± 2.02	23.51 ± 1.66	54.55 ± 5.78	0.50 ± 0.04	0.64 ± 0.02	0.45 ± 0.02
		120	48.17 ± 1.39	34.62 ± 2.09	24.69 ± 2.33	45.10 ± 3.15	0.48 ± 0.04	0.63 ± 0.03	0.48 ± 0.03
544	30	30	21.23 ± 0.53	15.00 ± 0.49	**9.93 ± 0.35**	82.45 ± 0.87	**0.76 ± 0.01**	**0.89 ± 0.00**	**0.21 ± 0.01**
		60	**20.66 ± 0.31**	**14.71 ± 0.43**	9.99 ± 0.53	**83.40 ± 0.50**	0.75 ± 0.01	0.88 ± 0.02	0.22 ± 0.01
		90	22.55 ± 0.45	15.56 ± 0.37	10.40 ± 0.27	80.21 ± 0.79	0.72 ± 0.01	0.88 ± 0.01	0.22 ± 0.00
		120	23.38 ± 2.94	16.49 ± 1.81	11.35 ± 1.30	78.51 ± 5.18	0.71 ± 0.04	0.84 ± 0.03	0.24 ± 0.03
	60	30	31.43 ± 0.05	23.19 ± 0.08	15.59 ± 0.16	61.46 ± 0.12	0.58 ± 0.01	0.76 ± 0.00	0.32 ± 0.00
		60	**30.45 ± 0.12**	**22.09 ± 0.45**	**14.81 ± 0.52**	**63.83 ± 0.29**	**0.59 ± 0.02**	**0.78 ± 0.01**	**0.31 ± 0.01**
		90	32.39 ± 0.61	22.91 ± 0.32	15.40 ± 0.39	59.04 ± 1.55	0.57 ± 0.01	0.76 ± 0.01	0.33 ± 0.01
		120	36.19 ± 1.38	25.61 ± 0.40	17.44 ± 0.10	48.85 ± 3.94	0.52 ± 0.04	0.74 ± 0.01	0.36 ± 0.01
552	30	30	**16.72 ± 0.44**	**10.31 ± 0.24**	**8.04 ± 0.22**	**80.45 ± 1.01**	**0.71 ± 0.02**	**0.90 ± 0.01**	**0.16 ± 0.01**
		60	21.54 ± 3.51	14.67 ± 3.62	11.21 ± 2.37	66.99 ± 10.53	0.59 ± 0.14	0.85 ± 0.04	0.22 ± 0.04
		90	18.81 ± 1.50	12.58 ± 1.52	9.73 ± 0.98	75.16 ± 3.97	0.69 ± 0.01	0.89 ± 0.01	0.19 ± 0.01
		120	20.91 ± 5.44	14.00 ± 4.23	11.01 ± 3.87	68.05 ± 17.09	0.69 ± 0.08	0.85 ± 0.10	0.22 ± 0.08
	60	30	**25.47 ± 0.30**	**16.27 ± 0.24**	**13.02 ± 0.27**	**54.73 ± 1.05**	**0.61 ± 0.01**	**0.83 ± 0.01**	**0.24 ± 0.01**
		60	27.15 ± 1.00	18.20 ± 0.92	15.02 ± 0.93	48.51 ± 3.76	0.58 ± 0.03	0.78 ± 0.02	0.28 ± 0.02
		90	27.51 ± 2.98	17.70 ± 1.96	14.55 ± 1.73	46.78 ± 11.78	0.56 ± 0.06	0.80 ± 0.04	0.27 ± 0.04
		120	40.75 ± 25.37	32.17 ± 26.99	26.17 ± 21.83	45.82 ± 170.04	0.33 ± 0.44	0.60 ± 0.38	0.53 ± 0.49
567	30	30	26.21 ± 1.00	18.74 ± 1.00	14.41 ± 1.01	79.74 ± 1.56	**0.61 ± 0.01**	0.77 ± 0.01	0.32 ± 0.02
		60	25.54 ± 0.32	18.38 ± 0.28	13.83 ± 0.55	80.78 ± 0.48	**0.61 ± 0.01**	**0.78 ± 0.00**	**0.31 ± 0.01**
		90	**24.64 ± 0.97**	**17.85 ± 0.81**	**13.48 ± 0.66**	**82.10 ± 1.41**	0.60 ± 0.01	0.78 ± 0.01	**0.31 ± 0.01**
		120	27.89 ± 3.45	20.96 ± 3.26	16.17 ± 2.94	76.86 ± 5.47	0.57 ± 0.05	0.74 ± 0.04	0.35 ± 0.06
	60	30	43.16 ± 1.27	32.69 ± 1.21	27.34 ± 1.23	45.19 ± 3.24	0.44 ± 0.02	0.60 ± 0.02	0.53 ± 0.02
		60	**40.13 ± 1.22**	**30.57 ± 1.14**	**25.05 ± 1.96**	**52.61 ± 2.86**	**0.45 ± 0.01**	**0.62 ± 0.02**	**0.50 ± 0.03**
		90	42.89 ± 2.29	32.84 ± 2.03	26.97 ± 2.57	45.79 ± 5.74	0.41 ± 0.01	0.60 ± 0.02	0.53 ± 0.03
		120	45.08 ± 4.52	34.30 ± 3.01	26.78 ± 0.56	39.83 ± 12.30	0.40 ± 0.06	0.58 ± 0.04	0.54 ± 0.04
584	30	30	26.87 ± 0.77	19.56 ± 0.72	13.10 ± 0.55	79.81 ± 1.16	0.72 ± 0.02	0.84 ± 0.01	0.26 ± 0.01
		60	**25.31 ± 1.32**	**18.27 ± 0.95**	**11.49 ± 0.52**	**82.05 ± 1.89**	**0.75 ± 0.01**	**0.86 ± 0.01**	**0.23 ± 0.01**
		90	25.93 ± 1.03	19.25 ± 0.82	13.00 ± 0.65	81.19 ± 1.47	0.74 ± 0.01	0.85 ± 0.01	0.26 ± 0.01
		120	27.62 ± 0.80	20.65 ± 1.21	13.36 ± 0.35	78.66 ± 1.24	0.72 ± 0.02	0.84 ± 0.01	0.27 ± 0.00
	60	30	**41.45 ± 1.58**	**31.50 ± 1.91**	**21.43 ± 2.17**	**51.75 ± 3.64**	0.55 ± 0.03	**0.67 ± 0.04**	**0.42 ± 0.04**
		60	42.14 ± 1.60	32.72 ± 1.78	23.12 ± 1.60	50.12 ± 3.74	0.55 ± 0.01	0.64 ± 0.04	0.45 ± 0.03
		90	41.75 ± 0.90	32.60 ± 0.83	22.86 ± 1.00	51.08 ± 2.11	**0.56 ± 0.01**	0.65 ± 0.02	0.44 ± 0.02
		120	47.83 ± 3.54	37.15 ± 4.34	25.97 ± 4.37	35.58 ± 9.66	0.46 ± 0.05	0.59 ± 0.07	0.50 ± 0.08
596	30	30	**19.96 ± 0.28**	**14.31 ± 0.03**	**10.83 ± 0.18**	**83.78 ± 0.45**	**0.70 ± 0.01**	**0.87 ± 0.00**	**0.23 ± 0.00**
		60	21.15 ± 0.65	15.31 ± 0.40	11.64 ± 0.41	81.77 ± 1.12	0.69 ± 0.01	0.86 ± 0.01	0.24 ± 0.01
		90	22.54 ± 0.82	16.38 ± 0.95	12.32 ± 0.90	79.29 ± 1.50	0.66 ± 0.04	0.85 ± 0.01	0.25 ± 0.01
		120	33.46 ± 10.29	25.29 ± 8.45	19.64 ± 6.92	51.54 ± 25.67	0.50 ± 0.16	0.75 ± 0.10	0.36 ± 0.11
	60	30	30.97 ± 0.19	22.79 ± 0.17	17.23 ± 0.22	61.02 ± 0.48	0.52 ± 0.01	0.78 ± 0.00	0.33 ± 0.00
		60	**30.28 ± 0.72**	**22.17 ± 0.71**	**16.97 ± 0.45**	**62.72 ± 1.77**	**0.56 ± 0.02**	**0.79 ± 0.00**	**0.32 ± 0.01**
		90	31.70 ± 1.25	23.44 ± 1.22	17.94 ± 1.21	59.12 ± 3.24	0.52 ± 0.03	0.78 ± 0.01	0.34 ± 0.02
		120	36.31 ± 9.68	27.21 ± 8.48	21.03 ± 6.87	43.87 ± 30.66	0.43 ± 0.21	0.71 ± 0.13	0.40 ± 0.11

Note. Values in bold indicate the best evaluation outcome for each metric in each learning scenario, and grey highlights denote the best model in each scenario based on the best-achieved evaluation metrics. Note. PID: patient identification; PH: prediction horizon; LL: lag length; RMSE: root mean square error; SD: standard deviation; MAE: mean absolute error; MAPE: mean absolute percentage error; r²: coefficient of determination; MCC: Matthew's correlation coefficient; SE: surveillance error; ASE: average surveillance error.

References

1. DiMeglio, L.A.; Evans-Molina, C.; Oram, R.A. Type 1 Diabetes. *Lancet* **2018**, *391*, 2449–2462. [CrossRef] [PubMed]
2. Melin, J.; Lynch, K.F.; Lundgren, M.; Aronsson, C.A.; Larsson, H.E.; Johnson, S.B.; Rewers, M.; Barbour, A.; Bautista, K.; Baxter, J.; et al. Is Staff Consistency Important to Parents' Satisfaction in a Longitudinal Study of Children at Risk for Type 1 Diabetes: The TEDDY Study. *BMC Endocr. Disord.* **2022**, *22*, 19. [CrossRef] [PubMed]
3. Khadem, H.; Nemat, H.; Elliott, J.; Benaissa, M. Interpretable Machine Learning for Inpatient COVID-19 Mortality Risk Assessments: Diabetes Mellitus Exclusive Interplay. *Sensors* **2022**, *22*, 8757. [CrossRef] [PubMed]
4. Yamada, T.; Shojima, N.; Noma, H.; Yamauchi, T.; Kadowaki, T. Sodium-Glucose Co-Transporter-2 Inhibitors as Add-on Therapy to Insulin for Type 1 Diabetes Mellitus: Systematic Review and Meta-Analysis of Randomized Controlled Trials. *Diabetes Obes. Metab.* **2018**, *20*, 1755–1761. [CrossRef] [PubMed]
5. Smith, A.; Harris, C. Type 1 Diabetes: Management Strategies. *Am. Fam. Physician* **2018**, *98*, 154–162.
6. Hamilton, K.; Stanton-Fay, S.H.; Chadwick, P.M.; Lorencatto, F.; de Zoysa, N.; Gianfrancesco, C.; Taylor, C.; Coates, E.; Breckenridge, J.P.; Cooke, D.; et al. Sustained Type 1 Diabetes Self-Management: Specifying the Behaviours Involved and Their Influences. *Diabet. Med.* **2021**, *38*, e14430. [CrossRef]
7. Campbell, F.; Lawton, J.; Rankin, D.; Clowes, M.; Coates, E.; Heller, S.; De Zoysa, N.; Elliott, J.; Breckenridge, J.P. Follow-Up Support for Effective Type 1 Diabetes Self-Management (The FUSED Model): A Systematic Review and Meta-Ethnography of the Barriers, Facilitators and Recommendations for Sustaining Self-Management Skills after Attending a Structured Education Programme. *BMC Health Serv. Res.* **2018**, *18*, 898. [CrossRef]
8. Cummings, C.; Benjamin, N.E.; Prabhu, H.Y.; Cohen, L.B.; Goddard, B.J.; Kaugars, A.S.; Humiston, T.; Lansing, A.H. Habit and Diabetes Self-Management in Adolescents With Type 1 Diabetes. *Health Psychol.* **2022**, *41*, 13–22. [CrossRef]
9. McCarthy, M.M.; Grey, M. Type 1 Diabetes Self-Management From Emerging Adulthood Through Older Adulthood. *Diabetes Care* **2018**, *41*, 1608–1614. [CrossRef]
10. Saoji, N.; Palta, M.; Young, H.N.; Moreno, M.A.; Rajamanickam, V.; Cox, E.D. The Relationship of Type 1 Diabetes Self-Management Barriers to Child and Parent Quality of Life: A US Cross-Sectional Study. *Diabet. Med.* **2018**, *35*, 1523–1530. [CrossRef]
11. Butler, A.M.; Weller, B.E.; Rodgers, C.R.R.; Teasdale, A.E. Type 1 Diabetes Self-Management Behaviors among Emerging Adults: Racial/Ethnic Differences. *Pediatr. Diabetes* **2020**, *21*, 979–986. [CrossRef]
12. Dai, X.; Luo, Z.C.; Zhai, L.; Zhao, W.P.; Huang, F. Artificial Pancreas as an Effective and Safe Alternative in Patients with Type 1 Diabetes Mellitus: A Systematic Review and Meta-Analysis. *Diabetes Ther.* **2018**, *9*, 1269–1277. [CrossRef]
13. Bekiari, E.; Kitsios, K.; Thabit, H.; Tauschmann, M.; Athanasiadou, E.; Karagiannis, T.; Haidich, A.B.; Hovorka, R.; Tsapas, A. Artificial Pancreas Treatment for Outpatients with Type 1 Diabetes: Systematic Review and Meta-Analysis. *BMJ* **2018**, *361*, 1310. [CrossRef]
14. Zhang, Y.; Sun, J.; Liu, L.; Qiao, H. A Review of Biosensor Technology and Algorithms for Glucose Monitoring. *J. Diabetes Complicat.* **2021**, *35*, 107929. [CrossRef]
15. Choudhary, P.; Amiel, S.A. Hypoglycaemia in Type 1 Diabetes: Technological Treatments, Their Limitations and the Place of Psychology. *Diabetologia* **2018**, *61*, 761–769. [CrossRef]
16. Tagougui, S.; Taleb, N.; Rabasa-Lhoret, R. The Benefits and Limits of Technological Advances in Glucose Management around Physical Activity in Patients Type 1 Diabetes. *Front. Endocrinol.* **2019**, *10*, 818. [CrossRef]
17. Laffel, L.M.; Kanapka, L.G.; Beck, R.W.; Bergamo, K.; Clements, M.A.; Criego, A.; Desalvo, D.J.; Goland, R.; Hood, K.; Liljenquist, D.; et al. Effect of Continuous Glucose Monitoring on Glycemic Control in Adolescents and Young Adults With Type 1 Diabetes: A Randomized Clinical Trial. *JAMA* **2020**, *323*, 2388–2396. [CrossRef]
18. Martens, T.; Beck, R.W.; Bailey, R.; Ruedy, K.J.; Calhoun, P.; Peters, A.L.; Pop-Busui, R.; Philis-Tsimikas, A.; Bao, S.; Umpierrez, G.; et al. Effect of Continuous Glucose Monitoring on Glycemic Control in Patients With Type 2 Diabetes Treated With Basal Insulin: A Randomized Clinical Trial. *JAMA* **2021**, *325*, 2262–2272. [CrossRef]
19. Pickup, J.C. Is Insulin Pump Therapy Effective in Type 1 Diabetes? *Diabet. Med.* **2019**, *36*, 269–278. [CrossRef]
20. Ranjan, A.G.; Rosenlund, S.V.; Hansen, T.W.; Rossing, P.; Andersen, S.; Nørgaard, K. Improved Time in Range Over 1 Year Is Associated With Reduced Albuminuria in Individuals With Sensor-Augmented Insulin Pump–Treated Type 1 Diabetes. *Diabetes Care* **2020**, *43*, 2882–2885. [CrossRef]
21. Mian, Z.; Hermayer, K.L.; Jenkins, A. Continuous Glucose Monitoring: Review of an Innovation in Diabetes Management. *Am. J. Med. Sci.* **2019**, *358*, 332–339. [CrossRef] [PubMed]
22. Aggarwal, A.; Pathak, S.; Goyal, R. Clinical and Economic Outcomes of Continuous Glucose Monitoring System (CGMS) in Patients with Diabetes Mellitus: A Systematic Literature Review. *Diabetes Res. Clin. Pract.* **2022**, *186*, 109825. [CrossRef] [PubMed]
23. Burckhardt, M.A.; Smith, G.J.; Cooper, M.N.; Jones, T.W.; Davis, E.A. Real-World Outcomes of Insulin Pump Compared to Injection Therapy in a Population-Based Sample of Children with Type 1 Diabetes. *Pediatr. Diabetes* **2018**, *19*, 1459–1466. [CrossRef] [PubMed]
24. Cardona-Hernandez, R.; Schwandt, A.; Alkandari, H.; Bratke, H.; Chobot, A.; Coles, N.; Corathers, S.; Goksen, D.; Goss, P.; Imane, Z.; et al. Glycemic Outcome Associated With Insulin Pump and Glucose Sensor Use in Children and Adolescents With Type 1 Diabetes. Data From the International Pediatric Registry SWEET. *Diabetes Care* **2021**, *44*, 1176–1184. [CrossRef]

25. Rytter, K.; Schmidt, S.; Rasmussen, L.N.; Pedersen-Bjergaard, U.; Nørgaard, K. Education Programmes for Persons with Type 1 Diabetes Using an Insulin Pump: A Systematic Review. *Diabetes. Metab. Res. Rev.* **2021**, *37*, e3412. [CrossRef]
26. Vashist, S.K. Non-Invasive Glucose Monitoring Technology in Diabetes Management: A Review. *Anal. Chim. Acta* **2012**, *750*, 16–27. [CrossRef]
27. Alrezj, O.; Benaissa, M.; Alshebeili, S.A. Digital Bandstop Filtering in the Quantitative Analysis of Glucose from Near-Infrared and Midinfrared Spectra. *J. Chemom.* **2020**, *34*, e3206. [CrossRef]
28. Khadem, H.; Nemat, H.; Elliott, J.; Benaissa, M. Signal Fragmentation Based Feature Vector Generation in a Model Agnostic Framework with Application to Glucose Quantification Using Absorption Spectroscopy. *Talanta* **2022**, *243*, 123379. [CrossRef]
29. Khadem, H.; Eissa, M.R.; Nemat, H.; Alrezj, O.; Benaissa, M. Classification before Regression for Improving the Accuracy of Glucose Quantification Using Absorption Spectroscopy. *Talanta* **2020**, *211*, 120740. [CrossRef]
30. Vettoretti, M.; Cappon, G.; Facchinetti, A.; Sparacino, G. Advanced Diabetes Management Using Artificial Intelligence and Continuous Glucose Monitoring Sensors. *Sensors* **2020**, *20*, 3870. [CrossRef]
31. Nemat, H.; Khadem, H.; Elliott, J.; Benaissa, M. Causality Analysis in Type 1 Diabetes Mellitus with Application to Blood Glucose Level Prediction. *Comput. Biol. Med.* **2023**, *153*, 106535. [CrossRef]
32. Xie, J.; Wang, Q. Benchmarking Machine Learning Algorithms on Blood Glucose Prediction for Type i Diabetes in Comparison with Classical Time-Series Models. *IEEE Trans. Biomed. Eng.* **2020**, *67*, 3101–3124. [CrossRef]
33. Nemat, H.; Khadem, H.; Elliott, J.; Benaissa, M. Data Fusion of Activity and CGM for Predicting Blood Glucose Levels. In *Knowledge Discovery in Healthcare Data 2020, Proceedings of the 5th International Workshop on Knowledge Discovery in Healthcare Data Co-Located with 24th European Conference on Artificial Intelligence (ECAI 2020), Santiago de Compostela, Spain (virtual), 29–30 August 2020*; Bach, K., Bunescu, R., Marling, C., Wiratunga, N., Eds.; CEUR Workshop Proceedings: Aachen, Germany, 2020; Volume 2675, pp. 120–124.
34. Woldaregay, A.Z.; Årsand, E.; Botsis, T.; Albers, D.; Mamykina, L.; Hartvigsen, G. Data-Driven Blood Glucose Pattern Classification and Anomalies Detection: Machine-Learning Applications in Type 1 Diabetes. *J. Med. Internet Res.* **2019**, *21*, e11030. [CrossRef]
35. Khadem, H.; Nemat, H.; Elliott, J.; Benaissa, M. Multi-Lag Stacking for Blood Glucose Level Prediction. In *Knowledge Discovery in Healthcare Data 2020, Proceedings of the 5th International Workshop on Knowledge Discovery in Healthcare Data Co-Located with 24th European Conference on Artificial Intelligence (ECAI 2020), Santiago de Compostela, Spain (virtual), 29–30 August 2020*; Bach, K., Bunescu, R., Marling, C., Wiratunga, N., Eds.; CEUR Workshop Proceedings: Aachen, Germany, 2020; Volume 2675, pp. 146–150.
36. Boughton, C.K.; Hovorka, R. Is an Artificial Pancreas (Closed-Loop System) for Type 1 Diabetes Effective? *Diabet. Med.* **2019**, *36*, 279–286. [CrossRef]
37. Bremer, A.A.; Arreaza-Rubín, G. Analysis of "Artificial Pancreas (AP) Systems for People With Type 2 Diabetes: Conception and Design of the European CLOSE Project". *J. Diabetes Sci. Technol.* **2019**, *13*, 268–270. [CrossRef]
38. Woldaregay, A.Z.; Årsand, E.; Walderhaug, S.; Albers, D.; Mamykina, L.; Botsis, T.; Hartvigsen, G. Data-Driven Modeling and Prediction of Blood Glucose Dynamics: Machine Learning Applications in Type 1 Diabetes. *Artif. Intell. Med.* **2019**, *98*, 109–134. [CrossRef]
39. Nemat, H.; Khadem, H.; Eissa, M.R.; Elliott, J.; Benaissa, M. Blood Glucose Level Prediction: Advanced Deep-Ensemble Learning Approach. *IEEE J. Biomed. Health Inform.* **2022**, *26*, 2758–2769. [CrossRef]
40. Felizardo, V.; Garcia, N.M.; Pombo, N.; Megdiche, I. Data-Based Algorithms and Models Using Diabetics Real Data for Blood Glucose and Hypoglycaemia Prediction—A Systematic Literature Review. *Artif. Intell. Med.* **2021**, *118*, 102120. [CrossRef]
41. Semenoglou, A.-A.; Spiliotis, E.; Assimakopoulos, V. Image-Based Time Series Forecasting: A Deep Convolutional Neural Network Approach. *Neural Netw.* **2023**, *157*, 39–53. [CrossRef]
42. Garg, A.; Zhang, W.; Samaran, J.; Savitha, R.; Foo, C.S. An Evaluation of Anomaly Detection and Diagnosis in Multivariate Time Series. *IEEE Trans. Neural Netw. Learn. Syst.* **2022**, *33*, 2508–2517. [CrossRef]
43. De Oliveira, J.F.L.; Silva, E.G.; De Mattos Neto, P.S.G. A Hybrid System Based on Dynamic Selection for Time Series Forecasting. *IEEE Trans. Neural Netw. Learn. Syst.* **2022**, *33*, 3251–3263. [CrossRef] [PubMed]
44. Cichos, F.; Gustavsson, K.; Mehlig, B.; Volpe, G. Machine Learning for Active Matter. *Nat. Mach. Intell.* **2020**, *2*, 94–103. [CrossRef]
45. Lim, B.; Zohren, S. Time-Series Forecasting with Deep Learning: A Survey. *Philos. Trans. R. Soc. A* **2021**, *379*, 20200209. [CrossRef]
46. Ismail Fawaz, H.; Forestier, G.; Weber, J.; Idoumghar, L.; Muller, P.A. Deep Learning for Time Series Classification: A Review. *Data Min. Knowl. Discov.* **2019**, *33*, 917–963. [CrossRef]
47. Zhu, T.; Wang, W.; Yu, M. A Novel Blood Glucose Time Series Prediction Framework Based on a Novel Signal Decomposition Method. *Chaos Solitons Fractals* **2022**, *164*, 112673. [CrossRef]
48. Tejedor, M.; Woldaregay, A.Z.; Godtliebsen, F. Reinforcement Learning Application in Diabetes Blood Glucose Control: A Systematic Review. *Artif. Intell. Med.* **2020**, *104*, 101836. [CrossRef]
49. Aiello, E.M.; Lisanti, G.; Magni, L.; Musci, M.; Toffanin, C. Therapy-Driven Deep Glucose Forecasting. *Eng. Appl. Artif. Intell.* **2020**, *87*, 103255. [CrossRef]

50. Asad, M.; Qamar, U. A Review of Continuous Blood Glucose Monitoring and Prediction of Blood Glucose Level for Diabetes Type 1 Patient in Different Prediction Horizons (PH) Using Artificial Neural Network (ANN). *Adv. Intell. Syst. Comput.* **2020**, *1038*, 684–695. [CrossRef]

51. Li, K.; Daniels, J.; Liu, C.; Herrero, P.; Georgiou, P. Convolutional Recurrent Neural Networks for Glucose Prediction. *IEEE J. Biomed. Health Inform.* **2020**, *24*, 603–613. [CrossRef]

52. Zhang, M.; Flores, K.B.; Tran, H.T. Deep Learning and Regression Approaches to Forecasting Blood Glucose Levels for Type 1 Diabetes. *Biomed. Signal Process. Control* **2021**, *69*, 102923. [CrossRef]

53. Tena, F.; Garnica, O.; Lanchares, J.; Hidalgo, J.I.; Cappon, G.; Herrero, P.; Sacchi, L.; Coltro, W. Ensemble Models of Cutting-Edge Deep Neural Networks for Blood Glucose Prediction in Patients with Diabetes. *Sensors* **2021**, *21*, 7090. [CrossRef]

54. Wadghiri, M.Z.; Idri, A.; El Idrissi, T.; Hakkoum, H. Ensemble Blood Glucose Prediction in Diabetes Mellitus: A Review. *Comput. Biol. Med.* **2022**, *147*, 105674. [CrossRef]

55. Daniels, J.; Herrero, P.; Georgiou, P. A Multitask Learning Approach to Personalized Blood Glucose Prediction. *IEEE J. Biomed. Health Inform.* **2022**, *26*, 436–445. [CrossRef]

56. Yang, T.; Yu, X.; Ma, N.; Wu, R.; Li, H. An Autonomous Channel Deep Learning Framework for Blood Glucose Prediction. *Appl. Soft Comput.* **2022**, *120*, 108636. [CrossRef]

57. Zhu, T.; Li, K.; Chen, J.; Herrero, P.; Georgiou, P. Dilated Recurrent Neural Networks for Glucose Forecasting in Type 1 Diabetes. *J. Healthc. Inform. Res.* **2020**, *4*, 308–324. [CrossRef]

58. Martinsson, J.; Schliep, A.; Eliasson, B.; Mogren, O. Blood Glucose Prediction with Variance Estimation Using Recurrent Neural Networks. *J. Healthc. Inform. Res.* **2020**, *4*, 1–18. [CrossRef]

59. Rodríguez-Rodríguez, I.; Rodríguez, J.V.; Molina-García-Pardo, J.M.; Zamora-Izquierdo, M.Á.; Martínez-Inglés, M.T. A Comparison of Different Models of Glycemia Dynamics for Improved Type 1 Diabetes Mellitus Management with Advanced Intelligent Analysis in an Internet of Things Context. *Appl. Sci.* **2020**, *10*, 4381. [CrossRef]

60. Marling, C.; Bunescu, R. The OhioT1DM Dataset for Blood Glucose Level Prediction: Update 2020. In Proceedings of the 5th International Workshop on Knowledge Discovery in Healthcare Data Co-Located with 24th European Conference on Artificial Intelligence, KDH@ECAI 2020, Santiago de Compostela, Spain & Virtually, 29–30 August 2020; NIH Public Access: Bethesda, MD, USA, 2020; Volume 2675, pp. 71–74.

61. Kwiatkowski, D.; Phillips, P.C.B.; Schmidt, P.; Shin, Y. Testing the Null Hypothesis of Stationarity against the Alternative of a Unit Root: How Sure Are We That Economic Time Series Have a Unit Root? *J. Econom.* **1992**, *54*, 159–178. [CrossRef]

62. Dickey, D.A.; Fuller, W.A. Distribution of the Estimators for Autoregressive Time Series with a Unit Root. *J. Am. Stat. Assoc.* **2012**, *74*, 427–431. [CrossRef]

63. Sagi, O.; Rokach, L. Ensemble Learning: A Survey. *Wiley Interdiscip. Rev. Data Min. Knowl. Discov.* **2018**, *8*, e1249. [CrossRef]

64. Breiman, L. Stacked Regressions. *Mach. Learn.* **1996**, *24*, 49–64. [CrossRef]

65. Zhu, Q. On the Performance of Matthews Correlation Coefficient (MCC) for Imbalanced Dataset. *Pattern Recognit. Lett.* **2020**, *136*, 71–80. [CrossRef]

66. Klonoff, D.C.; Lias, C.; Vigersky, R.; Clarke, W.; Parkes, J.L.; Sacks, D.B.; Kirkman, M.S.; Kovatchev, B. The Surveillance Error Grid. *J. Diabetes Sci. Technol.* **2014**, *8*, 658–672. [CrossRef] [PubMed]

67. Friedman, M. A Comparison of Alternative Tests of Significance for the Problem of m Rankings on JSTOR. *Ann. Math. Stat.* **1940**, *11*, 86–92. [CrossRef]

68. Fisher, R. Statistical Methods and Scientific Induction. *J. R. Stat. Soc. Ser. B* **1955**, *17*, 69–78. [CrossRef]

69. Nemenyi, P.B. *Distribution-Free Multiple Comparisons*; Princeton University: Princeton, NJ, USA, 1963.

70. Holm, S. A Simple Sequentially Rejective Multiple Test Procedure. *Scand. J. Stat.* **1979**, *6*, 65–70.

71. Demšar, J. Statistical Comparisons of Classifiers over Multiple Data Sets. *J. Mach. Learn. Res.* **2006**, *7*, 1–30.

72. Van Rossum, G.; Drake, F.L. *Python 3 Reference Manual*; CreateSpace: Scotts Valley, CA, USA, 2009; ISBN 1441412697.

73. Abadi, M.; Barham, P.; Chen, J.; Chen, Z.; Davis, A.; Dean, J.; Devin, M.; Ghemawat, S.; Irving, G.; Isard, M.; et al. Tensorflow: A System for Large-Scale Machine Learning. In Proceedings of the 12th Symposium on Operating Systems Design and Implementation, Savannah, GA, USA, 2–4 November 2016; pp. 265–283.

74. McKinney, W. Data Structures for Statistical Computing in Python. In Proceedings of the the 9th Python in Science Conference, Austin, TX, USA, 28 June–3 July 2010; Volume 445, pp. 51–56.

75. Harris, C.R.; Millman, K.J.; van der Walt, S.J.; Gommers, R.; Virtanen, P.; Cournapeau, D.; Wieser, E.; Taylor, J.; Berg, S.; Smith, N.J.; et al. Array Programming with {NumPy}. *Nature* **2020**, *585*, 357–362. [CrossRef]

76. Pedregosa, F.; Varoquaux, G.; Gramfort, A.; Michel, V.; Thirion, B.; Grisel, O.; Blondel, M.; Prettenhofer, P.; Weiss, R.; Dubourg, V.; et al. Scikit-Learn: Machine Learning in Python. *J. Mach. Learn. Res.* **2011**, *12*, 2825–2830.

77. Virtanen, P.; Gommers, R.; Oliphant, T.E.; Haberland, M.; Reddy, T.; Cournapeau, D.; Burovski, E.; Peterson, P.; Weckesser, W.; Bright, J.; et al. SciPy 1.0: Fundamental Algorithms for Scientific Computing in Python. *Nat. Methods* **2020**, *17*, 261–272. [CrossRef]

78. Seabold, S.; Perktold, J. Statsmodels: Econometric and Statistical Modeling with Python. In Proceedings of the 9th Python in Science Conference, Austin, TX, USA, 28 June–3 July 2010.

79. Terpilowski, M. Scikit-Posthocs: Pairwise Multiple Comparison Tests in Python. *J. Open Source Softw.* **2019**, *4*, 1169. [CrossRef]
80. Benavoli, A.; Corani, G.; Mangili, F. Should We Really Use Post-Hoc Tests Based on Mean-Ranks? *J. Mach. Learn. Res.* **2016**, *17*, 152–161.

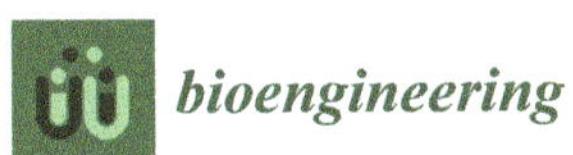 *bioengineering*

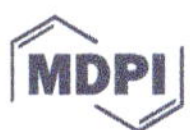

Article

Walking Stability and Risk of Falls

Arunee Promsri [1],*, Prasit Cholamjiak [2] and Peter Federolf [3]

1   Department of Physical Therapy, School of Allied Health Sciences, University of Phayao, Phayao 56000, Thailand
2   Department of Mathematics, School of Sciences, University of Phayao, Phayao 56000, Thailand
3   Department of Sport Science, University of Innsbruck, 6020 Innsbruck, Austria
*   Correspondence: arunee.pr@up.ac.th; Tel.: +66-54-466-666-(3817)

Abstract: Walking stability is considered a necessary physical performance for preserving independence and preventing falls. The current study investigated the correlation between walking stability and two clinical markers for falling risk. Principal component analysis (PCA) was applied to extract the three-dimensional (3D) lower-limb kinematic data of 43 healthy older adults (69.8 ± 8.5 years, 36 females) into a set of principal movements (PMs), showing different movement components/synergies working together to accomplish the walking task goal. Then, the largest Lyapunov exponent (LyE) was applied to the first five PMs as a measure of stability, with the interpretation that the higher the LyE, the lower the stability of individual movement components. Next, the fall risk was determined using two functional motor tests—a Short Physical Performance Battery (SPPB) and a Gait Subscale of Performance-Oriented Mobility Assessment (POMA-G)—of which the higher the test score, the better the performance. The main results show that SPPB and POMA-G scores negatively correlate with the LyE seen in specific PMs ($p \leq 0.009$), indicating that increasing walking instability increases the fall risk. The current findings suggest that inherent walking instability should be considered when assessing and training the lower limbs to reduce the risk of falling.

Keywords: gait; neuromuscular control; movement synergy; overground walking; principal component analysis (PCA); largest Lyapunov exponent (LyE)

Citation: Promsri, A.; Cholamjiak, P.; Federolf, P. Walking Stability and Risk of Falls. *Bioengineering* **2023**, *10*, 471. https://doi.org/10.3390/bioengineering10040471

Academic Editors: Pedro Miguel Rodrigues, João Paulo do Vale Madeiro and João Alexandre Lobo Marques

Received: 27 March 2023
Revised: 11 April 2023
Accepted: 11 April 2023
Published: 12 April 2023

1. Introduction

Falls have been linked to a loss of function and independence in older people, leading to injury-related hospitalizations in the aging population worldwide [1]. They usually occur according to degenerative changes of postural reflex impairment accompanied by the inherent aging process [2]. Approximately one-third of older adults (>65 years) living in the community fall yearly [3], leading to several types of injuries (e.g., pain, soft tissue injuries, fractures, dislocations, and functional impairment [4]) and impacting the quality of life [2]. As previously reported [5,6], several internal risk factors for falling have been reported, e.g., previous history of falls, balance impairment, functional limitations, visual impairment, gait impairment, decreased muscle strength, arthritis, diabetes, pain, using polypharmacy or psychoactive drugs, depression, dizziness, age over 80 years, female sex, and cognitive impairment. Analyzing the main fall risk factors, which is crucial for prevention, has frequently been performed [1,2,4,5].

One of the physical performances necessary for preserving independence and minimizing the risk of falls is the ability to walk successfully and safely on both stable and unstable surfaces [7]. Walking instability has been recognized as one of the leading contributors [5,6] among the several risk factors for falls. Commonly, stability is described as the intrinsic ability of a motor system to retain or recover to its initial condition in the face of internal (e.g., neuromuscular) and external (e.g., environmental) perturbations [8,9]. In this sense, stability measures yield relevant information on the intrinsic noise in motor task performance and directly quantify the performance of dynamic error correction [8,9]. Alternatively, variability measures have also been used to indirectly quantify how stable a person performs locomotion tasks due to inherent noise in the motor tasks or the environment that can bring an individual's dynamic state closer to their stability limits [8–10]. Furthermore, since human movement is believed to result from nonlinear interactions between multiple neuromuscular elements and internal and external factors [11], the largest Lyapunov exponent (LyE), one of the nonlinear methods to assess local dynamic stability, is frequently used to analyze the capacity to manage for small internal or external perturbations in order to maintain functional locomotion (i.e., used to measure walking stability) [9,12–14].

In order to complete any given motor activity (e.g., walking), the cooperative contribution of multi-body segments is needed, typically seen as different movement components/synergies forming together to accomplish the task goal [10,15,16]. Principal component analysis (PCA), one of the methods for reducing the number of dimensions, has widely been used on kinematic marker data to extract movement components or synergies, which have been called "principal movements" (PM), from the original, whole postural movements [15,17]. This method helps by minimizing the number of features (i.e., redundancy issues in motor apparatus) needed to finish the given task goal by forming fewer new variables, which still contain the most information regarding how people move or generate motions from the original feature set of postural movements [15,17–19]. Moreover, information about the position and acceleration of individual PMs reveals their direct association with system forces and myoelectric activity [20,21], confirming that PCA-based variables have an adequate probability of assessing neuromuscular control of individual movement components/strategies [15,20–22]. Regarding local dynamic stability as measured by the LyE, walking stability can be referred to as the neuromuscular system's ability to manage infinitesimal perturbations during locomotion [9,12–14]. Therefore, the LyE applied to individual PM positions can aid in quantifying the stability of individual movement components/strategies that come together to achieve locomotion tasks [10,16,23].

Several functional motor tests have been developed to assess physical performance, since poor physical performance, balance impairment, and gait alterations are among the leading causes of falls in older individuals [24]. When focusing on gait ability, functional motor tests assessing gait ability are commonly used to determine the risk of falling. For example, the Short Physical Performance Battery (SPPB) is a well-established tool for quantifiably assessing the lower extremity physical performance based on three tasks: repeated chair stand, standing balance, and walking speed [25]. Unlike the SPPB, the Gait Subscale of Performance Oriented Mobility Assessment (POMA-G) assesses the quality of walking by considering gait initiation, step length, step height, step symmetry, step continuity, path, trunk movement, and walking stance [26]. The results of these two tests are represented as ordinal scores, ranging from 0 to 12, considered the worst-to-best performance [25,26]. Both tests are reported to accurately discriminate between fallers and non-fallers in a large group of frail older adults [27]. Practically, fall risks are usually predicted using multi-item or functional motor assessment tools [28]. For example, it has been reported that SPPB [29] and POMA-G [30] have the practical ability to predict falls. In this sense, since the ability to maintain stability while walking is critical for avoiding falls, particularly in older adults [31], studying the relationship between falling risk and walking stability by considering movement patterns (i.e., movement strategies) can help to identify individuals who are at higher risk of falling and develop effective interventions to improve walking stability and reduce the falling risk.

In summary, the main purpose of the current study was to determine the correlation between walking stability and the risk of falling. Walking stability was defined in terms of individual PMs' local dynamic stability (Lyapunov stability), and fall risk was determined by two functional motor tests—SPPB and POMA-G. Since the stability of individual PMs reflects the neuromuscular control of individual movement components or movement synergies [10], it was hypothesized that the correlation between walking stability and the risk of falling would appear in the specific relevant PMs to the gait cycle.

2. Materials and Methods

2.1. Secondary Data Analysis

The lower-limb kinematic marker data of 43 healthy older adults (36 females and 7 males) used in the current study was derived from a peer-reviewed open-access dataset [32]. All participants had no neurological or musculoskeletal problems concerned with the risk of falling or affecting walking ability. The Mini-Mental State Examination (MMSE) was utilized to assess the mental status (i.e., mental health) to confirm that all participants could understand the experiment protocol and complete the tasks. In addition, two functional motor tests—SPPB and POMA-G—were performed on each participant by an experienced physiotherapist. The Ethics Committee of the Escuela Colombiana de Ingeniería and Clínica Universidad de la Sabana, Colombia, approved the study protocol in accordance with the ethical principles of the Helsinki Declaration, and all participants provided written informed consent before participation, as reported in Caicedo et al. [32]. The participant characteristics are represented in Table 1.

Table 1. Descriptive characteristics of participants (*n* = 43).

	Min	Max	Mean	SD
Age (years)	54.0	87.0	69.8	8.5
Mass (kg)	41.8	104.4	67.6	11.2
Height (m)	1.4	1.7	1.6	0.1
Body Mass Index (kg/m^2)	17.4	40.3	27.8	4.5
MMSE	22.0	30.0	26.6	2.5
SPPB	5.0	12.0	9.8	1.7
POMA-G	8.0	12.0	10.2	0.8
Walking speed (m/s)	0.6	1.2	0.8	0.2
Number of falls in the last month (time)	0	1	0.1	0.3

Experimental measurement procedures were detailed and explained in Caicedo et al. [32]. In brief, each participant was equipped with 24 reflective markers, ten at each leg and four around the hip, as shown in Caicedo et al. [32]. The optical motion capture system comprised seven cameras (Vantage V5, Vicon Motion Systems, Ltd., Oxford, UK), with the sample rate set at 100 Hz. Each camera was mounted on a tripod at 1.90 m above the floor. For each walking trial, a C3D file is generated by Nexus movement analysis software, version 2.9.3 (Vicon Motion Systems, Ltd., Oxford, UK), with an accuracy better than 0.3 mm. Each participant was instructed to walk ten times at a self-preferred speed between two points six meters apart, while one researcher walked beside them to ensure their safety during walking. However, the data of the best five walking trials of each participant were provided in the original data article. The current study selected only three walking trials in which all participants walked in the same direction (e.g., walking from point A to point B but not from point B to point A), as checked by running the C3D files for further analysis.

2.2. Movement Synergy Extraction

All data processing for the current study was conducted in MATLAB version 2022a (MathWorks Inc., Natick, MA, USA). For each dataset, 16 markers were placed on the main anatomical landmarks (ASIS, PSIS, thigh, knee, tibia, lateral malleolus, heel, and toe) of each leg. These markers gave 48 spatial coordinates (x, y, z), which were interpreted as 48-dimensional posture vectors [15]. Each participant's kinematic dataset of three walking trials was pre-processed, centered by subtracting the mean posture vector [15], and normalized to the mean Euclidean distance [15] before they were concatenated to form one input matrix (3 trials × 43 participants) for further PCA. Supplementary Video S1, an animated stick figure video, shows an example of the original overground walking movement obtained from one female participant.

PCA was carried out with a singular-value decomposition of the covariance matrix through the PManalyzer software [15] to extract all lower-limb kinematic data into a set of orthogonal eigenvectors, which has been called "principal components" (PC_k; k indicates the order of movement components). For each orthogonal eigenvector, an animated stick figure called "principal movement" (PM_k), can be created to characterize its movement pattern [15]. The use of the term "principal" in the variable names denotes that those variables were derived from PCA, of which (t) indicates that these variables are functions of time t [15]. Furthermore, the actual time evolution (i.e., time series) of each PM is quantified by the PC scores (i.e., principal positions; $PP_k(t)$), which represent the positions in posture space or the vector space spanned by the PC-eigenvectors [15]. In analogy to Newton's mechanics, PM_k-accelerations (i.e., principal accelerations; $PA_k(t)$), a second-time derivative, can be computed from the $PP_k(t)$ based on the conventional differentiation rules [15]. As previously reported in a postural control study [20], $PA_k(t)$ have associations with leg myoelectric activity, supporting the idea that PA-based variables could be used to determine the neuromuscular control of individual PM_k [21,33–35]. A Fourier analysis was performed on the raw $PP_k(t)$ [35] to detect noise amplification that occurred in the differentiation processes, showing that the highest power resided in a range of frequencies between 2 and 5 Hz, but that the visible power was still seen in the frequency range between 5 and 10 Hz. Hence, the PCA-based time series were filtered with a 3rd-order zero-phase 10-Hz low-pass Butterworth filter before performing the differentiation step. In addition, based on a previous study [15], leave-one-out cross-validation was performed to assess the vulnerability of individual PM_k and the PCA-based dependent variables that change the input data matrix to address validity considerations. In this regard, the current study selected the first five PCs that proved robust to test the hypotheses.

In order to describe the coordinative structure of PM_{1-5}, the compositions of overground walking movements were assessed based on their principal position ($PP_k(t)$) and acceleration ($PA_k(t)$) [35]. First, the participant-specific *relative explained variance* of $PP_k(t)$ (PP_k_rVAR) was computed to investigate the percentage of the contribution of each PM to the total variance in postural positions, quantifying how important each PM_k is for the overall coordinative movement structures of the overground walking movements [17,33]. Second, the *relative explained variance* of the $PA_k(t)$ (PA_k_rVAR) was computed, which quantifies the percentage of the contribution of each PM to the total variance in postural accelerations [20,22,36]. A greater PA_k_rVAR value reflects that a given movement component is performed fast enough to impact accelerations and forces acting in the system [36].

2.3. Investigating Walking Stability

Each $PP_k(t)$ was normalized to an individual's walking speed [23,37]. Then, the participant-specific *largest Lyapunov exponent* (LyE) of $PP_{1-5}(t)$ or PP_k_LyE was used to investigate walking stability by computing the rate of divergence of close trajectories in state space (i.e., the ability of the motor system to attenuate small perturbations revealed by the divergence of the trajectories in state space) [10,16,23,38].

PP_k_LyE was computed by applying Wolf's algorithm [39], with the time delay ($\tau = 10$) and embedding dimension ($m = 4$) determined using the average mutual information (AMI) [10,38] and the false nearest neighbor algorithms [40], respectively. A greater PP_k_LyE value indicates the inability of the motor system to reduce infinitesimal perturbations [13], resulting in a greater divergence of state space trajectories. In other words, a higher PP_k_LyE value reflects a lower individual's walking stability [16,23]. For statistical analysis, the current study used the average of individual PP_k_LyE values calculated from three walking trials.

2.4. Statistical Analysis

All statistical analyses were performed using the IBM SPSS Statistics software, version 26.0 (SPSS Inc., Chicago, IL, USA), with the alpha level set at $a = 0.05$. A Shapiro–Wilk test was used to determine the data's normality, suggesting using a Spearman's rho test to determine the correlation between participants' demographic data (age, BMI, MMSE, walking speed (WS), SPPB, and POMA-G) and individual PP_{1-5}_LyE. Pearson correlation was used to examine the relationship between individual PP_{1-5}_LyE. The correlation coefficient (r), which varies between -1 and $+1$, represents the strength of the relationship between the two variables in positive or negative directions, respectively. The absolute correlation ($|r|$) in the range of 0 to 0.4 is interpreted as a weak correlation, 0.4 to 0.8 as a moderate correlation, and 0.8 to 1 as a strong correlation [41].

3. Results

3.1. Movement Synergies

Table 2 shows the descriptive characteristics of the first five principal movements (PM_{1-5}), which together explained 99.9% of the total position variance (PP_k_rVAR) and 70.9% of the acceleration variance (PA_k_rVAR). In addition, the example visualizations of PM_{2-5} are shown in Figure 1.

Table 2. The relative explained variances (mean $\pm$ SD) of the principal positions (PP_k_rVAR) and the principal accelerations (PA_k_rVAR) of the first five principal movements (PM_{1-5}), amended with a qualitative description of the main features of each movement component. Note: k indicates the order of principal movements, and animated stick figures of PM_{2-5} are represented in Supplementary Video S2.

PM_k	Descriptive Characteristics	PP_k_rVAR	PA_k_rVAR
1	Movements of the lower extremities in the direction of walking	98.91 ± 0.33	4.90 ± 1.12
2	Resemble swing phase movement of the gait cycle: the anti-phase lower-limb movements in the anteroposterior direction	0.90 ± 0.25	31.67 ± 2.94
3	Movements of the lower extremities in the mediolateral direction (i.e., mediolateral sway) combined with anti-phase knee flexion and extension movements in the vertical direction	0.07 ± 0.12	0.43 ± 0.17
4	Both ankle and knee flexion and extension movements in the vertical direction	0.05 ± 0.01	24.65 ± 1.95
5	Resemble the mid-stance phase movement of the gait cycle: the anti-phase lower-limb movements in the vertical direction	0.04 ± 0.01	9.22 ± 1.95

As shown in Table 2, the highest value of PA_k_rVAR is observed for PM_2, resembling the swing phase movement, followed by PM_4, representing ankle and knee flexion and extension movements in the vertical direction; and PM_5, resembling the mid-stance phase movement, respectively.

3.2. Relationship between Walking Stability and Risk of Falls

As shown in Table 3, the main results show that correlations appear in specific pairs of two variables. Regarding the demographic data, the age of participants is negatively correlated with MMSE ($r = -0.449$ (moderate correlation), $p = 0.003$), POMA-G ($r = -0.450$ (moderate correlation), $p = 0.002$), and PP_3_LyE ($r = -0.306$ (weak correlation), $p = 0.046$). The BMI of participants is negatively correlated with SPPB ($r = -0.355$ (weak correlation), $p = 0.020$), but positively correlated with two walking stability variables: PP_2_LyE ($r = 0.343$ (weak correlation), $p = 0.024$) and PP_4_LyE ($r = 0.506$ (moderate correlation), $p = 0.001$). The MMSE value is positively correlated with POMA-G ($r = 0.379$ (weak correlation), $p = 0.012$).

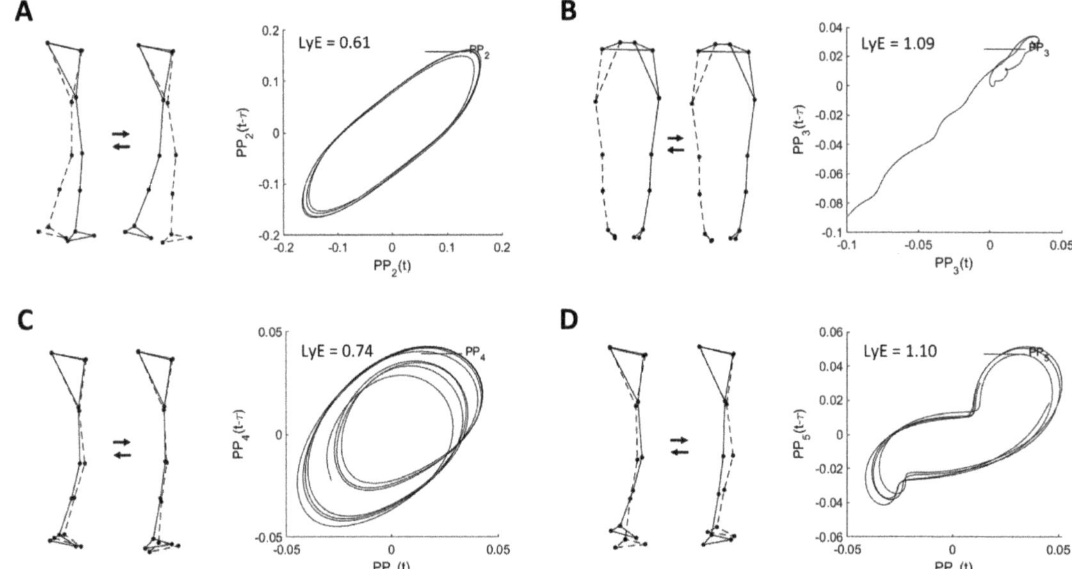

Figure 1. Example visualizations of (**A**) PM_2, (**B**) PM_3, (**C**) PM_4, and (**D**) PM_5 extracted from the overground walking movement and their corresponding space-time representation for computed largest Lyapunov exponent (LyE) of individual PP_k. Note: LyE data are derived from the first trial of one female participant. The dashed line indicates the left limb. Only PM_3 is shown in the back view.

Table 3. Correlation coefficients (r) between participants' demographic data (age, BMI, MMSE, SPPB, and POMA–G) and individual PP_{1-5}_LyE. Note: p-values smaller than 0.05 are printed in bold (n = 43; * $p < 0.050$; ** $p < 0.01$; and *** $p \leq 0.001$ (two-tailed)).

Variable	1	2	3	4	5	6	7	8	9	10	11
1. Age	1										
2. BMI	−0.063	1									
3. MMSE	**−0.449 ****	−0.290	1								
4. WS	0.242	0.206	−0.122	1							
5. SPPB	−0.205	**−0.355 ***	0.142	**−0.556 *****	1						
6. POMA–G	**−0.450 ****	−0.051	**0.379 ***	**−0.356 ***	0.146	1					
7. PP_1_LyE	0.178	0.173	−0.086	−0.001	−0.100	0.043	1				
8. PP_2_LyE	0.102	**0.343 ***	−0.145	**0.516 *****	−0.164	−0.249	0.032	1			
9. PP_3_LyE	**−0.306 ***	0.145	0.030	0.099	−0.097	0.003	0.066	0.075	1		
10. PP_4_LyE	0.145	**0.506 *****	−0.186	**0.635 *****	**−0.402 ****	**−0.417 ****	0.160	**0.718 *****	0.050	1	
11. PP_5_LyE	0.266	0.091	−0.097	**0.428 ****	−0.046	**−0.396 ****	0.021	**0.443 ****	−0.056	**0.386 ***	1

In addition, walking speed is negatively correlated with both two functional motor tests: SPPB ($r = -0.556$ (moderate correlation), $p < 0.001$) and POMA-G ($r = -0.356$ (weak correlation), $p = 0.019$), but is positively correlated with specific walking stability variables: PP_2_LyE ($r = 0.516$ (moderate correlation), $p < 0.001$), PP_4_LyE ($r = 0.635$ (moderate correlation), $p < 0.001$), and PP_5_LyE ($r = 0.428$ (moderate correlation), $p = 0.004$).

Regarding the functional motor tests, SPPB negatively correlates with the specific walking stability variable, PP_4_LyE ($r = -0.402$ (moderate correlation), $p = 0.008$). In addition, POMA-G negatively correlates with the specific walking stability variables: PP_4_LyE ($r = -0.417$ (moderate correlation), $p = 0.005$) and PP_5_LyE ($r = -0.396$ (weak correlation), $p = 0.009$).

Moreover, correlations within the individual PP_k_LyE are observed in the specific pairs of PP_k_LyE. Specifically, PP_2_LyE is positively correlated with PP_4_LyE ($r = 0.718$

(moderate correlation), $p < 0.001$), and PP_5_LyE ($r = 0.443$ (moderate correlation), $p = 0.003$). PP_4_LyE is positively correlated with PP_5_LyE ($r = 0.386$ (weak correlation), $p = 0.011$).

4. Discussion

The current study determined the correlation between walking stability and fall risk in healthy older adults. Walking stability defined in terms of local dynamic stability was assessed through the largest Lyapunov exponent (LyE) of individual movement components or movement synergies (i.e., called "principal movements," PMs) extracted by applying principal component analysis (PCA) to overground walking movements. The fall risk was determined by two functional motor tests—the Short Physical Performance Battery (SPPB) and the Gait Subscale of Performance-Oriented Mobility Assessment (POMA-G). The main results show that negative, small-to-moderate correlations between PP_k_LyE and two functional motor tests (SPPB and POMA-G) appear in the specific PMs, suggesting that the lower the PP_4-Lyapunov stability, the greater the risk of falling. Based on the empirical findings, two main points can be discussed.

First, the lower performance of the lower extremities possibly influences walking instability, especially in movement components resembling the ground contact phases of the gait cycle (PM_{4-5}). Walking instability can be caused by a degenerative change in the lower-limb muscle–tendon neuromechanics (e.g., a decline in muscle strength [42] and a degenerative muscle [43] and tendon [44] property), which usually happens as a normal part of the inherent aging process [45]. This degenerative physical decline could make it harder to control body weight while walking [46]. For example, in the PM_4, which represents the ankle and knee flexion and extension movements, the declining calf muscle strength (e.g., the gastrocnemius, as the two joint muscles associated with both ankle and knee movements) may be involved in the instability of this movement component. A previous review article reported age-related declines in the contribution of the Achilles tendon in recoiling to ankle power output during walking, leading to an increase in the metabolic cost of walking because of less economical calf muscle contractions and increased work of the proximal joint (e.g., the hip joints) [44]. This point is of interest and may need further analysis. In addition, in the PM_5, which resembles the mid-stance phase, the hamstring muscles are an essential group of muscles that play the main role in the weight-bearing and takeoff phases of the gait cycle for three functions [46]: (I) decelerating the knee extension through an eccentric contraction at the end of the swing phase to stabilize the weight-bearing knee dynamically; (II) facilitating the hip extension through an eccentric contraction at foot strike to stabilize the weight-bearing leg; and (III) supporting the gastrocnemius muscles through an eccentric contraction in extending the knee during the takeoff phase.

Second, since SPPB [29] and POMA-G [30] have the potential to predict the risk of falls in terms of measuring lower-limb physical performance, walking instability should be considered a potential fall risk. Although SPPB and POMA-G assess lower limb performance, they focus on different aspects. For example, the SPPS measures lower-limb performance in terms of time spent performing standing balance, walking speed, and chair stand tests [47]. Unlike the SPPB, the POMA-G focuses on the quality of walking, e.g., the ability of gait initiation, step length, step height, step symmetry, step continuity, walking path, trunk movement, and walking stance [26]. In this sense, the SPPB is one of the functional tests practically used to assess lower extremity strength [29] and used as a predictor of mortality in older adults by all causes [47].

Regarding the characteristics of participants, age has negatively correlated with the MMSE and POMA-G, indicating possible cognitive [48] and gait [26] impairments that may occur with advancing age. The BMI negatively correlates with SPPB, indicating that individuals with increasing body mass relative to height may have lower limb muscle strength [29] and physical performance [25]. The MMSE positively correlates with the POMA-G, indicating that individuals with possible cognitive impairment [48] may have been associated with gait impairments [26]. In addition, walking speed negatively correlates with both

SPPB and POMA-G, indicating that reduced walking speed reflects decreased physical performance in individuals. Moreover, walking speed has a positive correlation with walking instability, reflecting that increased walking speed increases walking instability. Based on these findings, it is suggested that individuals with an advancing age, an increasing BMI, a decreasing MMSE, and a reduced walking speed are associated with lower physical performance, possibly leading to an increased risk of falling.

When considering the correlation among the PP_k_LyE, a positive interrelationship between the walking stability variables is observed between PM_2 (PP_2_LyE) and PM_{4-5} (PP_{4-5}_LyE), indicating that the higher the instability of the swing phase, the greater the instability of the contact ground movements of the two legs. In addition, a positive interrelationship between PM_4 (PP_4_LyE) and PM_5 (PP_5_LyE) indicates that the higher the instability of the swing phase, the greater the instability of the mid-stance phase. Although these three movement components ($PM_{2,4-5}$) are movement components that are small in positional amplitude ($PP_{2,4-5}\_rVAR$), they are performed fast enough ($PA_{2,4-5}\_rVAR$) to influence accelerations considerably, and thus forces acting in the system [36]. In this sense, fall prevention programs should take into account how unstable a person is during both the swing and stance phases of a gait cycle.

In terms of practical application, the current study suggests that reducing walking Lyapunov stability, specifically in the ground contact movement components (PP_{4-5}), should be considered for fall prevention and rehabilitation, for which task-specific gait training to improve neuromuscular control of the lower extremities is recommended. For instance, the three subtasks of the SPPB—chair stand, standing balance, and walking speed [25]—can be applied as an exercise or training for fall prevention. Furthermore, exercising or training to improve walking quality by considering the POMA-G components—gait initiation, step length, step height, step symmetry, step continuity, walking path, trunk movement, and walking stance [26]—is of interest and can be practical in clinical settings.

Limitations and Future Study

One limitation of the current study was that only the lower limb movements provided by an open-access dataset were analyzed. Therefore, for future research, whole-body movement analysis is suggested since the effective contribution of all the body segments is required for achieving the given task goal [21], representing that the neuromuscular system controls posture and movement through multiple muscles that produce relative movements between multiple body segments [20]. Another limitation was that the characteristics of participants enrolled in the current study were not generalized, but mostly female. In this regard, considering the impact of the sexes [5,6] or investigating the age-related differences in walking stability is suggested for future research.

Since, in the current study, only the correlation test was performed to study the relationship between walking stability and the risk of falling, applying the regression analysis focused on modeling the relationship may be of interest. Moreover, the risk of falls is considered highly correlated to lower extremity muscle strength and joint moments [49,50], usually observed in frail, older adults [51] or individuals with neurological or musculoskeletal impairments [52]. Therefore, encouraging the collection of kinematics combined with kinetic or electromyographic (EMG) data is suggested [20], since it is highly informative and may offer insights into net muscle forces acting at the joints, especially during periods of the single support phase of the gait cycle.

5. Conclusions

In healthy older adults, the negative small-to-moderate correlations are observed between the Lyapunov instability of specific movement components (i.e., principal movements, PMs) extracted from the lower limb movements during overground walking with self-selected speed and the potential risk of falls assessed by two functional motor tests—the Short Physical Performance Battery (SPPB) and the Gait Subscale of Performance-Oriented Mobility Assessment (POMA-G), indicating the higher the LyE, the lower the physical performance with possibly increased risk of falling. Based on the current findings, it is, therefore, suggested that the inherent impacts of walking (Lyapunov) stability should be considered for fall investigation, prevention, and rehabilitation, not particularly in healthy older adults but also in frail, older adults and individuals with neurological or musculoskeletal impairments, possibly increasing the risk of falls.

Supplementary Materials: The following supporting information can be downloaded at: https://www.mdpi.com/article/10.3390/bioengineering10040471/s1, Video S1: An original walking movement derived from one female participant, Video S2: Visualization of the PM_{2-5}.

Author Contributions: Conceptualization, A.P. and P.F.; methodology, A.P.; software, A.P. and P.F.; validation, A.P. and P.F.; formal analysis, A.P.; data curation, A.P.; writing—original draft preparation, A.P.; writing—review and editing, A.P. and P.F.; visualization, A.P.; supervision, P.C. and P.F.; project administration, A.P.; funding acquisition, A.P. All authors have read and agreed to the published version of the manuscript.

Funding: This work (Grant No. RGNS 65–136) was supported by the Office of the Permanent Secretary, Ministry of Higher Education, Science, Research, and Innovation (OPS MHESI), Thailand Science Research and Innovation (TSRI), and University of Phayao.

Institutional Review Board Statement: The experiment was conducted in accordance with the Declaration of Helsinki, and approved by the Ethics Committee of both the Escuela Colombiana de Ingeniería and Clínica Universidad de la Sabana, Colombia [32].

Informed Consent Statement: Informed consent was obtained from all participants involved in the study [32].

Data Availability Statement: Not applicable.

Conflicts of Interest: The authors declare no conflict of interest.

References

1. Sturnieks, D.L.; St George, R.; Lord, S.R. Balance Disorders in the Elderly. *Neurophysiol. Clin.* **2008**, *38*, 467–478. [CrossRef] [PubMed]
2. Khalaf, S.; Morris, C. Falls in the Elderly. *Psychiatr. Bull.* **1996**, *20*, 501. [CrossRef]
3. Gillespie, L. Preventing Falls in Elderly People. *Br. Med. J.* **2004**, *328*, 653–654. [CrossRef] [PubMed]
4. Karlsson, M.K.; Vonschewelov, T.; Karlsson, C.; CÅster, M.; Rosengen, B.E. Prevention of Falls in the Elderly: A Review. *Scand. J. Public Health* **2013**, *41*, 442–454. [CrossRef] [PubMed]
5. Tinetti, M.E.; Kumar, C. The Patient Who Falls: "It's Always a Trade-Off". *JAMA-J. Am. Med. Assoc.* **2010**, *303*, 258–266. [CrossRef]
6. Tinetti, M.E. Preventing Falls in Elderly Persons. *N. Engl. J. Med.* **2003**, *348*, 42–49. [CrossRef]
7. Callisaya, M.L.; Blizzard, L.; Schmidt, M.D.; McGinley, J.L.; Srikanth, V.K. Ageing and Gait Variability—A Population-Based Study of Older People. *Age Ageing* **2010**, *39*, 191–197. [CrossRef]
8. Hamacher, D.; Singh, N.B.; Van Dieën, J.H.; Heller, M.O.; Taylor, W.R. Kinematic Measures for Assessing Gait Stability in Elderly Individuals: A Systematic Review. *J. R. Soc. Interface* **2011**, *8*, 1682–1698. [CrossRef]
9. Bruijn, S.M.; Meijer, O.G.; Beek, P.J.; Van Dieen, J.H.; van Dieën, J.H. Assessing the Stability of Human Locomotion: A Review of Current Measures. *J. R. Soc. Interface* **2013**, *10*, 20120999. [CrossRef]
10. Federolf, P.; Tecante, K.; Nigg, B. A Holistic Approach to Study the Temporal Variability in Gait. *J. Biomech.* **2012**, *45*, 1127–1132. [CrossRef]
11. Cavanaugh, J.T.; Guskiewicz, K.M.; Stergiou, N. A Nonlinear Dynamic Approach for Evaluating Postural Control: New Directions for the Management of Sport-Related Cerebral Concussion. *Sport. Med.* **2005**, *35*, 935–950. [CrossRef] [PubMed]
12. Dingwell, J.B.; Cusumano, J.P.; Cavanagh, P.R.; Sternad, D. Local Dynamic Stability Versus Kinematic Variability of Continuous Overground and Treadmill Walking. *J. Biomech. Eng.* **2001**, *123*, 27–32. [CrossRef] [PubMed]
13. Dingwell, J.B.; Marin, L.C. Kinematic Variability and Local Dynamic Stability of Upper Body Motions When Walking at Different Speeds. *J. Biomech.* **2006**, *39*, 444–452. [CrossRef] [PubMed]
14. England, S.A.; Granata, K.P. The Influence of Gait Speed on Local Dynamic Stability of Walking. *Gait Posture* **2007**, *25*, 172–178. [CrossRef] [PubMed]
15. Haid, T.H.; Zago, M.; Promsri, A.; Doix, A.-C.M.; Federolf, P.A. PManalyzer: A Software Facilitating the Study of Sensorimotor Control of Whole-Body Movements. *Front. Neuroinformat.* **2019**, *13*, 24. [CrossRef] [PubMed]
16. Promsri, A. Assessing Walking Stability Based on Whole-Body Movement Derived from a Depth-Sensing Camera. *Sensors* **2022**, *22*, 7542. [CrossRef]

17. Federolf, P.A. A Novel Approach to Study Human Posture Control: "Principal Movements" Obtained from a Principal Component Analysis of Kinematic Marker Data. *J. Biomech.* **2016**, *49*, 364–370. [CrossRef]

18. Troje, N.F. Decomposing Biological Motion: A Framework for Analysis and Synthesis of Human Gait Patterns. *J. Vis.* **2002**, *2*, 371–387. [CrossRef]

19. Daffertshofer, A.; Lamoth, C.J.C.; Meijer, O.G.; Beek, P.J. PCA in Studying Coordination and Variability: A Tutorial. *Clin. Biomech.* **2004**, *19*, 415–428. [CrossRef]

20. Promsri, A.; Mohr, M.; Federolf, P. Principal Postural Acceleration and Myoelectric Activity: Interrelationship and Relevance for Characterizing Neuromuscular Function in Postural Control. *Hum. Mov. Sci.* **2021**, *77*, 102792. [CrossRef]

21. Promsri, A.; Haid, T.; Federolf, P. Complexity, Composition, and Control of Bipedal Balancing Movements as the Postural Control System Adapts to Unstable Support Surfaces or Altered Feet Positions. *Neuroscience* **2020**, *430*, 113–124. [CrossRef]

22. Promsri, A.; Longo, A.; Haid, T.; Doix, A.-C.M.; Federolf, P. Leg Dominance as a Risk Factor for Lower-Limb Injuries in Downhill Skiers—A Pilot Study into Possible Mechanisms. *Int. J. Environ. Res. Public Health* **2019**, *16*, 3399. [CrossRef]

23. Promsri, A. Sex Difference in Running Stability Analyzed Based on a Whole-Body Movement: A Pilot Study. *Sports* **2022**, *10*, 138. [CrossRef] [PubMed]

24. Enderlin, C.; Rooker, J.; Ball, S.; Hippensteel, D.; Alderman, J.; Fisher, S.J.; McLeskey, N.; Jordan, K. Summary of Factors Contributing to Falls in Older Adults and Nursing Implications. *Geriatr. Nurs.* **2015**, *36*, 397–406. [CrossRef] [PubMed]

25. Guralnik, J.M.; Simonsick, E.M.; Ferrucci, L.; Glynn, R.J.; Berkman, L.F.; Blazer, D.G.; Scherr, P.A.; Wallace, R.B. A Short Physical Performance Battery Assessing Lower Extremity Function: Association with Self-Reported Disability and Prediction of Mortality and Nursing Home Admission. *J. Gerontol.* **1994**, *49*, M85–M94. [CrossRef]

26. Abbruzzese, L.D. The Tinetti Performance-Oriented Mobility Assessment Tool. *Am. J. Nurs.* **1998**, *98*, 16J. [CrossRef]

27. Lauretani, F.; Ticinesi, A.; Gionti, L.; Prati, B.; Nouvenne, A.; Tana, C.; Meschi, T.; Maggio, M. Short-Physical Performance Battery (SPPB) Score Is Associated with Falls in Older Outpatients. *Aging Clin. Exp. Res.* **2019**, *31*, 1435–1442. [CrossRef] [PubMed]

28. Perell, K.L.; Nelson, A.; Goldman, R.L.; Luter, S.L.; Prieto-Lewis, N.; Rubenstein, L.Z. Fall Risk Assessment Measures: An Analytic Review. *J. Gerontol. Ser. A Biol. Sci. Med. Sci.* **2001**, *56*, 761–766. [CrossRef]

29. Veronese, N.; Bolzetta, F.; Toffanello, E.D.; Zambon, S.; De Rui, M.; Perissinotto, E.; Coin, A.; Corti, M.C.; Baggio, G.; Crepaldi, G.; et al. Association between Short Physical Performance Battery and Falls in Older People: The Progetto Veneto Anziani Study. *Rejuvenation Res.* **2014**, *17*, 276–284. [CrossRef]

30. Faber, M.J.; Bosscher, R.J.; Van Wieringen, P.C.W. Clinimetric Properties of the Performance-Oriented Mobility Assessment. *Phys. Ther.* **2006**, *86*, 944–954. [CrossRef]

31. Menz, H.B.; Lord, S.R.; Fitzpatrick, R.C. Age-Related Differences in Walking Stability. *Age Ageing* **2003**, *32*, 137–142. [CrossRef] [PubMed]

32. Caicedo, P.E.; Rengifo, C.F.; Rodriguez, L.E.; Sierra, W.A.; Gómez, M.C. Dataset for Gait Analysis and Assessment of Fall Risk for Older Adults. *Data Br.* **2020**, *33*, 106550. [CrossRef] [PubMed]

33. Promsri, A.; Haid, T.; Federolf, P. How Does Lower Limb Dominance Influence Postural Control Movements during Single Leg Stance? *Hum. Mov. Sci.* **2018**, *58*, 165–174. [CrossRef]

34. Promsri, A.; Haid, T.; Werner, I.; Federolf, P. Leg Dominance Effects on Postural Control When Performing Challenging Balance Exercises. *Brain Sci.* **2020**, *10*, 128. [CrossRef] [PubMed]

35. Promsri, A.; Federolf, P. Analysis of Postural Control Using Principal Component Analysis: The Relevance of Postural Accelerations and of Their Frequency Dependency for Selecting the Number of Movement Components. *Front. Bioeng. Biotechnol.* **2020**, *8*, 480. [CrossRef]

36. Longo, A.; Haid, T.; Meulenbroek, R.; Federolf, P. Biomechanics in Posture Space: Properties and Relevance of Principal Accelerations for Characterizing Movement Control. *J. Biomech.* **2019**, *82*, 397–403. [CrossRef]

37. Ó'Reilly, D.; Federolf, P. Identifying Differences in Gait Adaptability across Various Speeds Using Movement Synergy Analysis. *PLoS ONE* **2021**, *16*, e0244582. [CrossRef]

38. Longo, A.; Federolf, P.; Haid, T.; Meulenbroek, R. Effects of a Cognitive Dual Task on Variability and Local Dynamic Stability in Sustained Repetitive Arm Movements Using Principal Component Analysis: A Pilot Study. *Exp. Brain Res.* **2018**, *236*, 1611–1619. [CrossRef]

39. Wolf, A.; Swift, J.B.; Swinney, H.L.; Vastano, J.A. Determining Lyapunov Exponents from a Time Series. *Phys. D Nonlinear Phenom.* **1985**, *16*, 285–317. [CrossRef]

40. Kantz, H. A Robust Method to Estimate the Maximal Lyapunov Exponent of a Time Series. *Phys. Lett. A* **1994**, *185*, 77–87. [CrossRef]

41. Akoglu, H. User's Guide to Correlation Coefficients. *Turk. J. Emerg. Med.* **2018**, *18*, 91–93. [CrossRef] [PubMed]

42. Cappellini, G.; Ivanenko, Y.P.; Poppele, R.E.; Lacquaniti, F. Motor Patterns in Human Walking and Running. *J. Neurophysiol.* **2006**, *95*, 3426–3437. [CrossRef] [PubMed]

43. Yasuda, T.; Ota, S.; Yamashita, S.; Tsukamoto, Y.; Onishi, E. Association of Preoperative Variables of Ipsilateral Hip Abductor Muscles with Gait Function after Total Hip Arthroplasty: A Retrospective Study. *Arthroplasty* **2022**, *4*, 23. [CrossRef]

44. Krupenevich, R.L.; Beck, O.N.; Sawicki, G.S.; Franz, J.R. Reduced Achilles Tendon Stiffness Disrupts Calf Muscle Neuromechanics in Elderly Gait. *Gerontology* **2022**, *68*, 241–251. [CrossRef]

45. Keller, K.; Coldewey, M.; Engelhardt, M. Muscle Mass and Strength Loss with Aging. *Gazz. Med. Ital. Arch. Sci. Med.* **2014**, *173*, 477–483.
46. Fredericson, M.; Moore, W.; Guillet, M.; Beaulieu, C. High Hamstring Tendinopathy in Runners Meeting the Challenges of Diagnosis, Treatment, and Rehabilitation. *Physician Sportsmed.* **2005**, *33*, 32–43. [CrossRef]
47. Pavasini, R.; Guralnik, J.; Brown, J.C.; di Bari, M.; Cesari, M.; Landi, F.; Vaes, B.; Legrand, D.; Verghese, J.; Wang, C.; et al. Short Physical Performance Battery and All-Cause Mortality: Systematic Review and Meta-Analysis. *BMC Med.* **2016**, *14*, 215. [CrossRef]
48. Creavin, S.T.; Wisniewski, S.; Noel-Storr, A.H.; Trevelyan, C.M.; Hampton, T.; Rayment, D.; Thom, V.M.; Nash, K.J.E.; Elhamoui, H.; Milligan, R.; et al. Mini-Mental State Examination (MMSE) for the Detection of Dementia in Clinically Unevaluated People Aged 65 and over in Community and Primary Care Populations. *Cochrane Database Syst. Rev.* **2016**, *2016*, CD011145. [CrossRef]
49. Pijnappels, M.; van der Burg, J.C.E.; Reeves, N.D.; van Dieën, J.H. Identification of Elderly Fallers by Muscle Strength Measures. *Eur. J. Appl. Physiol.* **2008**, *102*, 585–592. [CrossRef]
50. Pijnappels, M.; Reeves, N.D.; Maganaris, C.N.; van Dieën, J.H. Tripping without Falling; Lower Limb Strength, a Limitation for Balance Recovery and a Target for Training in the Elderly. *J. Electromyogr. Kinesiol.* **2008**, *18*, 188–196. [CrossRef]
51. Torpy, J.M.; Lynm, C.; Glass, R.M. Frailty in Older Adults. *JAMA* **2006**, *296*, 2280. [CrossRef] [PubMed]
52. Larson, S.T.; Wilbur, J. Muscle Weakness in Adults: Evaluation and Differential Diagnosis. *Am. Fam. Physician* **2020**, *101*, 95–108. [PubMed]

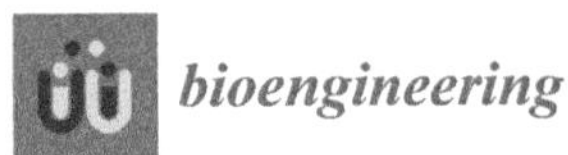

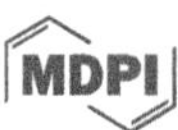

Article

Automated Quantification of Pneumonia Infected Volume in Lung CT Images: A Comparison with Subjective Assessment of Radiologists

Seyedehnafiseh Mirniaharikandehei [1,*], Alireza Abdihamzehkolaei [1], Angel Choquehuanca [2], Marco Aedo [2], Wilmer Pacheco [2], Laura Estacio [2], Victor Cahui [2], Luis Huallpa [2], Kevin Quiñonez [2], Valeria Calderón [2], Ana Maria Gutierrez [2], Ana Vargas [3], Dery Gamero [3], Eveling Castro-Gutierrez [2], Yuchen Qiu [1], Bin Zheng [1] and Javier A. Jo [1]

[1]   School of Electrical and Computer Engineering, University of Oklahoma, Norman, OK 73019-1102, USA
[2]   School of Systems Engineering and Informatics, Universidad Nacional de San Agustín de Arequipa, Arequipa 04000, Peru
[3]   Medical School, Universidad Nacional de San Agustín de Arequipa, Arequipa 04002, Peru
*   Correspondence: snmirnia@ou.edu

Abstract: Objective: To help improve radiologists' efficacy of disease diagnosis in reading computed tomography (CT) images, this study aims to investigate the feasibility of applying a modified deep learning (DL) method as a new strategy to automatically segment disease-infected regions and predict disease severity. Methods: We employed a public dataset acquired from 20 COVID-19 patients, which includes manually annotated lung and infections masks, to train a new ensembled DL model that combines five customized residual attention U-Net models to segment disease infected regions followed by a Feature Pyramid Network model to predict disease severity stage. To test the potential clinical utility of the new DL model, we conducted an observer comparison study. First, we collected another set of CT images acquired from 80 COVID-19 patients and process images using the new DL model. Second, we asked two chest radiologists to read images of each CT scan and report the estimated percentage of the disease-infected lung volume and disease severity level. Third, we also asked radiologists to rate acceptance of DL model-generated segmentation results using a 5-scale rating method. Results: Data analysis results show that agreement of disease severity classification between the DL model and radiologists is >90% in 45 testing cases. Furthermore, >73% of cases received a high rating score ($\geq$4) from two radiologists. Conclusion: This study demonstrates the feasibility of developing a new DL model to automatically segment disease-infected regions and quantitatively predict disease severity, which may help avoid tedious effort and inter-reader variability in subjective assessment of disease severity in future clinical practice.

Keywords: infected lung segmentation; quantification of lung disease severity; comparison between manual and automated image segmentation; deep neural network; COVID-19 detection; COVID-19 severity assessment

Citation: Mirniaharikandehei, S.; Abdihamzehkolaei, A.; Choquehuanca, A.; Aedo, M.; Pacheco, W.; Estacio, L.; Cahui, V.; Huallpa, L.; Quiñonez, K.; Calderón, V.; et al. Automated Quantification of Pneumonia Infected Volume in Lung CT Images: A Comparison with Subjective Assessment of Radiologists. *Bioengineering* **2023**, *10*, 321. https://doi.org/10.3390/bioengineering10030321

Academic Editors: Pedro Miguel Rodrigues, João Alexandre Lobo Marques and João Paulo do Vale Madeiro

Received: 10 February 2023
Revised: 26 February 2023
Accepted: 28 February 2023
Published: 2 March 2023

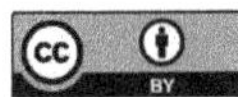

1. Introduction

Computed tomography (CT) is the most popular medical imaging modality used in clinical practice to detect lung diseases (i.e., lung cancer, chronic obstructive pulmonary disease, interstitial lung diseases, pneumonia, and others). To more accurately assess the severity of many lung diseases and predict patients' prognosis, estimation of disease-infected volume and/or its percentage to the total lung volume plays an important role. However, subjective estimation of disease-infected regions or volume by radiologists is quite difficult, tedious, and inaccurate (due to the large intra- and inter-reader variability), which makes it often infeasible in busy clinical practice. Thus, to help solve this clinical challenge, developing computer-aided detection (CAD) schemes or methods has been attracting broad research interest. For example, the CAD-generated lung density mask has been well developed and tested to quantify percentages of emphysema-infected lung volume [1] or degree of lung inflammation [2]. However, quantifying other lung diseases, such as the pneumonia-infected lung volume, has not been well developed and evaluated. Thus, we propose to investigate the feasibility of developing new CAD schemes that can automatically segment pneumonia-infected regions depicted on CT image slices and quantify the percentage of the diseased lung volume, which has the potential to assist radiologists in more accurately and efficiently reading and interpreting chest CT images in diagnosis of pneumonia-infected disease diagnosis and assessment of its severity.

In the last 3 years, SARS-CoV-2 virus named COVID-19 has infected millions of people globally [3] and it produces pneumonia-type diseases. Chest X-ray radiography and CT are two imaging modalities to assist diagnosis of COVID-19 induced pneumonia and/or monitor its severity [4]. While chest X-ray images are easier and faster to take, with lower cost, the CT scan is highly preferred mainly due to its three-dimensional nature and additional information to improve diagnostic accuracy [5,6]. Due to the wide and rapid spread of the COVID-19 virus, a large volume of chest X-ray images including CT images have been acquired in clinical practice. Meanwhile, several research image datasets with manual annotation masks have also become publicly available for researchers to develop new CAD schemes aiming to assist radiologists in more accurately and efficiently reading chest CT images to detect and diagnose COVID-19 induced pneumonia.

Recently, in developing CAD schemes of medical images, deep learning (DL) models have been well recognized and widely used to perform the tasks of segmenting the disease-infected regions of interest (ROIs) [7,8] and detecting or classifying diseases using the automatically extracted image features [9,10]. In using COVID-19 image datasets to develop CAD schemes, most of the previous studies focused on developing DL models to detect COVID-19 cases or classify between the COVID-19 and normal or other types of pneumonia cases [11–14]. Although many previous studies reported the extremely high accuracy of using DL models to detect and/or classify the COVID-19 infected cases (i.e., ranging from 90–100% accuracy [15]), no previous DL model is robust and clinically acceptable due to training bias and a "black-box" type approach [16]. Thus, the motivation of this study is to overcome disadvantages of previous DL models and investigate how to optimally use DL models to assist radiologists through increasing their accuracy and efficiency of disease diagnosis in future clinical practice. For these purposes, we propose a hypothesis that, in the technology aspect, it is important to add an interactive graphic user interface (GUI) to the DL model as a visual aid tool to increase the transparency of the DL model and allow radiologists to visually inspect results of DL model-segmented infected lesions or regions. In this application aspect, it is important to perform more observer performance or preference studies using DL models, which can help researchers better understand how to optimally develop and apply DL models to the future clinical practice to assist radiologists.

The objective of this study is to test our hypothesis. The study includes three steps or procedures. First, we build a novel ensembled DL model implemented with an interactive GUI to segment pneumonia-infected disease regions. Second, we conduct an observer reading and preference study that asks radiologists to estimate percentages of disease-infected volumes, assess disease severity, and rate their acceptance level for DL-generated lesion segmentation results. Third, we perform data analysis to compare agreement between the DL model and radiologists in the disease-infected region segmentation and disease severity assessment. The details of our study methods and results followed by discussions and conclusions are reported in this article. Specifically, Section 2 describes study datasets and the details of study methods to build a new DL model with a GUI tool and conduct the proposed observer study and data comparison analysis. Section 3 reports and explains study results. Section 4 discusses the unique characteristics or novelties and new observations or contributions of this study, as well as the limitations. Second 5 concludes this study and provides the take-home messages to the readers of this article.

2. Materials and Methods

2.1. Datasets

In this study, three chest CT image datasets were used, which include two public datasets, namely, "COVID-19 CT scans" and "COVID-19 CT segmentation dataset "https://www.kaggle.com/andrewmvd/covid19-ct-scans (accessed on 17 May 2021)". The first public dataset includes 20 CT scans of patients diagnosed with COVID-19 from two sources, Coronacases "https://coronacases.org/ (accessed on 17 May 2021)" and Radiopedia "https://radiopaedia.org/ (accessed on 17 May 2021)". Although numerous COVID-19 image datasets are publicly available, one unique characteristic of the datasets selected in this study is that all CT images have been annotated by experts providing three separate masks for the left lung, right lung, and infection regions. The second public dataset contains 100 axial CT images acquired from more than 40 COVID-19 patients. A mask with three labels is provided by a radiologist for each CT image indicating ground-glass opacity (GGO), pleural effusion and consolidation regions. These two datasets were used to build and/or train the DL model of segmenting and qualifying the disease infected regions or volumes. Additionally, another independent testing dataset including 80 CT scans of COVID-19 patients acquired from "Hospital Regional III Hanorio Delgado" Arequipa, Peru, was also assembled. This dataset is used to test and evaluate the trained DL models and conduct the proposed observer reading and preference study.

2.2. Image Preprocessing

To achieve higher reliability or robustness of the DL model, several image preprocessing techniques were employed to initially remove clinically unrelated images and normalize the remaining images. First, the "COVID-19 CT scans" dataset includes whole CT images of COVID-19 patients. However, some slices of each CT scan (i.e., in the beginning, and near the end of scan) usually contain very little lung area, thus not providing helpful information. Including these CT slices in the training data leads to a more unbalanced dataset. Thus, we removed up to 10% of CT images at the beginning and near the end of each CT scan. Generally, all lung infection datasets are unbalanced since the number of infection mask pixels is significantly less than the pixels of the healthy lung and other normal tissues presented in the image. To create a more balanced training dataset, we removed all healthy CT slices with no infection mask.

Second, since image normalization or standardization has been considered as an important preprocessing step when training deep neural networks to achieve high robustness or scientific rigor [17], we normalized all CT images by clipping the intensities outside the range [−1024, 600] HU. Specifically, if $x > max$, $x' = max$, if $x < min$, $x' = min$, and the remaining values are scaled between zero and one using a linear mapping equation: $x' = (x\text{-}x_{min})/(x_{max}\text{-}x_{min})$.

Third, we applied the data augmentation technique to generalize and enlarge the dataset and mitigate overfitting. The main augmentation method adopted in this study is Elastic Transform [18] which is commonly applied in biomedical image analysis. The python library Albumentations [19] was used to perform the Elastic Transform and other affine transformations. Along with the elastic Transform, we also applied other common methods of horizontal and vertical flipping and random rotation to increase the size of training images. Figure 1 demonstrates the changes in a CT slice after applying an augmentation method in this study.

Last, we applied another image preprocessing technique using several filters to further enhance image features detected on the CT image. In this step, several filters have been tested with various channel arrangements to enhance different textures and structures and consequently achieve better discrimination between healthy and infected regions. For example, contrast Limited Adaptive Histogram Equalization (CLAHE) is one of the filters that has been applied as a channel to the CT images. CLAHE is a variant of adaptive histogram equalization that limits contrast amplification to reduce noise amplification. This filter performs histogram equalization in small patches with high accuracy and contrast limiting. Figure 2 illustrates the effect of applying a CLAHE filter on a CT image.

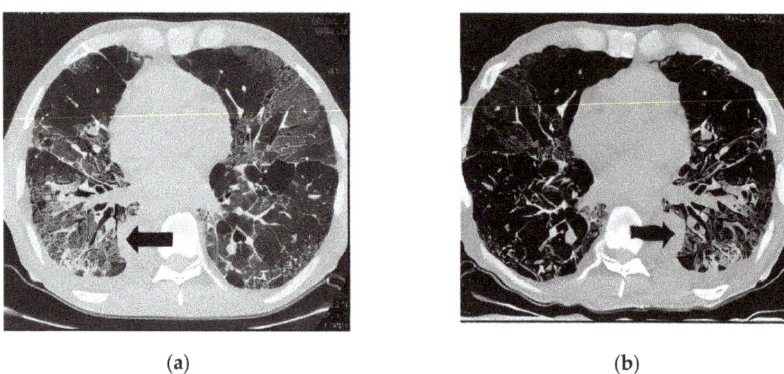

(a)   (b)

Figure 1. An example of applying an augmentation method. (**a**) The original image; (**b**) After applying an augmentation method.

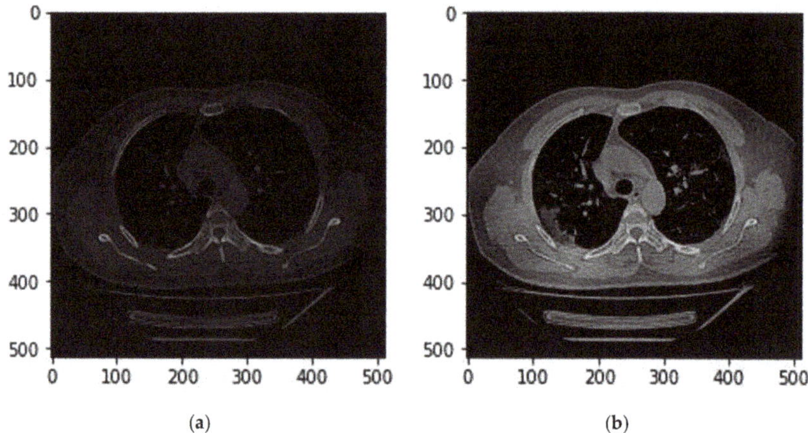

(a)   (b)

Figure 2. (**a**) Before applying a CLAHE filter; (**b**) After applying a CLAHE filter.

2.3. Image Segmentation Models and Output

Several common deep neural network models were selected and used in this study, including UNet [20], Feature Pyramid Network (FPN) [21], and Attention Residual UNet (AR-UNet) [22]. The Segmentation Models library [23] available on GitHub was also used to test various segmentation models with different backbones and parameters more conveniently. For each model, many parameters have been tested and modified, including loss functions, fixed and variable learning rates, encoders and decoders, and dropout rates.

2.3.1. Lung Segmentation

The first step is to segment the lung area depicted on each CT slide. For this purpose, a publicly available model for lung parenchyma segmentation was used to create lung masks and segment the lung area [24]. In brief, this model used the UNet, with the only adaption being batch normalization after each layer. Figure 3 demonstrates an example of the created lung mask and the lung segmentation result using this mask.

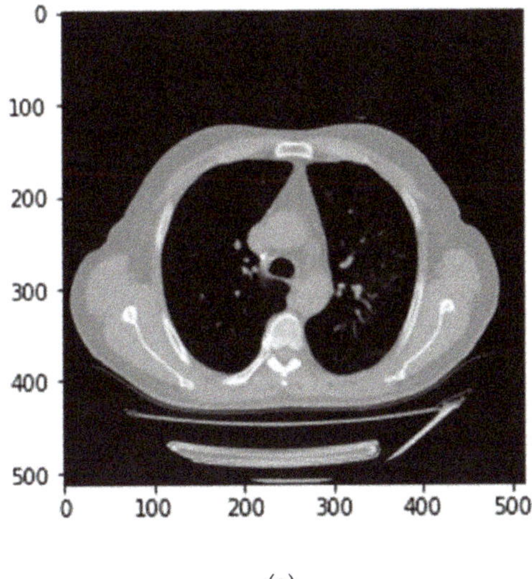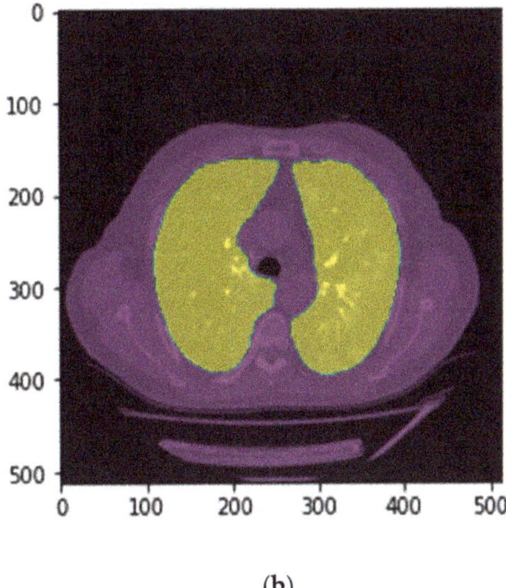

(a)   (b)

Figure 3. An example of the lung segmentation. (**a**) Raw CT image; (**b**) CT image and lung mask.

2.3.2. Infection Area Segmentation

The next step is to segment the disease infected lung regions (from fuzzy ground glass to consolidation patterns). For this purpose, various object detection and segmentation models with different hyper-parameters have been tested and employed to achieve the highest accuracy. First, the AR-UNet is selected to build the ensembled model in this step. AR-UNet model is an end-to-end infection segmentation network, which embeds an attention mechanism and residual block simultaneously into the UNet architecture. Hence, this model efficiently balances the limited training data. In this model, the attention path employs the attention mechanism to capture spatial feature details. The residual block involves the semantic information flow through a 1×1 convolution [25].

Based on the literature search and our experiments, we recognize that among many tested loss functions, the Binary cross-entropy loss and the Tversky loss [24] led to the best predictions. Binary cross-entropy is calculated as the following Formula (1) [26].

$$L_{BCE} = -\sum_{i=1}^{2} t_i \log(p_i) \tag{1}$$

where t_i is the truth value (either 0 or 1), and p_i is the SoftMax probability for the ith class.

To compute the Tversky loss function, a SoftMax along each voxel is applied [24]. Let P and t be the predicted and truth binary labels, respectively. The Dice similarity coefficient (D) between two binary volumes is identified and computed using Formula (2):

$$D\,(P, t) = 2\,|\,Pt\,|\,/\,(\,|\,P\,| + |\,t\,|) \tag{2}$$

Since, in most cases, non-lesion voxels outnumber the lesion voxels, one of the main challenges in medical imaging is imbalanced data, especially in lesion segmentation. Therefore, using the unbalanced data in training lead to predictions that are severely biased towards low sensitivity (recall) and high precision, which is not desired, particularly in medical applications where false-positive (FP) detections are much more tolerable than false negatives (FNs). To achieve an optimum balance between sensitivity and precision (FPs vs. FNs), we used a loss layer based on the Tversky index. This index allows us to put emphasis on FNs and leads to high sensitivity. Using the formula (2) in a training loss layer, it equally weighs recall and precision, FN and FP, respectively [24]. To weigh FNs more than FPs in the training of a network with highly imbalanced data where small lesions' detection is essential, a loss layer based on the Tversky index is efficient. The Tversky index is computed as the Formula (3) [24]:

$$\text{Ti}(P,t,\alpha,\beta) = |Pt| / (|Pt| + \beta|P\!\!\!/t| + \alpha|t\!\!\!/P|) \tag{3}$$

where α and β control the magnitude of penalties for FNs and FPs, respectively. Hence, the finally used Tversky loss function is defined as follows using Formula (4) [24]:

$$L_T(\alpha, \beta) = \frac{\sum_{i=1}^{N} p_{0i} v_{0i}}{\sum_{i=1}^{N} p_{0i} v_{0i} + \beta \sum_{i=1}^{N} p_{0i} v_{1i} + \alpha \sum_{i=1}^{N} p_{1i} v_{0i}} \tag{4}$$

In the above equation, p_{0i} and p_{1i} are the probability of voxel i lesion and non-lesion, respectively. Additionally, v_{0i} is 1 for a lesion and 0 for a non-lesion voxel and vice versa for the v_{1i}.

Since image segmentation accuracy and robustness depend on choosing and use of DL models along with optimal training parameters, to more accurately and robustly segment disease infection areas or blobs depicting on chest CT images, we developed, tested, and compared five models based on AR-UNet with different training parameters, as summarized in Table 1. Additionally, based on the hypothesis that if the five models contain complementary prediction scores of pixels belonging to a disease infected area, the fusion of the predictions of all five selected models can further improve image segmentation results (i.e., prevent under-segmentation as much as possible). While involving several models comes with a longer processing time, the more reliable and precise prediction is worth the extra time. For each of these models, we have used Adam optimizer with a learning rate of 0.01.

Table 1. The detail of the ensembled model for infection detection.

	Loss Function	**Augmentation**	**Dropout**
Model 1	Binary Cross Entropy	5 times	0
Model 2	Tversky	10 times	0
Model 3	Tversky	10 times	0.10
Model 4	Binary Cross Entropy	10 times	0
Model 5	Binary Focal Loss	5 times	0.10

2.3.3. Segmentation of GGO and Consolidation Patches

Moreover, besides the overall infected region segmentation, it is of great importance to distinguish between different stages of COVID-19-infected pneumonia developments in the lung and provide better assistance to radiologists to assess disease severity levels. The "COVID-19 CT segmentation dataset" provides manual annotations with 3 infection types, the ground glass opacity (GGO), pleural effusion, and consolidation. Since the pleural effusion type is not of great interest in this study, we only included the GGO and consolidation labels in the training dataset.

Like the infection region segmentation model, we tested various neural network architectures and hyperparameters aiming to achieve the best predictions. We applied a FPN model to categorize different stages of the COVID-19 in the infected area. This model has 23,915,590 trainable parameters. As depicted in Figure 4, the patch segmentation is based on Residual-Network (ResNet) and FPN model. ResNet34 is the backbone, and FPN is the feature extractor network. The loss function for this model is the categorical cross entropy which computes the cross entropy between the labels and predictions. This loss function is common when there are two or more label classes.

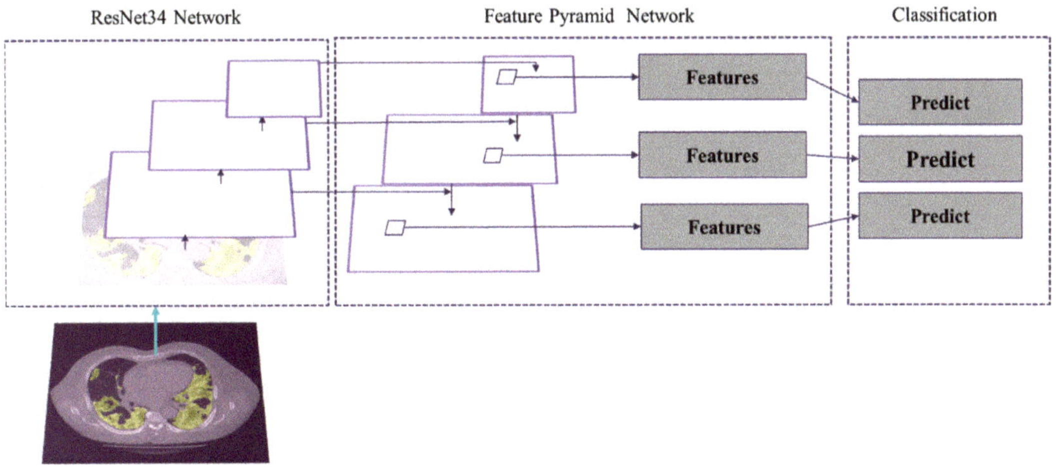

Figure 4. Overview of deep learning architecture for the patch segmentation model.

Although the staging model tends to over-segment the GGO regions, the consolidation segmentation is very accurate. To prevent the over-segmentation of the GGO area, the infection segmentation model is used to constrain the staging model. This model classifies each patch to three classes of normal tissue background, GGO, and consolidation.

2.3.4. Integrated Model and GUI

In summary, three common deep neural network architectures were trained and employed in this study. For lung segmentation, we applied a publicly available model for lung parenchyma segmentation based on the UNet model. Additionally, an ensembled AR-UNet was developed for infection segmentation since the attention blocks have been shown to be very beneficial in image segmentation [22]. Moreover, an FPN model was applied to categorize the severity of the COVID-19 infected area. For each model, many parameters were tested and modified, including loss functions, fixed and variable learning rates, different encoders and decoders, and dropout rates. All models are written in Python, and the TensorFlow library is used to train and test the models.

After extracting the lung and infected lesions by the two segmentation models, the percentage of the infected lung volume is reported along with the average Hounsfield units (HU) inside the infected region, which can indicate the density of the lesion of interest and hence the severity of infection. This information is reported for the left and right lungs for each CT slice as well as the whole CT.

Finally, to assist radiologists in the diagnosis of COVID-19 infected pneumonia using the DL model generated quantitative results or predictive scores, we also designed a stand-alone graphical user interface (GUI) as an interactive "visual-aid" tool, which can be installed on any Windows-based computers without the need for any specific programing language or library. Figure 5 illustrates the flow diagram of the developed DL model method and GUI tool.

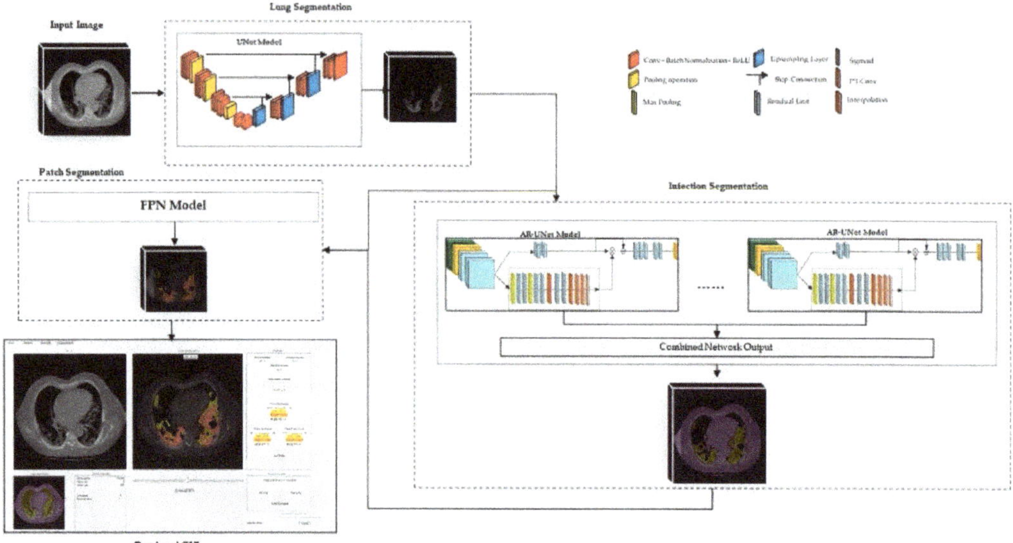

Figure 5. The flowchart of the proposed method.

2.4. Image Postprocessing and Correction

After observing the output of the lung segmentation model, it was noted that in several cases with severe disease infection, a small percentage of the lung may be missing from the segmentation as shown in Figure 6a, which typically represents the disease infection area. To recover the missed lung area if the lung segmentation error is visually observed from our GUI, the user (i.e., radiologist) can call a specially-designed image post-processing function that applies a unique conventional image processing algorithm inspired by the rolling ball algorithm [27] to automatically correct segmentation error. This algorithm starts with extracting the lung contours followed by several steps and morphological filters such as disk drawing, filling holes, median, and erosion operations. As shown in Figure 6, it can convert a jagged and rough lung boundary, as shown in Figure 6a, to a smooth one that covers the previously missed lung area, as shown in Figure 6b. While it might lead to a small over-segmentation in some cases, the previously missed area contains very important infected lesions that can significantly affect the assessment of severe cases.

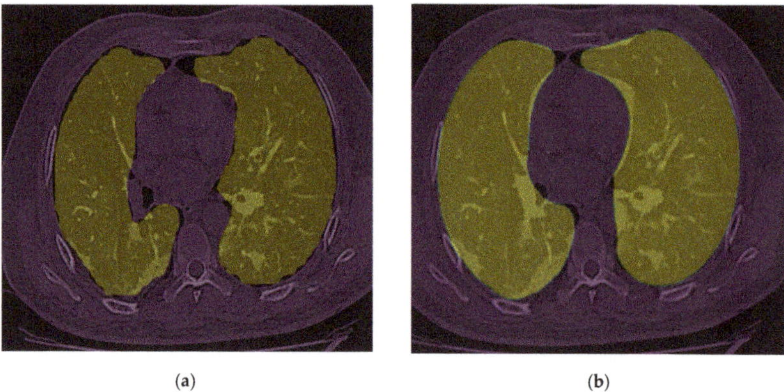

(a)   (b)

Figure 6. (**a**) Lung segmentation mask; (**b**) Post-processing lung segmentation.

2.5. Evaluation

To evaluate new DL model performance, the model was first tested "as is" using an independent testing dataset of 80 CT scans. Next, we asked two expert chest radiologists to retrospectively read and review these 80 sets of CT images. Each radiologist read and examined half of the CT scans (40 patients) and reported the patient infection spread in percentage based on their judgment of the percentage of infected lung volume. These subjectively assessed values were then collected and compared to the values generated by the DL model. It is important to note that in this new testing image dataset of 80 clinical cases, there are no manually annotated lung and disease infection area segmentation marks. Thus, no Dice coefficients can be computed, and we only compared the agreement between the radiologists and the DL model in predicting the percentage of disease infected lung area (or volume) based on the predicted result of infection area ratio or spread scores between radiologists' assessment and DL models.

Moreover, in order to test radiologists' confidence level to accept DL-generated infection area segmentation results, we showed radiologists the DL segmentation results displayed on the developed GUI and asked them to rate their acceptance level of the infection area segmentation of each CT slice with a score of 1 (poor segmentation) to 5 (excellent segmentation).

Last, we asked the radiologists to assign each patient to the group of mild infection cases that are dominated by GGO or the group of severe infection cases that have a significant fraction of consolidation areas or blobs. We then compared the agreement between the DL model generated case classification results and the radiologists' classification results. A corresponding confusion matrix was generated for the comparison and diagnostic accuracy computation.

3. Results

Figure 7 shows several image examples of DL-model generated lung and infection segmentation results. The left column illustrates the raw CT images, while the second and third columns illustrate the masks of the segmented lung and disease infection areas, respectively. In addition, Figure 8 shows the patch segmentation results of GGO and consolidation areas (or blobs), respectively. By using the commonly used evaluation index in image segmentation namely, the intersection over union (IOU), the quantitative data analysis results show that IOUs are 0.78 and 0.88 for the disease-infection region segmentation model and for the patch model, respectively.

Figure 9 shows a snapshot of the GUI window used in this study to obtain the subjective ratings from the radiologists. Using this GUI tool, radiologists can observe the raw CT image and the predicted segmentation side by side for better comparison. The radiologists can also rate the accuracy or acceptance level of the DL-generated disease infection area segmentation on each slice using a rating scale from 1 to 5, as well as provide their overall assessment of lung infection spread. Additionally, the lung segmentation is also visualized to make sure that the predicted spread scores are reliable. If a significant portion of the lung is missing, the radiologist can call and run the function to correct the segmentation errors as described in the Methods section of this paper.

Figure 10 shows two diagrams that illustrate the distribution of our data analysis results to compare the agreement between the DL-model and radiologists in segmentation or estimation of disease-infected volumes, and acceptance level by radiologists of DL model generated disease region segmentation results. From these two summary or comparison diagrams, we observe the following study results.

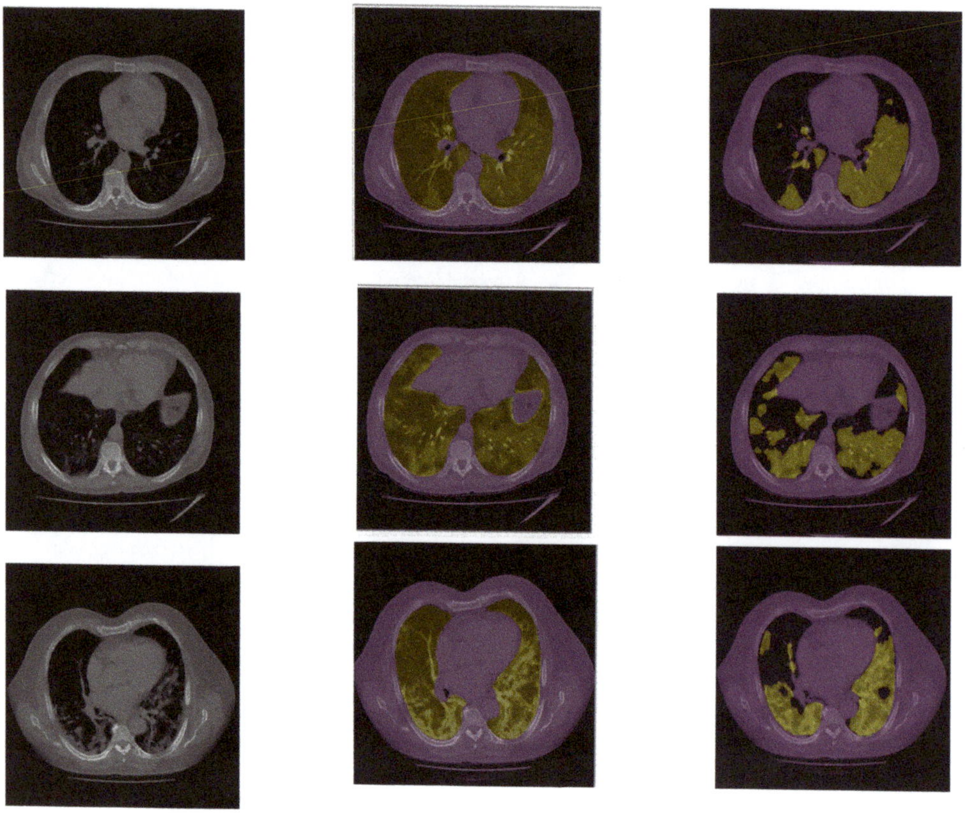

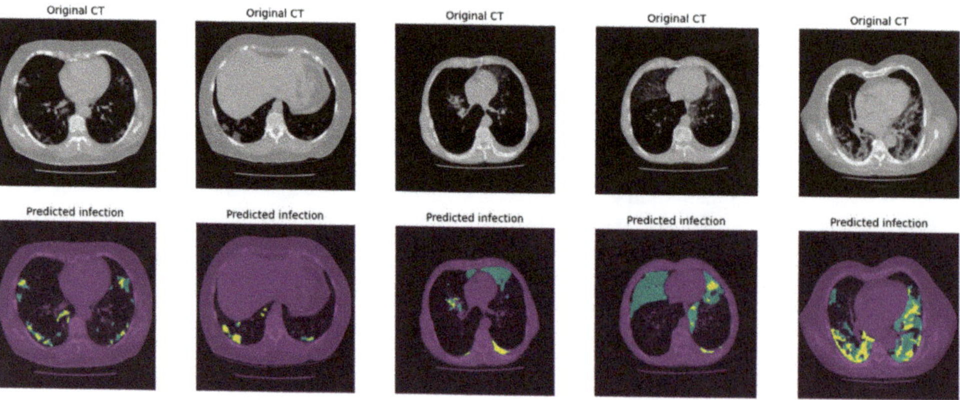

Figure 7. (**a**) Raw CT image; (**b**) Lung mask; (**c**) Infection Segmentation.

Figure 8. Patch segmentation results. The green area represents the GGO and Crazy Paved pattern. The yellow area shows the Consolidation area.

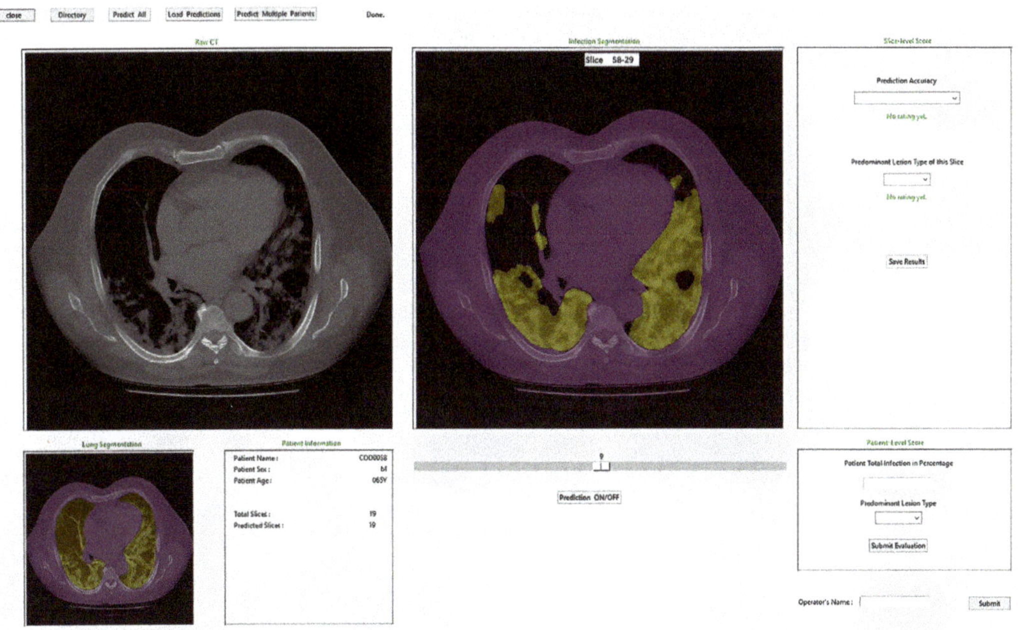

Figure 9. Illustration of the developed GUI for lung and COVID-19 infection segmentation.

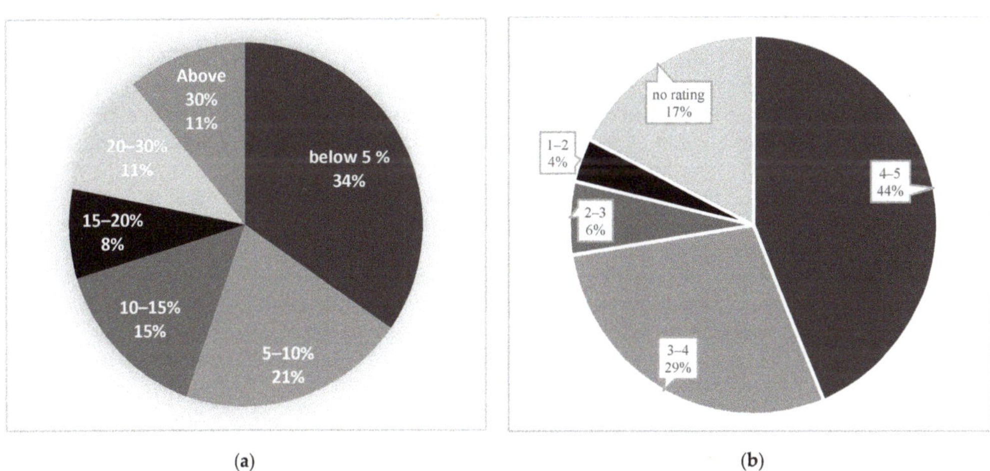

(**a**)   (**b**)

Figure 10. Part (**a**) illustrates the difference between the spread score of radiologists and the predicted score by the model; part (**b**) presents the average ratings of radiologists on the test dataset.

(1) From Figure 10a, we observe that in 34% (27/80) of testing cases, the difference between the DL model generated diseased region segmentation and radiologist's estimation is less than 5% (indicating the accuracy > 95%).

(2) In 55% (44/80) of testing cases, the difference between the DL model generated diseased region segmentation and radiologist's estimation is less than 10% (or accuracy > 90%).

(3) In 90% (72/80) of testing cases, the difference between the DL model generated diseased region segmentation and radiologist's estimation is less than 30% (or accuracy > 70%).

(4)   From Figure 10b, we observe that in 73% (58/80) of testing cases, radiologists rated a score of 3 or higher indicating an acceptable lung and disease-infection region segmentation results generated by the DL model.

Additionally, the ratings of the testing cases with high spread score accuracy have been carefully analyzed to ensure that the high accuracy is not by chance. For example, among the testing cases with more than 95% spread accuracy, the radiologists rated an acceptance score higher than 3 in over 78% of cases, and among the testing cases with >90% accuracy, 84% of cases received an acceptance rating higher than 3 indicating the DL segmentation is acceptable, and the spread score is reliable.

Moreover, to evaluate the performance of our DL model in identifying different stages of COVID-19, the radiologists also put a label on the infected regions. Then, the results of our model and radiologists were compared together. Table 2 shows the confusion matrix of the disease staging performance. When using radiologists' rating or disease level classification results as a reference ("ground-truth"), our DL model yields an 85% (68/80) accuracy in predicting or classifying disease infection severity levels in this testing dataset.

Table 2. Confusion matrix illustrating the developed model's stage detection. The cases dominated with GGO and crazy paved pattern area are classified as "A" group, and "C" represents the cases with significant consolidation area (blobs).

Radiologists\Model	A	C
A	61	2
C	10	7

4. Discussion

In the last three years, large number of studies have been reported in the literature to develop DL-based models of detection and classification of COVID-19 infected pneumonia using chest X-ray radiographs and/or CT images. However, as reported in a comprehensive review study [16], no previous DL model was accepted in clinical practice to effectively assist radiologists. To effectively address or solve this challenge and make the DL model acceptable to radiologists, we conducted a unique model development and observer-involved comparison study. This study has the following unique characteristics and/or new observations.

First, we tested a new hypothesis to quantify percentages of COVID-19 infected volume and demonstrated a potential application of a novel DL model in the segmentation of the COVID-19 generated pneumonia infection in chest CT images. One of the innovations of this study is that we developed a combined five AR-UNet models for the infected region segmentation and a novel lung segmentation correcting algorithm based on conventional image processing techniques to ensure all infected lesions are included in the prediction. Furthermore, we applied an FPN model to identify different stages of the COVID-19 infected area.

Second, since physicians including radiologists have low confidence in accepting results generated by current "black box" type artificial intelligence (AI) or DL models, developing "explainable AI" tools [28] has been attracting broad research interest in the medical imaging field. Thus, we designed and implemented a graphic user interface (GUI) as an interactive "visual-aid" tool (Figure 9) that shows DL segmented disease infection areas. This stand-alone GUI allows radiologists to easily navigate through all generated outputs, rate each CT slice automatic segmentation, and submit their assessment of the percentage of lung volume with COVID-19 infection. Additionally, the radiologist can also call a supplementary image postprocessing algorithm to automatically correct the possibly identified segmentation errors. Our experience and results of the observer reading and preference study demonstrate that using this interactive GUI-based "visual-aid" supporting tool can provide radiologists with the reasoning of DL model generated prediction results and thus increase their confidence to use the DL model in their decision-making process of disease diagnosis.

Third, based on our interaction with the radiologists, we learned that radiologists typically assign the patients into 3 classes of disease severity, namely, mild, moderate, and severe diseases, based on the distribution or domination of GGO, pleural effusion, and consolidation patterns. Thus, we believe that to increase its clinical utility, the DL model should also have a function or capability to assign each testing case to one of these three classes. Since in three image datasets used in this study, very few pleural effusion patterns exist, we developed a patch segmentation-based model to identify GGO and consolidation areas depicted on each CT image slice and then predict or classify the cases into either mild/moderate (A) and severe (C) classes as shown in Table 2. In this way, we were able to compare disease severity prediction results between the radiologists and DL model. In future studies, we need to collect more study cases with more diversity. Thus, we can apply the same DL concept to train the model that enables us to classify 3 classes of disease severity.

Fourth, we conducted a unique observer reading and preference study involving two chest radiologists and reported data comparison results. Thus, unlike many previous studies in this field, which only reported Dice coefficients of agreement between DL model generated image segmentation results and the manual segmentation results of one radiologist, which does not have a real clinical impact due to the large inter-reader variability in manual image segmentation or annotation, we used a simple and more efficient or practical method to evaluate DL model segmentation results by asking radiologists to rate the acceptance level of DL model segmentation using a 5 rating scale. This practical approach has proved quite effective and higher clinically relevant in the medical imaging field [29]. Our study generates quite encouraging results or observations of the higher agreement between the DL-model generated segmentation and radiologists' estimation of the COVID-19 infected region or volume, as well as the higher acceptance rate of radiologists to the DL model-segmented results (Figure 10).

The above observations also demonstrate a new contribution of this study, which provides the research community with new scientific data or evidence. (1) Our study demonstrates a higher acceptance rate of radiologists to DL model generated results of disease-infected region segmentation. This supports the feasibility of improving the efficacy of radiologists in reading CT images to diagnose disease because the DL model can not only replace the tedious and time-consuming process of subjectively estimating the percentages of the pneumonia regions or volume, but also avoid or reduce the large inter-reader variability. (2) Our study also supports the importance of future evaluation studies to better investigate and find the optimal interaction between DL models and radiologists to reduce the application gaps and facilitate the process to make DL models or technology clinically useful or acceptable tools in future clinical practice. (3) Although this study only used COVID-19 cases to segment and quantify pneumonia regions or volume, if successful, the demonstrated new DL model and evaluation approach can be easily adapted to segment and quantify other types of virus infection pneumonia or other interstitial lung diseases (ILD) in future research studies.

Last, we also recognize the limitations of this study, including the small image datasets and involving only two radiologists. Thus, this is a very preliminary study. The developed DL model along with the GUI tool needs to be further optimized and validated using large and diverse image cases. We also need to recruit more radiologists to evaluate model performance and potential clinical utility in future studies. Despite the limitations, we believe that this is a unique and valid study.

5. Conclusions

In this study, we developed a new ensembled DL model to automatically segment and quantify the COVID-19 infected pneumonia region or volume and predict disease severity level. To increase the model transparency and radiologists' confidence in considering or accepting DL model generated results, we designed and integrated an interactive GUI as a "visual aid" tool to the DL model. The most important novelty or contribution of this study is that we conducted a unique observer reading and preference study. The data analysis and comparison results demonstrate the higher agreement between DL model and radiologists in disease region segmentation or estimation and disease severity level prediction. However, this is a preliminary and concept-approval type study. More evaluation studies involving more radiologists and more diverse image cases are needed in future research. If successful, such DL-based disease quantification models with interactive visual-aid tools will have promising potential to provide radiologists with useful decision-making supporting tools to improve the accuracy of lung disease diagnosis in future clinical practice.

Author Contributions: Conceptualization, S.M., A.A., J.A.J. and B.Z.; methodology, S.M. and A.A.; validation, A.V. and D.G.; formal analysis, A.C., M.A., W.P., V.C. (Victor Cahui), L.E., V.C. (Valeria Calderón), L.H. and K.Q.; writing—original draft preparation, S.M. and A.A.; writing—review and editing, B.Z., E.C.-G. and J.A.J.; supervision, J.A.J., B.Z., A.M.G., Y.Q. and E.C.-G.; funding acquisition, J.A.J. All authors have read and agreed to the published version of the manuscript.

Funding: This research was funded by the Universidad Nacional de San Agustin (UNSA), Arequipa, Peru, through the Latin America Sustainability Initiative (LASI) and the OU-UNSA Global Change and Human Health Institute, grant number A21-0257-IN-UNSA, as well as supported in part by grants from the National Institutes of Health (NIH) of USA (R01CA218739 and P20GM135009).

Data Availability Statement: Publicly available datasets were analyzed in this study. This data can be found here: [https://www.kaggle.com/andrewmvd/covid19-ct-scans] (accessed on 17 May 2021), [https://coronacases.org/] (accessed on 17 May 2021), [https://radiopaedia.org/] (accessed on 17 May 2021).

Conflicts of Interest: The authors declare no conflict of interest.

References

1. Müller, N.L.; Staples, C.A.; Miller, R.R.; Abboud, R.T. "Density mask": An objective method to quantitate emphysema using computed tomography. *Chest* **1988**, *94*, 782–787. [CrossRef]
2. Karimi, R.; Tornling, G.; Forsslund, H.; Mikko, M.; Wheelock, M.; Nyrén, S.; Sköld, C.M. Lung density on high resolution computer tomography (HRCT) reflects degree of inflammation in smokers. *Respir. Res.* **2014**, *15*, 23. [CrossRef]
3. Ciotti, M.; Ciccozzi, M.; Terrinoni, A.; Jiang, W.C.; Wang, C.B.; Bernardini, S. The COVID-19 pandemic. *Crit. Rev. Clin. Lab. Sci.* **2020**, *57*, 365–388. [CrossRef]
4. Heidari, M.; Mirniaharikandehei, S.; Khuzani, A.Z.; Danala, G.; Qiu, Y.; Zheng, B. Improving the performance of CNN to predict the likelihood of COVID-19 using chest X-ray images with preprocessing algorithms. *Int. J. Med. Inform.* **2020**, *144*, 104284. [CrossRef]
5. Fan, D.-P.; Zhou, T.; Ji, G.-P.; Zhou, Y.; Chen, G.; Fu, H.; Shen, J.; Shao, L. Inf-net: Automatic COVID-19 lung infection segmentation from CT images. *IEEE Trans. Med. Imaging* **2020**, *39*, 2626–2637. [CrossRef]
6. Wang, S.; Kang, B.; Ma, J.; Zeng, X.; Xiao, M.; Guo, J.; Cai, M.; Yang, J.; Li, Y.; Meng, X.; et al. A deep learning algorithm using CT images to screen for Corona Virus Disease (COVID-19). *Eur. Radiol.* **2021**, *31*, 6096–6104. [CrossRef]
7. Porwal, P.; Pachade, S.; Kokare, M.; Deshmukh, G.; Son, J.; Bae, W.; Liu, L.; Wang, J.; Liu, X.; Gao, L.; et al. IDRid: Diabetic retinopathy—Segmentation and grading challenge. *Med. Image Anal.* **2020**, *59*, 101561. [CrossRef]
8. Shi, T.; Jiang, H.; Zheng, B. C2MA-Net: Cross-modal cross-attention network for acute ischemic stroke lesion segmentation based on CT perfusion scans. *IEEE Trans. Biomed. Eng.* **2022**, *69*, 108–118. [CrossRef]
9. Jones, M.A.; Islam, W.; Faiz, R.; Chen, X.; Zheng, B. Applying artificial intelligence technology to assist with breast cancer diagnosis and prognosis prediction. *Front. Oncol.* **2022**, *12*, 980793. [CrossRef]
10. Islam, W.; Jones, M.; Faiz, R.; Sadeghipour, N.; Qiu, Y.; Zheng, B. Improving performance of breast lesion classification using a ResNet50 model optimized with a novel attention mechanism. *Tomography* **2022**, *8*, 2411–2425. [CrossRef]
11. Wu, Y.-H.; Gao, S.-H.; Mei, J.; Xu, J.; Fan, D.-P.; Zhang, R.-G.; Cheng, M.-M. JCS: An explainable COVID-19 diagnosis system by joint classification and segmentation. *IEEE Trans. Image Process.* **2021**, *30*, 3113–3126. [CrossRef]
12. Abbas, A.; Abdelsamea, M.M.; Gaber, M.M. 4S-DT: Self-supervised super sample decomposition for transfer learning with application to COVID-19 detection. *IEEE Trans. Neural Netw. Learn. Syst.* **2021**, *32*, 2798–2808. [CrossRef]
13. Ozturk, T.; Talo, M.; Yildirim, E.A.; Baloglu, U.B.; Yildirim, O.; Acharya, U.R. Automated detection of COVID-19 cases using deep neural networks with X-ray images. *Comput. Biol. Med.* **2020**, *121*, 103792. [CrossRef]
14. Zhuang, Y.; Rahman, M.F.; Wen, Y.; Pokojovy, M.; McCaffrey, P.; Vo, A.; Walser, E.; Moen, S.; Xu, H.; Tseng, T.L. An interpretable multi-task system for clinically applicable COVID-19 diagnosis using CXR. *J. X-Ray Sci. Technol.* **2022**, *30*, 847–862. [CrossRef]

Similarly, Chintalapudi et al. in [13] investigated the importance of utilizing machine learning techniques such as cascaded neural network models, recurrent neural networks (RNN), multilayer perception (MLP), and long short-term memory (LSTM) in the correct diagnosis of Parkinson's disease (PD).

We can also cite the work of [14] who proposed a public challenge based on the Physionet PCG dataset to improve the recognition score, which was initially 0.71 (sensitivity = 0.65, specificity = 0.76). During the competition, 48 teams submitted 348 open source entries and the highest score achieved was 0.86 (sensitivity = 0.94, specificity = 0.78). In the work of [15], the authors proposed a CVD classification technique using the Physionet dataset, which consisted of only 400 heart sound recordings. They relied on the time and frequency domain transformation of the phonocardiogram signal and used a logistic regression hidden semi-Markov model for PCG segmentation. For the classification task, they used and compared three different classifiers: support vector machines, convolutional neural network, and random forest.

In the study of [16], the authors proposed a classification method for cardiovascular diseases (CVD) using deep convolutional neural networks (CNNs) and time/frequency representations of the signals. In the work of [17], the authors used AdaBoost and CNNs to classify normal and abnormal PCG signals from the Physionet dataset. They achieved a sensitivity, specificity, and overall score of 0.9424, 0.7781, and 0.8602 respectively. In [18], the authors proposed a CVD classification based on preprocessing, feature extraction, and training with the Physionet dataset. They used neural networks to classify normal and abnormal signals and obtained a sensitivity of 0.812 and a specificity of 0.860 with an overall accuracy of 0.836.

The study in [19] used the Physionet dataset to perform anomaly detection using signal-to-noise ratio (SNR) and 1D Convolutional Neural Networks. In [20], the researchers presented a heart sound classification technique using multidomain features instead of heartbeat segmentation. They achieved an accuracy of 92.47% with improved sensitivity of 94.08% and specificity of 91.95%. The researchers in [20] used a Butterworth bandpass filter and a pretrained CNN model for CVD classification. In [21], the authors used deep neural network architectures and one-dimensional convolutional neural networks (1D-CNN) with a feed-forward neural network (F-NN) to classify normal and abnormal PCG signals from the Physionet dataset.

In the work of [22], the authors used Logistic Regression-Hsmm for PCG segmentation and feature extraction for CVD classification of normal and abnormal PCG signals from the Physionet dataset. They obtained an accuracy of 79%. In the study of [23], the authors used a pretrained CNN model (AlexNet) and achieved 87% recognition accuracy. The study in [24] aimed to use a nonlinear autoregressive network of exogenous inputs (NARX) for normal/abnormal classification of PCG signals from Physionet. In [25], the authors proposed a deep CNNs framework for heart acoustic classification using short segments of individual heartbeats. They used a 1D-CNN to learn features from raw heartbeats and a 2D-CNN to take inputs from two-dimensional time-frequency features.

3. Dataset

In this section, two different PCG datasets are presented. First, the raw Physionet dataset without any data selection process is described. Then, three different data selection methods applied on the original dataset are presented. The goal is to experiment with the impact of selection on the classification results.

3.1. Raw Dataset

The publicly available Physionet dataset [14] is a not balanced PCG dataset which contains 665 normal sample and 2575 abnormal sample in WAV format. As shown in Figure 1, the majority of PCG samples are concentrated in the duration range between 8 and 40 s for normal and abnormal class.

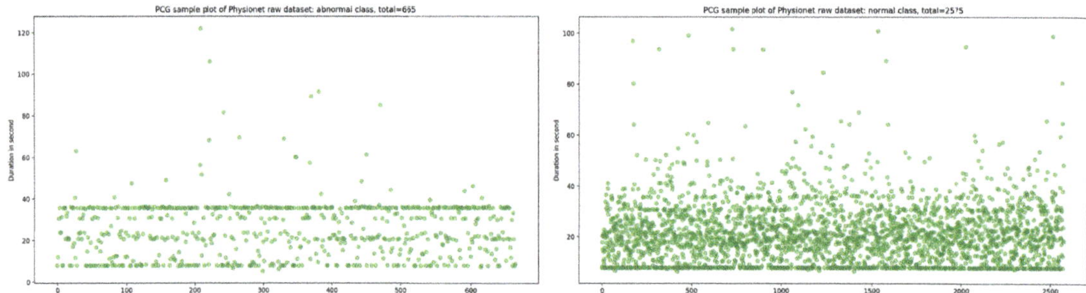

Figure 1. An overview of normal and abnormal sample distribution in function of duration in second.

If we look at Figure 2, we can deduce that for abnormal class, the highest density of PCG samples is defined at duration 35 s. Concerning the normal class, we can also deduce that the largest concentration of PCG samples are in signal duration 20 s.

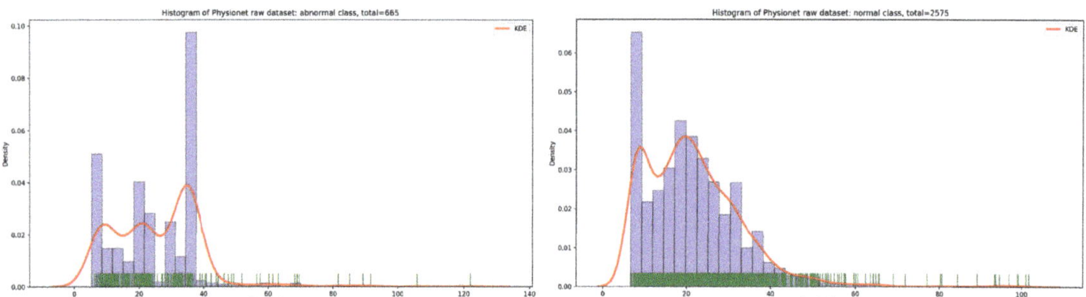

Figure 2. An overview of the kernel density estimation function using Gaussian kernel for normal and abnormal classes.

Concerning the signal-to-noise ratio (SNR) sample distribution in the function of density (as seen in Figure 3), we can deduce that the highest KDE value of SNR for normal and abnormal classes is zero. This means that the majority of Physionet PCG samples are approximately clean with an acceptable noise signal.

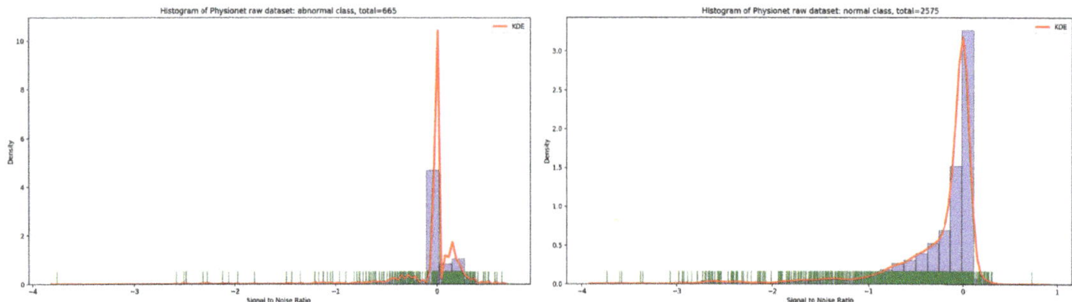

Figure 3. Signal-to-noise ratio in function of density related to normal and abnormal classes.

In the same manner, if we look at the Figure 4, it is visually clear that the highest concentration of PCG sample distribution related to normal and abnormal classes in function of SNR is approximately zero.

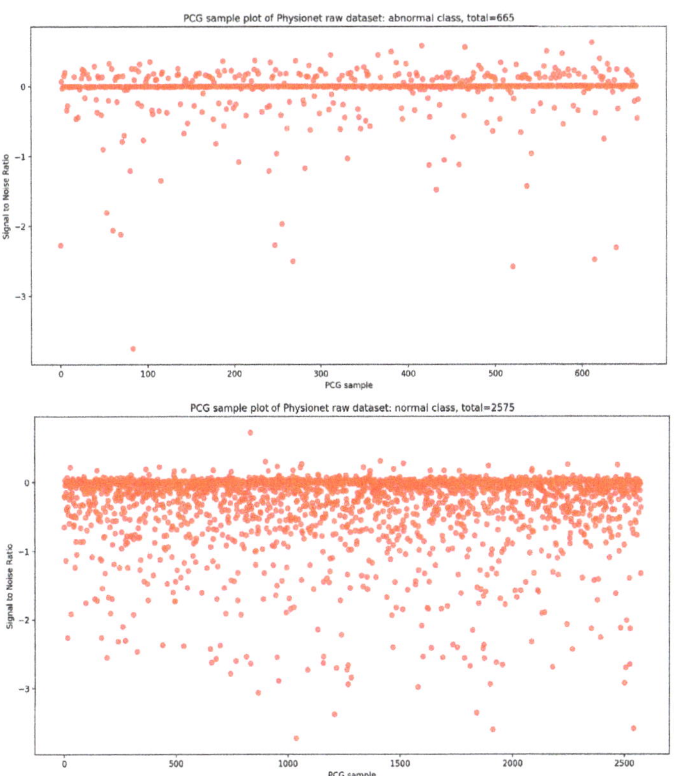

Figure 4. PCG sample distribution in function of signal-to-noise ratio of normal and abnormal classes.

3.2. PCG Data Selection

Based on the different results issued in the previous subsection, in this subsection, we present three main data selection process: data selection based on KDE for optimal signal duration determination, data selection based on optimal SNR, and data selection based on clustering. Notice that we will experiment the impact of these three data selection process on the classification results in the experimentation section.

3.2.1. Data Selection Based on Kernel Density Estimation for Optimal Signal Duration Determination

Kernel density estimation (KDE) [26] is a non-parametric method for estimating the probability density function of a random variable. Given a set of points X_i with $i = 1...n$ in a d dimension space R^d, the kernel multivariate density estimation is obtained with a kernel $K(x)$ and with window width h as following:

$$\hat{f}(x) = \frac{1}{nh^d} \sum_{i=1}^{n} K\left(\frac{|X_i - x|}{h}\right) \tag{1}$$

With $K(u)$: is a kernel function (using a Gaussian kernel (Formula (2)). The estimator $\hat{f}(x)$ determines the percentage of observations closest to a given x. If there are several observations close to x then $\hat{f}(x)$ widens. Conversely, if there are only a few X_i close to x

then $\hat{f}(x)$ remains weak. In other words, the h parameter of the Equation (1), determines the degree of smoothing of the KDE function.

$$k(u) = e^{-\frac{u^2}{2\sigma^2}}$$

(2)

Based on the discovery issued from the KDE curve shown in Figure 2, the idea is to select all the PCG samples for normal classes with signal duration equal to 20 s and 35 s for abnormal class. As seen in Figure 5, after applying this simple selection process, we obtain 238 PCG samples from abnormal class and 1291 PCG samples from normal class. If we look at the Figures 6 and 7, the obtained PCG samples after the KDE duration selection process for normal and abnormal classes have acceptable SNR values with a high SNR concentration, very close to zero.

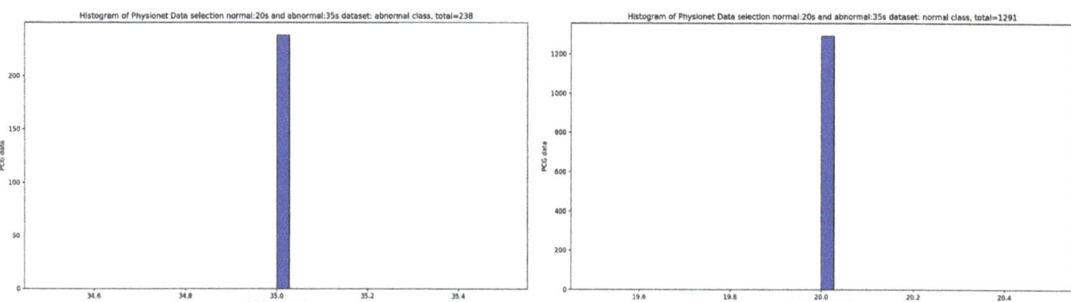

Figure 5. An overview of the PCG sample distribution in function of duration after selecting samples: 35 s from abnormal class and 20 s from normal class.

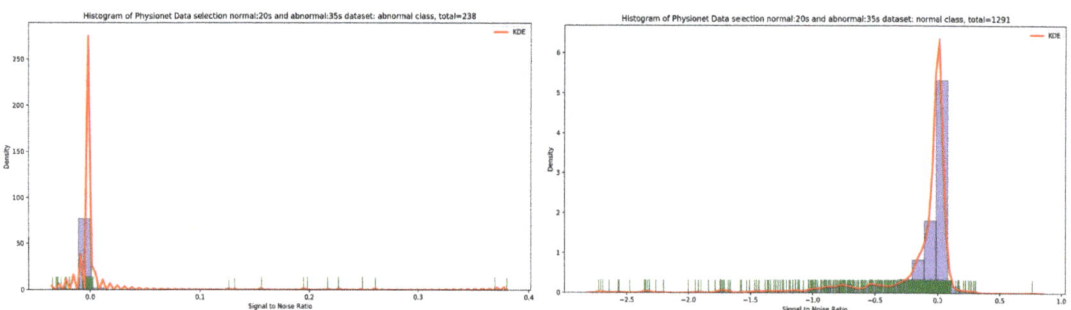

Figure 6. An overview of the SNR distribution in function of KDE density related to normal and abnormal samples after applying the KDE duration selection process.

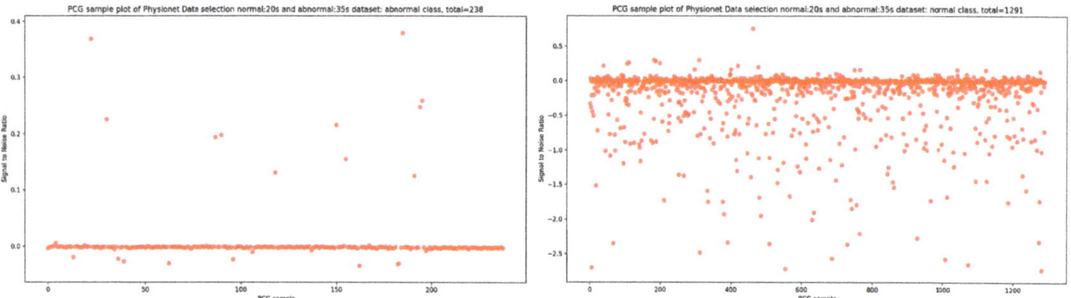

Figure 7. The PCG sample distribution in function of SNR of normal and abnormal classes after KDE duration selection process.

3.2.2. Data Selection Based on Optimal SNR

Signal-to-noise ratio (SNR) is defined as the ratio of signal power to the background noise power [27]. Based on the analysis of Figures 3 and 4, which show the highest concentration of SNR related to PCG samples for both normal and abnormal classes, we decided to select PCG samples with SNR greater than or equal to zero. As a result of this selection process, we obtained 221 PCG samples for the abnormal class and 822 PCG samples for the normal class, as shown in Figure 8. Additionally, Figures 9–11 provide an overview of the PCG sample distribution in terms of duration after the data selection process with SNR greater than or equal to 0, the KDE curve of PCG samples related to normal and abnormal classes in terms of duration after the SNR greater than or equal to zero in the data selection process, and the PCG sample distribution of normal and abnormal classes in terms of SNR greater than or equal to zero.

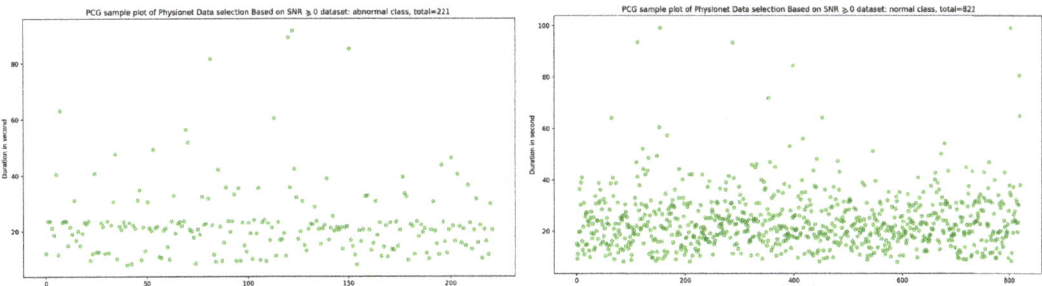

Figure 8. PCG sample distribution in function of duration after SNR greater than or equal to 0 in data selection process.

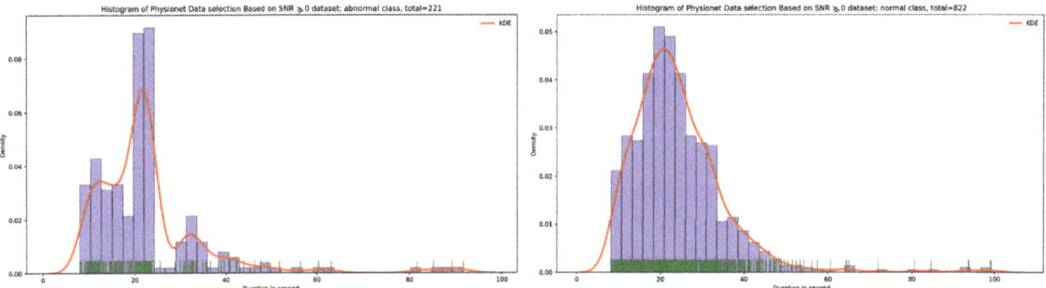

Figure 9. KDE curve of PCG samples related to normal and abnormal classes in function of duration after SNR greater than or equal to 0 in data selection process.

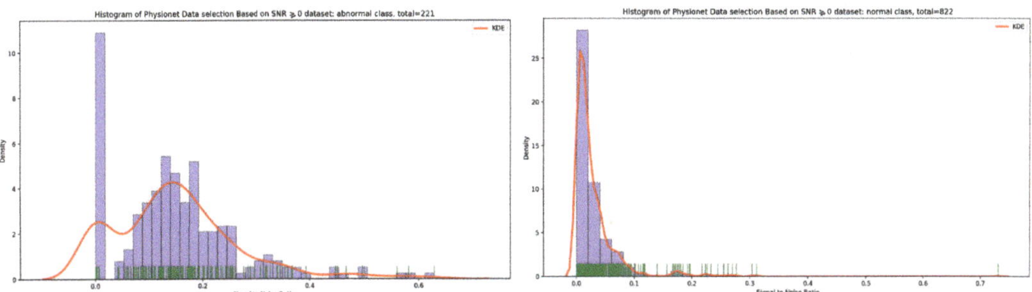

Figure 10. KDE curve of PCG samples related to normal and abnormal classes in function of SNR greater than or equal to 0.

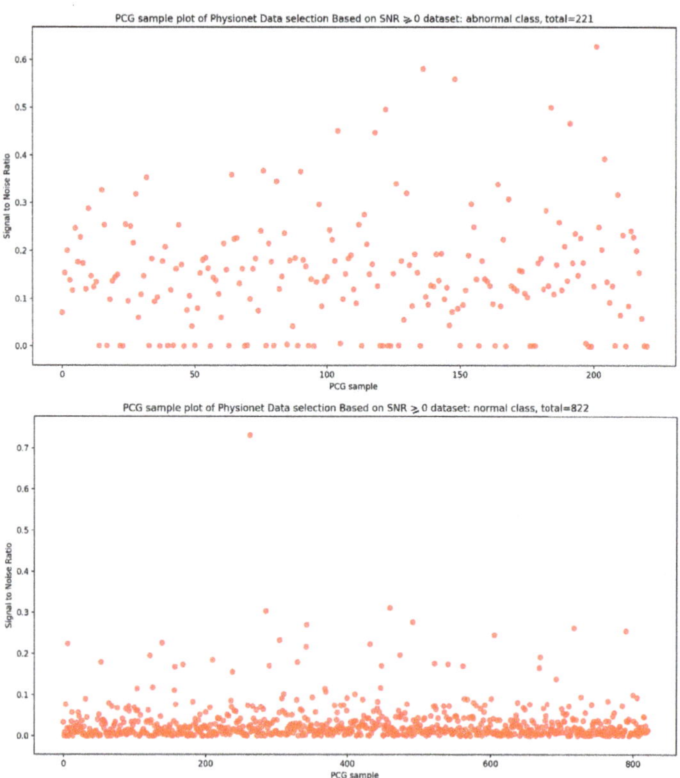

Figure 11. PCG samples distribution of normal and abnormal classes in function of SNR greater than or equal to 0.

3.2.3. Data Selection Based on Clustering

In this part, we chose to use biclustering as our data selection process. The main idea behind biclustering data selection is to suppose that the highest dense cluster constitutes our useful PCG data. In other words, we discard the remaining noise cluster and we preserve only the PCG samples belonging to the big cluster.

For this aim, we have chosen the mixture Gaussian model (GMM) [28] which is a parametric unsupervised clustering model. This model is used for data partitioning into several groups according to the probabilities of belonging and association to each Gaussian characteristics. GMM is based on a mixture of Gaussian models relying on learning the laws of probability that generated the observation data x_n (see Equation (3)).

$$f(x_n|\theta_k) = \sum_{k=1}^{M} \pi_k N(x_n|\mu_k, \sigma_k^2) \tag{3}$$

$N(x_n|\mu_k, \sigma_k^2) = \frac{1}{(2\pi)^{d/2}\sigma^{1/2}} e^{\left(-\frac{1}{2\sigma_k^2}(x_n-\mu_k)^2\right)}$, $\pi_k \in 1..M$ is the probability of belonging to a Gaussian k; $k \in 1..M$), $\mu_k \in 1..M$ is the set of the M Gaussian averages, $\sigma_k^2 \in 1..M$ the set of covariances matrices, and $\theta_k = \pi_k, \mu_k, \sigma_k^2$. Similarly, the multidimensional version of the Gaussian is as follows: $N(x_n|\mu_k, \Sigma_k) = \frac{1}{(2\pi)^{d/2}\Sigma^{1/2}} e^{\left(-\frac{1}{2}(x_n-\mu_k)^T-\Sigma_k^{-1}(x_n-\mu_k)\right)}$. The best-known method for estimating the GMM parameters (π_k, μ_k and σ_k^2), is the iterative method of maximum likelihood calculation (expectation-maximization algorithm or EM [29]). The EM algorithm could be defined through 3 steps:

- Step 1: Parameter initialization $\theta_k : \pi_k, \mu_k, \sigma_k^2$
- Step 2: Repeat until convergence

- Estimation step: Calculation of conditional probabilities t_{ik} that the sample i comes from the Gaussian k. $t_{(i,k)} = \dfrac{\pi_k N\left(x_i | \mu_k, \sigma_k^2\right)}{\sum_{j=1}^{m} \pi_k N\left(x_i | \mu_j, \sigma_j^2\right)}$ with $j \in 1, \ldots, m$: the set of Gaussians.

- Maximization step : Update settings $\theta_k^{estim} = argmax_{\theta_k}\left(\theta_k, \theta_k^{old}\right)$ and $\pi_k^{estim} = \frac{1}{n} \sum_{i=1}^{N} t_{i,k}$, $\sigma_k^{2estim} = \dfrac{\sum_{i=1}^{N} t_{i,k}\left(x_i - \mu_k^{estim}\right)^2}{\sum_{i=1}^{N} t_{i,k}}$, $\mu_k^{estim} = \dfrac{\sum_{i=1}^{N} t_{i,k} x_i}{\sum_{i=1}^{N} t_{i,k}}$

The time complexity of EM algorithm for GMM parameters estimation [28–31] is as following: If X : is the dataset size, M: the Gaussian number, and D: the dataset dimension.

EM estimation step $O(XMD + XM)$.

EM maximization step $O(2XMD)$.

As seen in Figure 12, the result of the selection process based on the highest dense cluster issued from GMM biclustering gives us a 334 PCG sample for the abnormal class and a 1626 PCG sample for the abnormal class. The KDE curve in the function of duration and SNR related to normal and abnormal PCG samples is shown, respectively, in Figures 13 and 14. Furthermore, Figure 15 gives us an overview of the KDE curve in function of SNR for normal and abnormal PCG classes after the GMM data selection process.

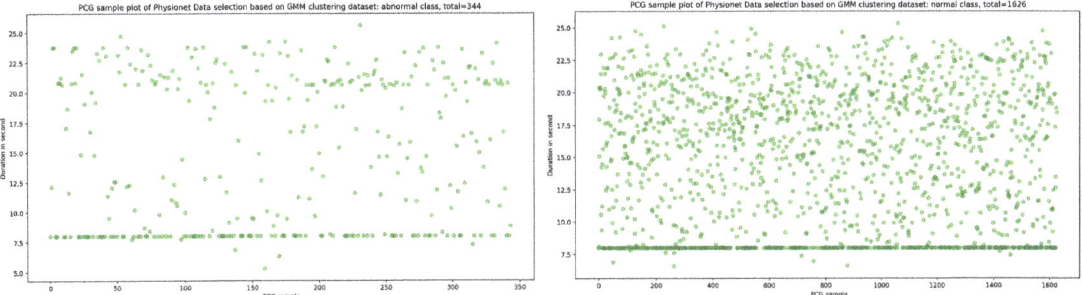

Figure 12. The PCG data distribution of normal and abnormal classes after selecting the highest dense cluster issued from GMM biclustering.

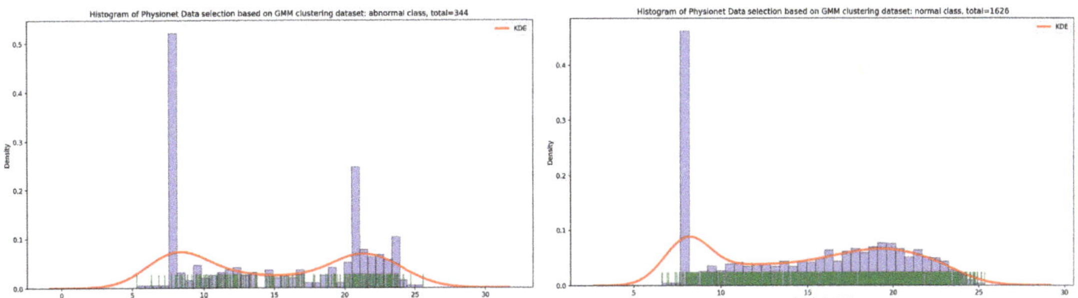

Figure 13. An overview of KDE curve in function of duration for normal and abnormal PCG classes after GMM data selection process.

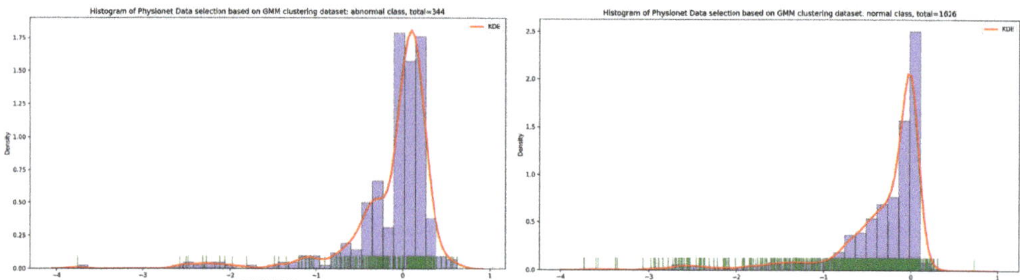

Figure 14. An overview of KDE curve in function of SNR for normal and abnormal PCG classes after GMM data selection process.

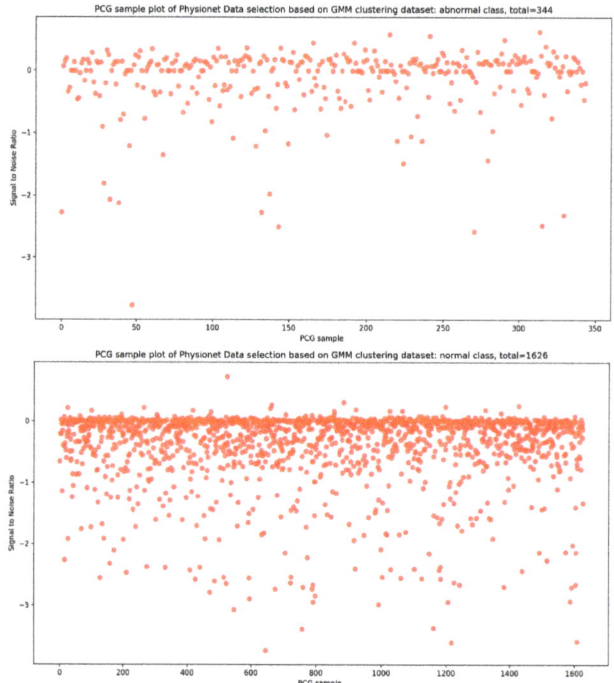

Figure 15. PCG data distribution in function of SNR for normal and abnormal classes after GMM data selection process.

4. The Process of Our CNN Benchmark

In this paper, we present a CNN classification system based on transfer learning and fine-tuning. Our system starts with the Physionet dataset, which we use to train the model. Figure 16 shows the architecture of our system, which is built on pretrained CNN models from ImageNet dataset. The first step involves transforming the wav PCG signals into mel spectrogram images using an FFT window of 1024 and a sample rate of 44,100. The second step defines the CNN parameters, including a two-class recognition, an input image size of width = 640 and height = 480, a batch size of 5, 30 epochs, and stochastic gradient descent as the optimizer with a learning rate of 0.0001. In the third step, we fine-tune the layers by using convolutional layers from the pretrained CNN models as feature extraction layers. Additionally, we add six layers including a GlobalAveragePooling2D layer for averaging and better representation of our training vector, three dense layers for the full connected network, a BatchNormalization layer to limit covariate shift, and a dense layer with a sigmoid activation function to obtain a classification value between 0 and 1 (probability).

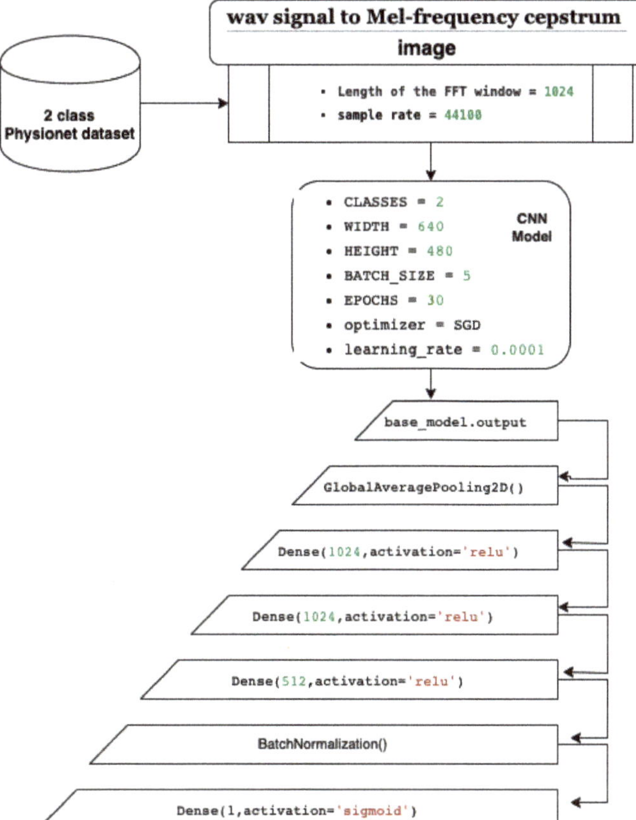

Figure 16. The architecture of our CNN system.

4.1. Mel Spectrogram Representation

The fast Fourier transform is a powerful method to decompose acoustic signal amplitude over time into a multifrequency non periodic signal. However, if we need to represent the spectrum of these frequencies in function of time, we need to perform FFT over several windowed partitioned segments of the input signal. In fact, inspired by measured responses from the human auditory system, studies [32–35] have shown that humans perception does not perceive the frequencies on a linear scale. For this reason, a dedicated unit to transform frequencies was proposed by Stevens, Volkmann, and Newmann in 1937. This is called the mel scale, which performs mathematical operation on frequencies to convert them to mel scale. In order to obtain the mel spectrogram, we perform the following steps (as seen in Figure 17:

1. Specify the signal into short frames.
2. Windowing in order to reduce spectral leakage.
3. Work out the discrete Fourier transformation.
4. Applying filter banks.
5. Applying the log of the spectrogram values to obtain the log filter-bank energies.
6. Applying discrete cosine transform to decorrelate the filter bank coefficients.

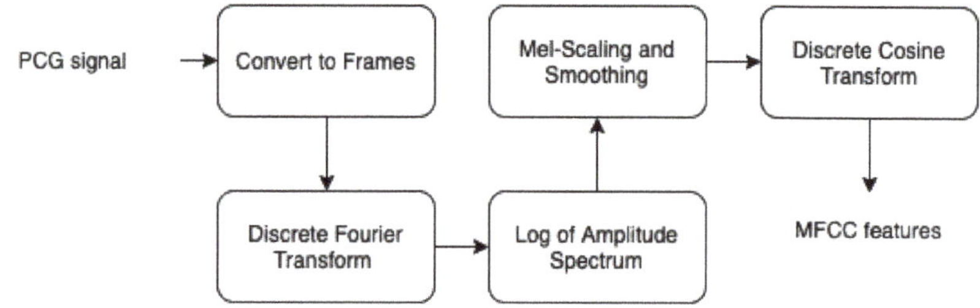

Figure 17. Mel spectrogram steps.

In this work, we have chosen MFCC signal by converting the output features into a png image, which will be applied to the CNN classifier. Figure 18 gives an overview of a normal and abnormal MFCC representation of the input PCG signal.

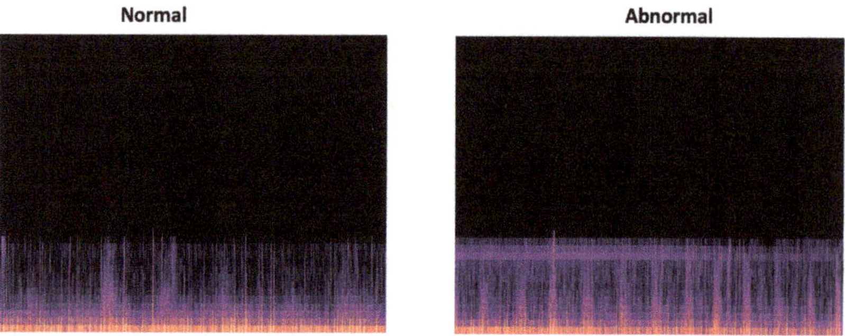

Figure 18. Overview of PCG spectrogram output (normal and abnormal, respectively).

4.2. CNN Models

Recently, deep learning and more especially convolutional neural network (CNN) has trended as an image analysis and classification tool. In fact, many research has [36–39] have been conducted using CNN to propose neural network models that enable powerful image classification results. Moreover, it is known that CNNs can perform high-level feature extraction while tolerating image distortion conditions and illumination changes, and can provide invariance of image translation. For these reasons, we chose to adopt CNN as our PCG image trainer and classifier.

In fact, in 1998 LeCun [40] introduced the first CNN architecture, designed to recognize handwritten characters. Since the last decade, due to their satisfactory results in computer vision tasks such as face detection [41–43], handwritten recognition [44–46], and image classification [47–49], CNNs are the most-used technology for classifying images. However, in order to design new powerful CNN models, CNN requires large training datasets. Thanks to the knowledge-transfer technique also known as transfer learning appellation [50], it becomes possible to take the advantages of the already trained CNN models on ImageNet by applying some modifications called fine-tuning. Therefore, we can customize these pretrained CNN models in order to be trained on a small dataset without a huge drop in the classification results.

In our work, we used several pretrained CNN models to classify normal/abnormal PCG spectrogram images. Based on the small public dataset PhysioNet, we fine-tuned and trained the 17 pretrained Keras CNN models (see Table 1). We preserved the convolutional layers which will be used for feature extraction then the additional layers are added:

1. GlobalAveragePooling2D layer for averaging and better representation of our training vector.
2. Three dense layers to define our full connected network.

3. BatchNormalization layer to limit covariate shift by normalizing the activations of each layer.
4. Dense layer with sigmoid activation function in order to obtain classification values between 0 and 1 (probability).

Keras CNN models are trained on the following dataset using the Google Colab plateform to allow the use of dedicated GPU facilities: $1 \times$ Tesla K80 , having 2496 CUDA cores, compute 3.7, 12 GB (11.439 GB Usable) GDDR5 VRAM:

1. Raw PhysioNet dataset.
2. PhysioNet dataset with data selection using KDE for duration extraction.
3. PhysioNet dataset with data selection using optimal SNR.
4. PhysioNet dataset with data selection using GMM biclustering.

Table 1. Keras CNN models.

Model	Citation	Layers	Size	Parameters
Xception	[51]	71	85 MB	44.6 million
VGG19	[52]	26	549 MB	143.6 million
VGG16	[52]	23	528 MB	138.3 million
ResNet152V2	[53]	-	98 MB	25.6 million
ResNet152	[53]	-	232 MB	60.4 million
ResNet101V2	[53]	-	171 MB	44.6 million
ResNet101	[53]	101	167 MB	44.6 million
ResNet50V2	[53]		98 MB	25.6 million
ResNet50	[53]	-	98 MB	25.6 million
NASNetMobile	[54]	-	20 MB	5.3 million
MobileNetV2	[55]	53	13 MB	3.5 million
MobileNet	[56]	88	16 MB	4.25 million
InceptionV3	[57]	48	89 MB	23.9 million
InceptionResNetV2	[58]	164	209 MB	55.9 million
DenseNet201	[59]	201	77 MB	20 million
DenseNet169	[59]	169	57 MB	14.3 million
DenseNet121	[59]	121	33 MB	8.06 million

5. Experiments and Results

The effect of selecting data on the accuracy of the classification is being studied. First, we concentrate on training and classifying CNN models using the raw dataset without any data selection. Next, we train our CNN models on the data that has been selected based on a 20 s duration for normal PCG signals and 35 s for abnormal PCG signals. Finally, we examine the impact of selecting data based on SNR greater than 0 in the third section. It is worth mentioning that all the classification results have been obtained by taking the average of the results from the three-fold cross validation.

5.1. Classification Using Raw Dataset

After performing CNN training on the raw Physionet dataset, we can notice that VGG19 gives the best classification results with accuracy = 0.854, sensitivity = 0.860, precision = 0.794, and specificity = 0.860 (as seen in Table 2).

Table 2. Average metric results related to the raw dataset.

Average	Accuracy	TPR (Sensitivity)	Precision (PPV)	TNR (Specificity)
VGG16	0.6	0.527	0.502	0.527
VGG19	**0.854**	**0.860**	**0.794**	**0.860**
Xception	0.783	0.797	0.714	0.797
ResNet152V2	0.659	0.679	0.665	0.679
ResNet152	0.580	0.689	0.634	0.689
ResNet101V2	0.282	0.537	0.575	0.537
ResNet101	0.404	0.585	0.596	0.585
ResNet50v2	0.792	0.702	0.702	0.702
ResNet50	0.538	0.624	0.638	0.624
NasNetMobile	0.619	0.496	0.347	0.496
MobileNetV2	0.435	0.476	0.460	0.476
MobileNet	0.558	0.595	0.653	0.595
Inceptionv3	0.676	0.758	0.673	0.758
InceptionResNetV2	0.825	0.807	0.748	0.807
DenseNet201	0.576	0.657	0.658	0.657
DenseNet169	0.704	0.771	0.715	0.771
DenseNet121	0.424	0.622	0.620	0.622

In addition, we can see that the classification results related to InceptionResNetV2 are close VGG19 with accuracy = 0.825, sensitivity = 0.807, precision = 0.748, and specificity = 0.807. Similarly, Figure 19 gives an overview of the validation and training curves related to VGG19 and InceptionResNEtV2. If we look at Figure 20, we can see that, if we consider the training step duration, mobileNet is the fastest CNN model and ResNet101 is the lowest CNN model. On the other hand, we can see that despite the number of layer of VGG19 (best accuracy result) which is 26 (as seen in Table 1) compared to deeper architecture (such as DenseNet201 with 201 layers) VGG19 is slower than DenseNet201 and is ranked as the fourth-slowest CNN model in term of training time.

Classification Using Kernel Density Estimation as Data Selection Method for Signal Duration 20 s Normal and 35 s Abnormal

After performing data selection on Physionet through the use of signal duration extraction with 20 s for normal PCG signals and 35 s for abnormal PCG signals, we trained all the 17 pretrained CNN models (see Table 1 and we obtained the classification results presented in Table 3. We can notice that through the use of this simple data selection, we obtained an enhancement of all the classification results compared to those without any data selection. As seen in Table 3, we obtained an improvement of VGG19 accuracy from 0.854 (raw dataset) to 0.970, for sensitivity from 0.860 to 0.946, for precision from 0.794 to 0.944, and for specificity from 0.860 to 0.946. Similarly, Figure 21 gives an overview of the validation and training curves related to VGG19 and VGG16. In addition, as seen in Figure 22, the training phase related to VGG19 becomes faster (fourth position after mobilenet, inceptionV3 and resnet50) than the one without data selection. This means that this data selection method allows us to speed up the training phase related to VGG19. On the other hand, we performed an experimental test in order to argue the choice of 20 s and 35 s signal duration extraction, respectively, for normal and abnormal signals. In this test we chose a random signal duration extraction value equal to 50 s for normal and abnormal signals. The classification results related to this experiment is shown in Table 4. If we compare the classification results presented in Tables 3 and 4, we can see that for VGG19 (best model), the accuracy decreases from 0.970 to 0.870, sensitivity decreases from 0.946 to 0.851, precision decreases from 0.944 to 0.801, and specificity decreases from 0.946 to 0.851. All these results support the idea behind our duration selection method (explained in data selection based on kernel density estimation for optimal signal duration determination subsection).

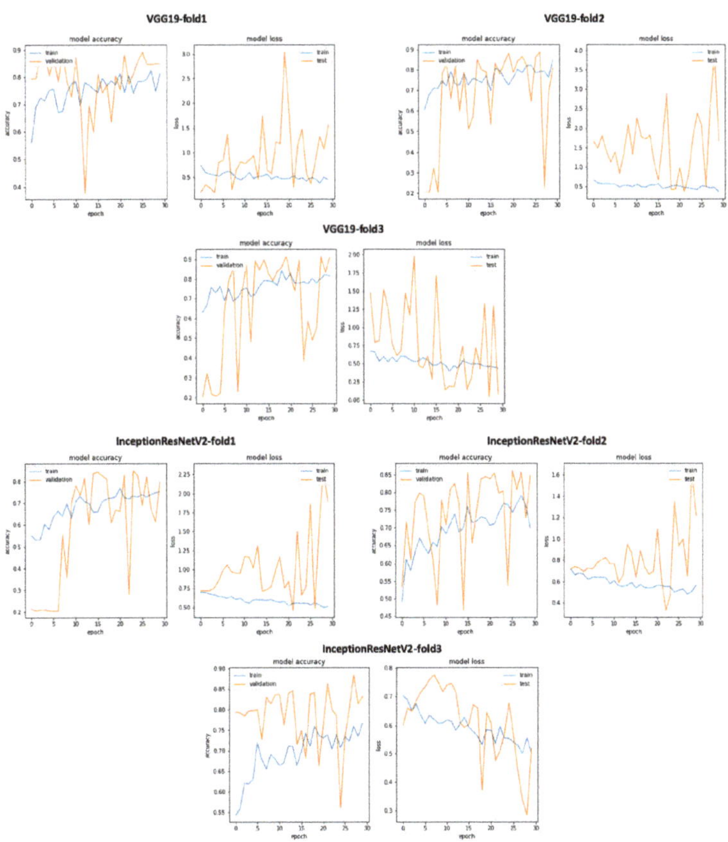

Figure 19. VGG19 and InceptionResNetV2 training and validation curves using raw dataset.

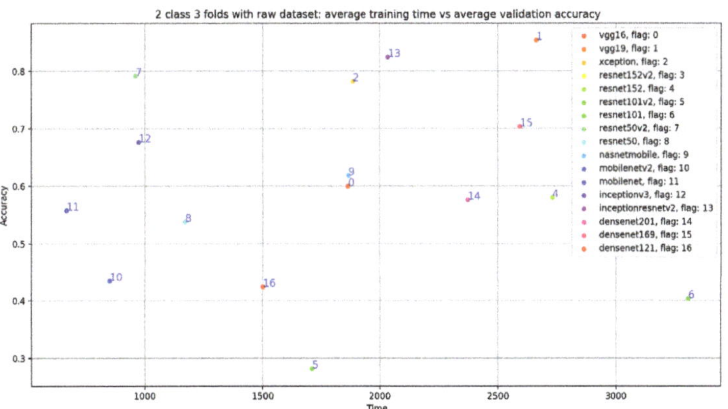

Figure 20. Training time vs. validation accuracy using raw dataset.

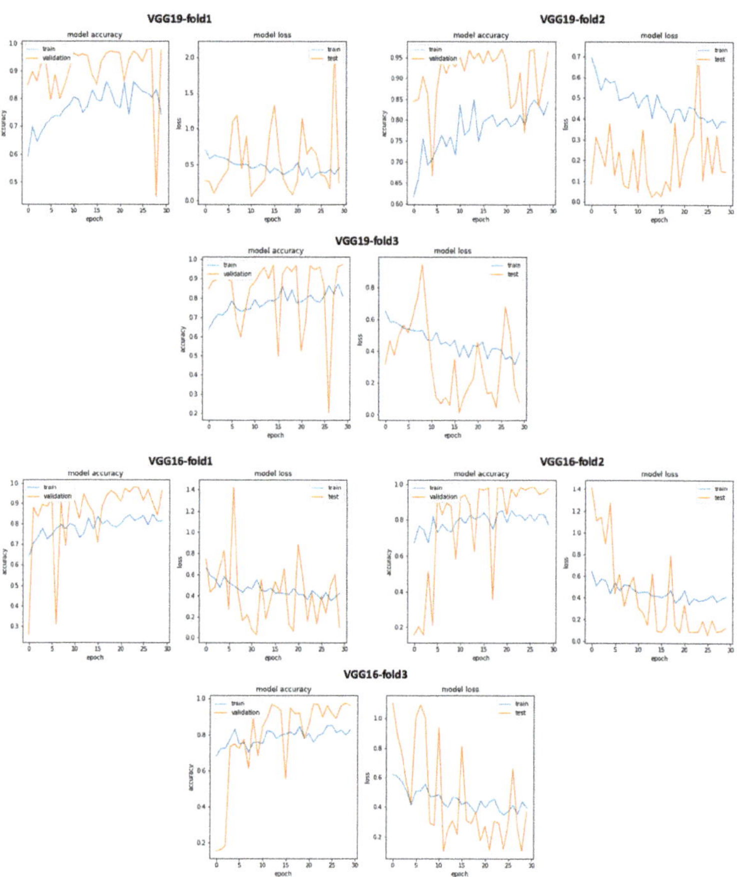

Figure 21. VGG19 and VGG16 training and validation curves using data selection based on KDE.

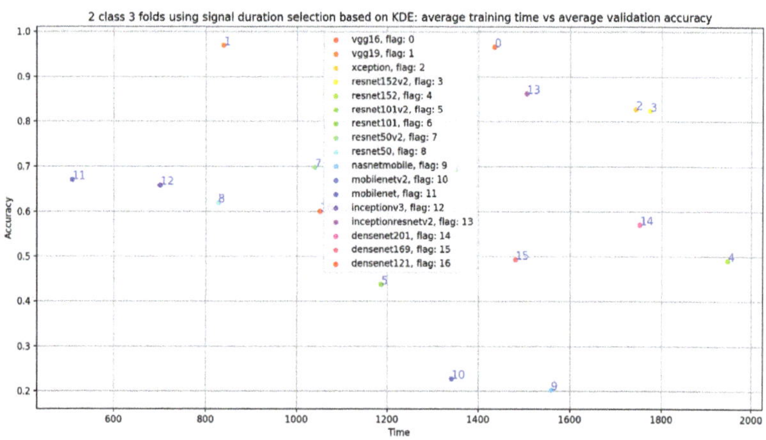

Figure 22. Training time vs. validation accuracy using signal-duration selection based on KDE.

Table 3. Average metric results related to KDE (duration = 20 s normal, duration = 35 s abnormal) datasets.

Average	Accuracy	TPR (Sensitivity)	Precision (PPV)	TNR (Specificity)
VGG16	0.966	0.930	0.946	0.930
VGG19	**0.970**	**0.946**	**0.944**	**0.946**
Xception	0.828	0.877	0.732	0.877
ResNet152V2	0.824	0.873	0.730	0.873
ResNet152	0.490	0.667	0.640	0.667
ResNet101V2	0.438	0.665	0.422	0.665
ResNet101	0.690	0.592	0.812	0.592
ResNet50v2	0.698	0.736	0.728	0.736
ResNet50	0.620	0.763	0.685	0.763
NasNetMobile	0.203	0.489	0.350	0.489
MobileNetV2	0.228	0.497	0.526	0.497
MobileNet	0.671	0.679	0.673	0.679
Inceptionv3	0.659	0.791	0.686	0.791
InceptionResNetV2	0.863	0.908	0.765	0.908
DenseNet201	0.571	0.725	0.719	0.725
DenseNet169	0.493	0.675	0.606	0.675
DenseNet121	0.601	0.734	0.714	0.734

Table 4. Average metric results related to duration = 50 s dataset.

Average	Accuracy	TPR (Sensitivity)	Precision (PPV)	TNR (Specificity)
VGG16	0.668	0.747	0.703	0.747
VGG19	**0.870**	**0.851**	**0.801**	**0.851**
Xception	0.702	0.781	0.689	0.781
ResNet152V2	0.501	0.669	0.636	0.669
ResNet152	0.785	0.677	0.687	0.677
ResNet101V2	0.457	0.628	0.606	0.628
ResNet101	0.600	0.616	0.674	0.616
ResNet50v2	0.433	0.626	0.611	0.626
ResNet50	0.473	0.581	0.636	0.581
NasNetMobile	0.451	0.494	0.329	0.494
MobileNetV2	0.576	0.535	0.541	0.535
MobileNet	0.562	0.680	0.657	0.680
Inceptionv3	0.751	0.740	0.729	0.740
InceptionResNetV2	0.667	0.687	0.687	0.687
DenseNet201	0.694	0.744	0.713	0.744
DenseNet169	0.609	0.703	0.699	0.703
DenseNet121	0.495	0.637	0.621	0.637

5.2. Classification Using Data Selection Based on Optimal SNR

The idea behind this data selection method is to select all the PCG signals with a signal-to-noise ratio greater than or equal to 0. In other words, we experiment the impact of selecting signals with SNR ≥ 0 on the classification result without performing any prepocessing steps or denoising methods. After applying this data selection method, we trained all the 17 pretrained CNN models (Figure 23 gives an overview of training and validation curves related to VGG19, VGG16, DenseNet169, and InceptionResNetV2). As seen in Table 5, we obtained very good classification results with VGG19, VGG16, DenseNet169, and InceptionResNetV2. The best result was obtained with VGG19 (accuracy = 0.96, sensitivity = 0.943, precision = 0.94 and specificity = 0.943). This result is very close to the classification result obtained after applying data selection based on signal duration.

In fact, if we look at Figure 24, we notice that the VGG19 training time is at the fifth position compared to the fourth position obtained with VGG19, trained on 20 s and 35 s normal and abnormal PCG signals. In other words, the best results in term of training time and classification results was obtained using VGG19 trained on 20 s and 35 s normal and abnormal PCG signals.

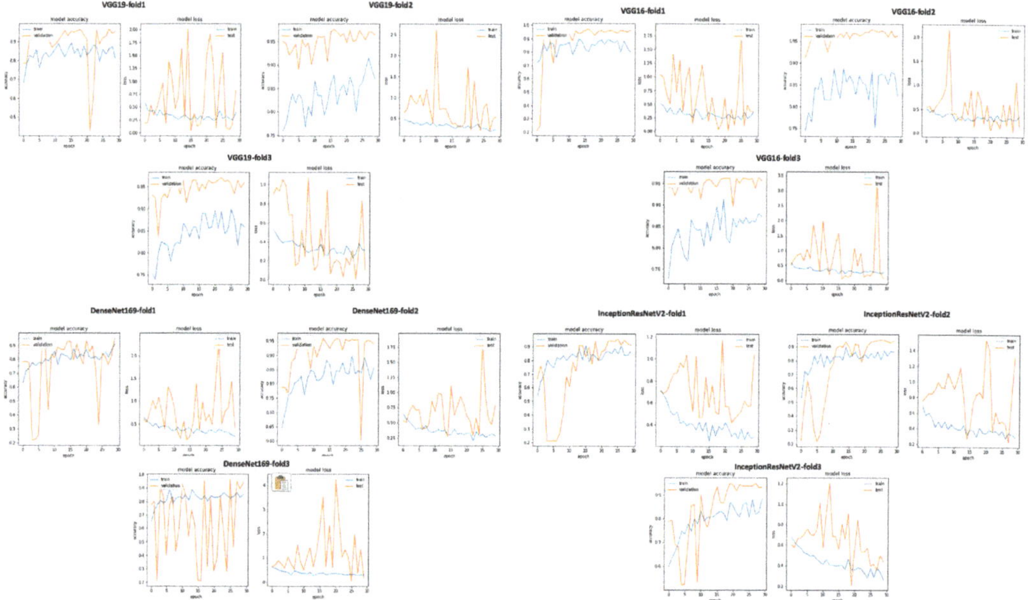

Figure 23. VGG19, VGG16, DenseNet169, and InceptionResNetV2 training and validation curves using data selection based on SNR ≥ 0.

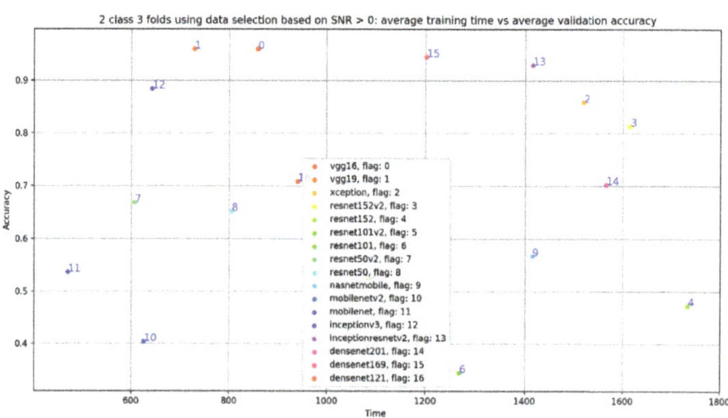

Figure 24. Training time vs. validation accuracy using data selection based on SNR ≥ 0.

Table 5. Average metric results related to SNR $\geq$ 0 dataset.

Average	Accuracy	Sensitivity	Precision	Specificity
VGG16	0.960	0.938	0.944	0.938
VGG19	**0.960**	**0.943**	**0.940**	**0.943**
Xception	0.860	0.895	0.807	0.895
ResNet152V2	0.815	0.845	0.790	0.845
ResNet152	0.474	0.660	0.665	0.660
ResNet101V2	0.525	0.687	0.561	0.687
ResNet101	0.346	0.581	0.611	0.581
ResNet50v2	0.669	0.773	0.745	0.773
ResNet50	0.653	0.746	0.566	0.746
NasNetMobile	0.568	0.492	0.344	0.492
MobileNetV2	0.405	0.561	0.521	0.561
MobileNet	0.537	0.696	0.712	0.696
Inceptionv3	0.885	0.893	0.855	0.893
InceptionResNetV2	0.930	0.939	0.880	0.939
DenseNet201	0.703	0.789	0.612	0.789
DenseNet169	0.945	0.938	0.907	0.938
DenseNet121	0.709	0.800	0.810	0.800

5.2.1. Classification Using Clustering as Data Selection Method

In this subsection, we investigate the impact of selecting training data using unsupervised biclustering. We used GMM biclustering with the hypothesis to consider the cluster with the maximum number of sample as our training data. As shown in Table 6 and in Figure 25, we obtained good classification results compared to results without using any data selection method. However, if we compare with the previous results, we can conclude that the best results are obtained using signal selection, based on duration 20 s for normal and 35 s for abnormal PCG data. In this configuration, VGG16 gives the best classification metrics compared to the remaining 16 CNN models with an acceptable training time (sixth position) as seen in Figure 26.

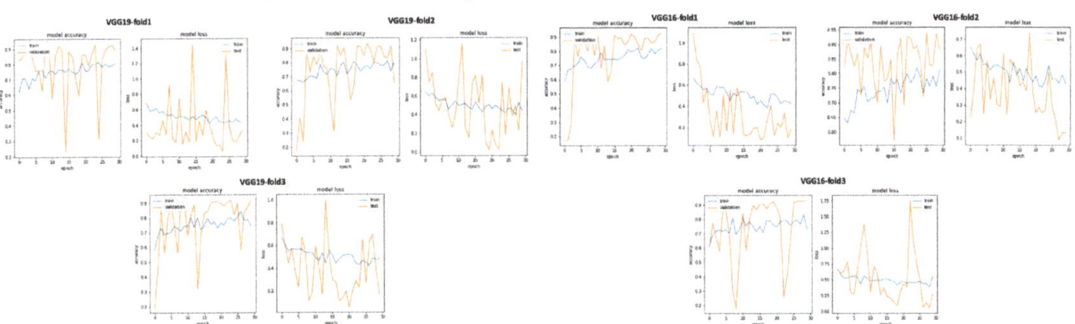

Figure 25. VGG19 abd VGG16 training and validation curves using data selection based on clustering.

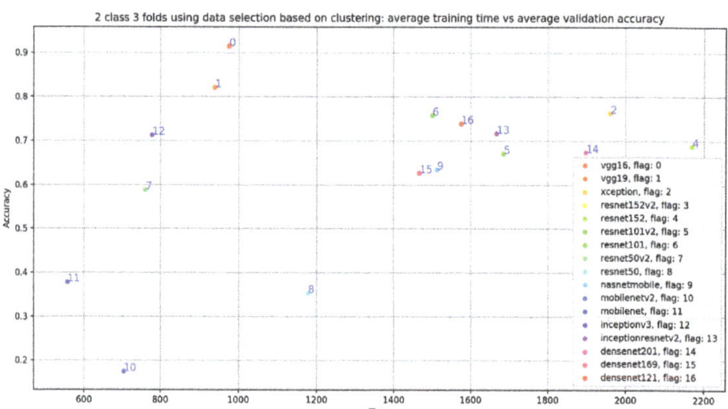

Figure 26. Training time vs. validation accuracy using data selection based on clustering.

Table 6. Average metric results related to clustered dataset.

Average	Accuracy	TPR (Sensitivity)	Precision (PPV)	TNR (Specificity)
VGG16	**0.915**	**0.873**	**0.860**	**0.873**
VGG19	0.821	0.808	0.787	0.808
Xception	0.763	0.795	0.690	0.795
ResNet152V2	0.283	0.561	0.590	0.561
ResNet152	0.688	0.712	0.728	0.712
ResNet101V2	0.671	0.702	0.674	0.702
ResNet101	0.758	0.765	0.682	0.765
ResNet50v2	0.589	0.666	0.633	0.666
ResNet50	0.353	0.576	0.396	0.576
NasNetMobile	0.635	0.498	0.561	0.498
MobileNetV2	0.175	0.500	0.195	0.500
MobileNet	0.378	0.606	0.422	0.606
Inceptionv3	0.713	0.773	0.668	0.773
InceptionResNetV2	0.717	0.717	0.761	0.717
DenseNet201	0.674	0.746	0.672	0.746
DenseNet169	0.627	0.758	0.656	0.758
DenseNet121	0.739	0.683	0.762	0.683

5.2.2. Synthesis

We have undergone a general comparative study against the state-of-the-art methods, as summarized in Table 7. As seen in this table, Dominguez et al. [60] achieved good classification results (accuracy of 0.97, sensitivity of 0.93, specificity of 0.95) using a complex recognition methodology based on heartbeat segmentation and a modified version of the CNN AlexNet model. Philip et al. [61] obtained the worst classification results in Table 7, and this is due to the elimination of the complex heart-cycle segmentation step. The majority of the research work presented in this table employed complex segmentation steps in their classification approach, and they obtained accuracy varying from 0.80 to 0.97, sensitivity from 0.76 to 0.96, and specificity from 0.72 to 0.95. In this work, our main contribution is to obtain very good classification results using a simple classification approach without any complex preprocessing steps, without any segmentation process, and without the use of any new CNN architecture. As seen in Table 7, compared to the work of Dominguez et al. [60], we have achieved similar results with an accuracy equal to 0.97, a slightly better sensitivity result of 0.946, and a slightly lower specificity result of 0.946.

Table 7. Comparative analysis of our method with state-of-the-art methods using whole datasets from PhysioNet 2016.

Average	Accuracy	TPR (Sensitivity)	Precision (PPV)	TNR (Specificity)
our approach	**0.970**	**0.946**	**0.944**	**0.946**
[62]	0.8697	0.964	-	0.726
[17]	-	0.942	-	0.778
[63]	0.824	-	-	-
[18]	-	0.8095	-	0.839
[16]	-	0.84	-	0.957
[64]	0.852	-	-	-
[65]	-	0.885	-	0.921
[20]	0.879	0.885	-	0.878
[60]	0.97	0.932	-	0.951
[66]	0.915	0.983	-	0.846
[67]	0.892	0.90	-	0.884
[68]	0.88	0.88	-	0.87
[69]	0.85	0.89	-	0.816
[70]	0.826	0.769	-	0.883
[71]	0.801	0.796	-	0.806
[72]	0.9	0.93	-	0.9
[61]	0.79	0.77	-	0.8

6. Conclusions and Perspectives

In this work, we presented a simple classification architecture based on a data-selection process designed to recognize normal and abnormal Physionet PCG signals. We compared our work with the state-of-the-art approaches and concluded that using a data selection process based on a signal duration of 20 s for normal and 35 s for abnormal PCG signals obtained very good CNN classification results with an overall accuracy equal to 0.97, an overall sensitivity equal to 0.946, an overall precision equal to 0.944, an overall specificity equal to 0.946. This work was tested only on the most-used binary class dataset Physionet, which can be considered as a limiting factor. We plan to test it on other public or private multiclass datasets. In addition, the feature-selection process can be improved through the exploitation of a large set of ML feature extraction/selection methods. Furthermore, we plan to create our own multiclass PCG dataset which will be trained on a new CNN model created especially for PCG spectrogram images.

Author Contributions: Conceptualization, A.B. and M.B.; methodology, A.B., M.B. and R.S.; software, M.B. and R.S.; validation, A.B. and M.B.; formal analysis, M.B. and R.S.; investigation, A.B. and M.B.; writing—original draft preparation, A.B., M.B. and R.S.; writing—review and editing, M.B. and A.B.; supervision, A.B.; project administration, A.B. and M.B. All authors have read and agreed to the published version of the manuscript.

Funding: This research work was funded by Institutional Fund Projects under grant no (IFPIP: 574-611-1442). Therefore, the authors gratefully acknowledge technical and financial support from the Ministry of Education and King Abdelaziz University, DSR, Jeddah, Saudi Arabia.

Institutional Review Board Statement: Not applicable.

Informed Consent Statement: Not applicable.

Data Availability Statement: Not applicable.

Acknowledgments: This research work was funded by Institutional Fund Projects under grant no (IFPIP: 574-611-1442). Therefore, the authors gratefully acknowledge technical and financial support from the Ministry of Education and King Abdelaziz University, DSR, Jeddah, Saudi Arabia.

Conflicts of Interest: The authors declare no conflict of interest.

References

1. World Health Organization World Health Ranking. 2020. Available online: https://www.who.int/health-topics/cardiovascular-diseases#tab=tab_1 (accessed on 15 February 2021).
2. Yang, Z.J.; Liu, J.; Ge, J.P.; Chen, L.; Zhao, Z.G.; Yang, W.Y. Prevalence of Cardiovascular Disease Risk Factor in the Chinese Population: The 2007–2008 China National Diabetes and Metabolic Disorders Study. *Eur. Heart J.* **2011**, *33*, 213–220. [CrossRef] [PubMed]
3. Mangione, S.; Nieman, L.Z. Cardiac Auscultatory Skills of Internal Medicine and Family Practice Trainees: A Comparison of Diagnostic Proficiency. *JAMA* **1997**, *278*, 717–722. [CrossRef] [PubMed]
4. Lam, M.; Lee, T.; Boey, P.; Ng, W.; Hey, H.; Ho, K.; Cheong, P. Factors influencing cardiac auscultation proficiency in physician trainees. *Singap. Med. J.* **2005**, *46*, 11–14.
5. Roelandt, J. The decline of our physical examination skills: Is echocardiography to blame? *Eur. Heart J. Cardiovasc. Imaging* **2013**, *15*, 249–252. [CrossRef]
6. Grzegorczyk, I.; Soliński, M.; Łepek, M.; Perka, A.; Rosiński, J.; Rymko, J.; Stępień, K.; Gierałtowski, J. PCG classification using a neural network approach. In Proceedings of the 2016 Computing in Cardiology Conference (CinC), Vancouver, BC, Canada, 11–14 September 2016; pp. 1129–1132.
7. Liu, C.; Springer, D.; Li, Q.; Moody, B.; Juan, R.A.; Chorro, F.J.; Castells, F.; Roig, J.M.; Silva, I.; Johnson, A.E.; et al. An open access database for the evaluation of heart sound algorithms. *Physiol. Meas.* **2016**, *37*, 2181. [CrossRef]
8. Nouraei, H.; Nouraei, H.; Rabkin, S.W. Comparison of Unsupervised Machine Learning Approaches for Cluster Analysis to Define Subgroups of Heart Failure with Preserved Ejection Fraction with Different Outcomes. *Bioengineering* **2022**, *9*, 175. [CrossRef]
9. Aruleba, R.T.; Adekiya, T.A.; Ayawei, N.; Obaido, G.; Aruleba, K.; Mienye, I.D.; Aruleba, I.; Ogbuokiri, B. COVID-19 Diagnosis: A Review of Rapid Antigen, RT-PCR and Artificial Intelligence Methods. *Bioengineering* **2022**, *9*, 153. [CrossRef]
10. Elaziz, M.A.; Hosny, K.M.; Salah, A.; Darwish, M.M.; Lu, S.; Sahlol, A.T. New machine learning method for image-based diagnosis of COVID-19. *PLoS ONE* **2020**, *15*, e0235187. [CrossRef]
11. Magar, R.; Yadav, P.; Barati Farimani, A. Potential neutralizing antibodies discovered for novel corona virus using machine learning. *Sci. Rep.* **2021**, *11*, 5261. [CrossRef]
12. Sujath, R.A.A.; Chatterjee, J.M.; Hassanien, A.E. A machine learning forecasting model for COVID-19 pandemic in India. *Stoch. Environ. Res. Risk Assess.* **2020**, *34*, 959–972. [CrossRef]
13. Chintalapudi, N.; Battineni, G.; Hossain, M.A.; Amenta, F. Cascaded Deep Learning Frameworks in Contribution to the Detection of Parkinson's Disease. *Bioengineering* **2022**, *9*, 116. [CrossRef] [PubMed]
14. Clifford, G.D.; Liu, C.; Moody, B.; Springer, D.; Silva, I.; Li, Q.; Mark, R.G. Classification of normal/abnormal heart sound recordings: The PhysioNet/Computing in Cardiology Challenge 2016. In Proceedings of the 2016 Computing in Cardiology Conference (CinC), Vancouver, BC, Canada, 11–14 September 2016; pp. 609–612.
15. Nogueira, D.M.; Ferreira, C.A.; Gomes, E.F.; Jorge, A.M. Classifying heart sounds using images of motifs, MFCC and temporal features. *J. Med. Syst.* **2019**, *43*, 168. [CrossRef] [PubMed]
16. Rubin, J.; Abreu, R.; Ganguli, A.; Nelaturi, S.; Matei, I.; Sricharan, K. Recognizing abnormal heart sounds using deep learning. *arXiv* **2017**, arXiv:1707.04642.
17. Potes, C.; Parvaneh, S.; Rahman, A.; Conroy, B. Ensemble of feature-based and deep learning-based classifiers for detection of abnormal heart sounds. In Proceedings of the 2016 Computing in Cardiology Conference (CinC), Vancouver, BC, Canada, 11–14 September 2016; pp. 621–624.
18. Tang, H.; Chen, H.; Li, T.; Zhong, M. Classification of normal/abnormal heart sound recordings based on multi-domain features and back propagation neural network. In Proceedings of the 2016 Computing in Cardiology Conference (CinC), Vancouver, BC, Canada, 11–14 September 2016; pp. 593–596.
19. Kiranyaz, S.; Zabihi, M.; Rad, A.B.; Ince, T.; Hamila, R.; Gabbouj, M. Real-time Phonocardiogram Anomaly Detection by Adaptive 1D Convolutional Neural Networks. *Neurocomputing* **2020**, *411*, 291–301. [CrossRef]
20. Singh, S.A.; Majumder, S. Short unsegmented PCG classification based on ensemble classifier. *Turk. J. Electr. Eng. Comput. Sci.* **2020**, *28*, 875–889. [CrossRef]
21. Krishnan, P.T.; Balasubramanian, P.; Umapathy, S. Automated heart sound classification system from unsegmented phonocardiogram (PCG) using deep neural network. *Phys. Eng. Sci. Med.* **2020**, *43*, 505–515. [CrossRef]

22. Garg, V.; Mathur, A.; Mangla, N.; Rawat, A.S. Heart Rhythm Abnormality Detection from PCG Signal. In Proceedings of the 2019 Twelfth International Conference on Contemporary Computing (IC3), Noida, India, 8–10 August 2019; pp. 1–5.
23. Alaskar, H.; Alzhrani, N.; Hussain, A.; Almarshed, F. The Implementation of Pretrained AlexNet on PCG Classification. In Proceedings of the International Conference on Intelligent Computing, Nanchang, China, 3–6 August 2019; pp. 784–794.
24. Khaled, S.; Fakhry, M.; Mubarak, A.S. Classification of PCG Signals Using A Nonlinear Autoregressive Network with Exogenous Inputs (NARX). In Proceedings of the 2020 International Conference on Innovative Trends in Communication and Computer Engineering (ITCE), Aswan, Egypt, 8–9 February 2020; pp. 98–102.
25. Noman, F.; Ting, C.M.; Salleh, S.H.; Ombao, H. Short-segment heart sound classification using an ensemble of deep convolutional neural networks. In Proceedings of the ICASSP 2019—2019 IEEE International Conference on Acoustics, Speech and Signal Processing (ICASSP), Brighton, UK, 12–17 May 2019; pp. 1318–1322.
26. Parzen, E. On estimation of a probability density function and mode. *Ann. Math. Stat.* **1962**, *33*, 1065–1076. [CrossRef]
27. Hoult, D.I.; Richards, R. The signal-to-noise ratio of the nuclear magnetic resonance experiment. *J. Magn. Reson. (1969)* **1976**, *24*, 71–85. [CrossRef]
28. McLachlan, G.; Peel, D. *Finite Mixture Models*; John Wiley & Sons: Hoboken, NJ, USA, 2004.
29. McLachlan, G.; Krishnan, T. *The EM Algorithm and Extensions*; John Wiley & Sons: Hoboken, NJ, USA, 2007; Volume 382.
30. Bishop, C.M. *Pattern Recognition and Machine Learning*; Springer: Berlin/Heidelberg, Germany, 2006.
31. Hastie, T.; Tibshirani, R.; Friedman, J.; Franklin, J. The elements of statistical learning: Data mining, inference and prediction. *Math. Intell.* **2005**, *27*, 83–85.
32. Fayek, H.M. Speech Processing for Machine Learning: Filter Banks, Mel Frequency Cepstral Coefficients (MFCCs) and What's In-Between. 2016. Available online: https://haythamfayek.com/2016/04/21/speech-processing-for-machine-learning.html (accessed on 15 February 2021).
33. Dave, N. Feature extraction methods LPC, PLP and MFCC in speech recognition. *Int. J. Adv. Res. Eng. Technol.* **2013**, *1*, 1–4.
34. Han, W.; Chan, C.F.; Choy, C.S.; Pun, K.P. An efficient MFCC extraction method in speech recognition. In Proceedings of the 2006 IEEE International Symposium on Circuits and Systems, Kos, Greece, 21–24 May 2006; p. 4.
35. Al Marzuqi, H.M.O.; Hussain, S.M.; Frank, A. Device Activation based on Voice Recognition using Mel Frequency Cepstral Coefficients (MFCC's) Algorithm. *Int. Res. J. Eng. Technol.* **2019**, *6*, 4297–4301.
36. Milletari, F.; Ahmadi, S.A.; Kroll, C.; Plate, A.; Rozanski, V.; Maiostre, J.; Levin, J.; Dietrich, O.; Ertl-Wagner, B.; Bötzel, K.; et al. Hough-CNN: Deep learning for segmentation of deep brain regions in MRI and ultrasound. *Comput. Vis. Image Underst.* **2017**, *164*, 92–102. [CrossRef]
37. Bar, Y.; Diamant, I.; Wolf, L.; Lieberman, S.; Konen, E.; Greenspan, H. Chest pathology detection using deep learning with non-medical training. In Proceedings of the 2015 IEEE 12th iNternational Symposium On Biomedical Imaging (ISBI), Brooklyn, NY, USA, 16–19 April 2015; pp. 294–297.
38. Yan, L.; Yoshua, B.; Geoffrey, H. Deep learning. *Nature* **2015**, *521*, 436–444.
39. Li, W.; Wu, G.; Du, Q. Transferred deep learning for anomaly detection in hyperspectral imagery. *IEEE Geosci. Remote. Sens. Lett.* **2017**, *14*, 597–601. [CrossRef]
40. LeCun, Y.; Bottou, L.; Bengio, Y.; Haffner, P. Gradient-based learning applied to document recognition. *Proc. IEEE* **1998**, *86*, 2278–2324. [CrossRef]
41. Jiang, H.; Learned-Miller, E. Face detection with the faster R-CNN. In Proceedings of the 2017 12th IEEE International Conference on Automatic Face & Gesture Recognition (FG 2017), Washington, DC, USA, 30 May–3 June 2017; pp. 650–657.
42. Zhu, C.; Zheng, Y.; Luu, K.; Savvides, M. Cms-rcnn: Contextual multi-scale region-based cnn for unconstrained face detection. In *Deep Learning for Biometrics*; Springer: Berlin/Heidelberg, Germany, 2017; pp. 57–79.
43. Li, H.; Lin, Z.; Shen, X.; Brandt, J.; Hua, G. A convolutional neural network cascade for face detection. In Proceedings of the IEEE Conference on Computer Vision and Pattern Recognition, Boston, MA, USA, 7–12 June 2015; pp. 5325–5334.
44. Niu, X.X.; Suen, C.Y. A novel hybrid CNN—SVM classifier for recognizing handwritten digits. *Pattern Recognit.* **2012**, *45*, 1318–1325. [CrossRef]
45. Matsumoto, T.; Chua, L.O.; Suzuki, H. CNN cloning template: Connected component detector. *IEEE Trans. Circuits Syst.* **1990**, *37*, 633–635. [CrossRef]
46. Wu, C.; Fan, W.; He, Y.; Sun, J.; Naoi, S. Handwritten character recognition by alternately trained relaxation convolutional neural network. In Proceedings of the 2014 14th International Conference on Frontiers in Handwriting Recognition, Crete Island, Greece, 1–4 September 2014; pp. 291–296.
47. Wang, J.; Yang, Y.; Mao, J.; Huang, Z.; Huang, C.; Xu, W. Cnn-rnn: A unified framework for multi-label image classification. In Proceedings of the IEEE Conference on Computer Vision and Pattern Recognition, Las Vegas, NV, USA, 27–30 June 2016; pp. 2285–2294.
48. Lee, H.; Kwon, H. Going deeper with contextual CNN for hyperspectral image classification. *IEEE Trans. Image Process.* **2017**, *26*, 4843–4855. [CrossRef]
49. Yu, S.; Jia, S.; Xu, C. Convolutional neural networks for hyperspectral image classification. *Neurocomputing* **2017**, *219*, 88–98. [CrossRef]
50. Tan, C.; Sun, F.; Kong, T.; Zhang, W.; Yang, C.; Liu, C. A survey on deep transfer learning. In Proceedings of the International Conference on Artificial Neural Networks, Rhodes, Greece, 4–7 October 2018; pp. 270–279.

51. Chollet, F. Xception: Deep learning with depthwise separable convolutions. In Proceedings of the IEEE Conference on Computer Vision and Pattern Recognition, Honolulu, HI, USA, 21–26 June 2017; pp. 1251–1258.
52. Simonyan, K.; Zisserman, A. Very deep convolutional networks for large-scale image recognition. *arXiv* **2014**, arXiv:1409.1556.
53. He, K.; Zhang, X.; Ren, S.; Sun, J. Deep residual learning for image recognition. In Proceedings of the IEEE Conference on Computer Vision and Pattern Recognition, Las Vegas, NV, USA, 27–30 June 2016; pp. 770–778.
54. Zoph, B.; Vasudevan, V.; Shlens, J.; Le, Q.V. Learning transferable architectures for scalable image recognition. In Proceedings of the IEEE Conference on Computer Vision and Pattern Recognition, Salt Lake City, UT, USA, 18–22 June 2018; pp. 8697–8710.
55. Sandler, M.; Howard, A.; Zhu, M.; Zhmoginov, A.; Chen, L.C. Mobilenetv2: Inverted residuals and linear bottlenecks. In Proceedings of the IEEE Conference on Computer Vision and Pattern Recognition, Salt Lake City, UT, USA, 18–22 June 2018; pp. 4510–4520.
56. Howard, A.G.; Zhu, M.; Chen, B.; Kalenichenko, D.; Wang, W.; Weyand, T.; Andreetto, M.; Adam, H. Mobilenets: Efficient convolutional neural networks for mobile vision applications. *arXiv* **2017**, arXiv:1704.04861.
57. Szegedy, C.; Vanhoucke, V.; Ioffe, S.; Shlens, J.; Wojna, Z. Rethinking the inception architecture for computer vision. In Proceedings of the IEEE Conference on Computer Vision and Pattern Recognition, Las Vegas, NV, USA, 27–30 June 2016; pp. 2818–2826.
58. Szegedy, C.; Ioffe, S.; Vanhoucke, V.; Alemi, A.A. Inception-v4, inception-resnet and the impact of residual connections on learning. In Proceedings of the Thirty-First AAAI Conference on Artificial Intelligence, San Francisco, CA, USA, 4–9 February 2017.
59. Huang, G.; Liu, Z.; Van Der Maaten, L.; Weinberger, K.Q. Densely connected convolutional networks. In Proceedings of the IEEE Conference on Computer Vision and Pattern Recognition, Honolulu, HI, USA, 21–26 June 2017; pp. 4700–4708.
60. Dominguez-Morales, J.P.; Jimenez-Fernandez, A.F.; Dominguez-Morales, M.J.; Jimenez-Moreno, G. Deep neural networks for the recognition and classification of heart murmurs using neuromorphic auditory sensors. *IEEE Trans. Biomed. Circuits Syst.* **2017**, *12*, 24–34. [CrossRef] [PubMed]
61. Langley, P.; Murray, A. Heart sound classification from unsegmented phonocardiograms. *Physiol. Meas.* **2017**, *38*, 1658. [CrossRef] [PubMed]
62. Nogueira, D.M.; Ferreira, C.A.; Jorge, A.M. Classifying heart sounds using images of MFCC and temporal features. In Proceedings of the EPIA Conference on Artificial Intelligence, Porto, Portugal, 5–8 September 2017; pp. 186–203.
63. Ortiz, J.J.G.; Phoo, C.P.; Wiens, J. Heart sound classification based on temporal alignment techniques. In Proceedings of the 2016 Computing in Cardiology Conference (CinC), Vancouver, BC, Canada, 11–14 September 2016; pp. 589–592.
64. Kay, E.; Agarwal, A. DropConnected neural networks trained on time-frequency and inter-beat features for classifying heart sounds. *Physiol. Meas.* **2017**, *38*, 1645. [CrossRef] [PubMed]
65. Abdollahpur, M.; Ghiasi, S.; Mollakazemi, M.J.; Ghaffari, A. Cycle selection and neuro-voting system for classifying heart sound recordings. In Proceedings of the 2016 Computing in Cardiology Conference (CinC), Vancouver, BC, Canada, 11–14 September 2016; pp. 1–4.
66. Han, W.; Yang, Z.; Lu, J.; Xie, S. Supervised threshold-based heart sound classification algorithm. *Physiol. Meas.* **2018**, *39*, 115011. [CrossRef] [PubMed]
67. Whitaker, B.M.; Suresha, P.B.; Liu, C.; Clifford, G.D.; Anderson, D.V. Combining sparse coding and time-domain features for heart sound classification. *Physiol. Meas.* **2017**, *38*, 1701. [CrossRef] [PubMed]
68. Tang, H.; Dai, Z.; Jiang, Y.; Li, T.; Liu, C. PCG classification using multidomain features and SVM classifier. *Biomed Res. Int.* **2018**, *2018*, 4205027. [CrossRef]
69. Plesinger, F.; Viscor, I.; Halamek, J.; Jurco, J.; Jurak, P. Heart sounds analysis using probability assessment. *Physiol. Meas.* **2017**, *38*, 1685. [CrossRef]
70. Abdollahpur, M.; Ghaffari, A.; Ghiasi, S.; Mollakazemi, M.J. Detection of pathological heart sounds. *Physiol. Meas.* **2017**, *38*, 1616. [CrossRef]
71. Homsi, M.N.; Warrick, P. Ensemble methods with outliers for phonocardiogram classification. *Physiol. Meas.* **2017**, *38*, 1631. [CrossRef]
72. Singh, S.A.; Majumder, S. Classification of unsegmented heart sound recording using KNN classifier. *J. Mech. Med. Biol.* **2019**, *19*, 1950025. [CrossRef]

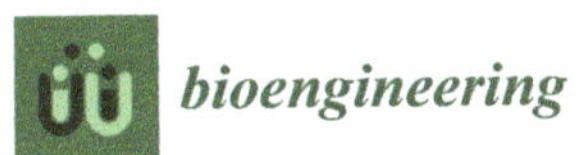 *bioengineering*

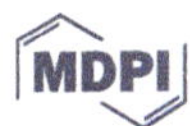

Article

A Novel and Noninvasive Risk Assessment Score and Its Child-to-Adult Trajectories to Screen Subclinical Renal Damage in Middle Age

Chen Chen [1,2], Guanzhi Liu [3], Chao Chu [1,2], Wenling Zheng [1,2], Qiong Ma [1,2], Yueyuan Liao [1,2], Yu Yan [1,2], Yue Sun [1,2], Dan Wang [1,2] and Jianjun Mu [1,2,*]

1   Department of Cardiovascular Medicine, First Affiliated Hospital of Xi'an Jiaotong University, Xi'an 710061, China
2   Key Laboratory of Molecular Cardiology of Shaanxi Province, Xi'an 710061, China
3   Department of Orthopedics, The First Affiliated Hospital, Zhejiang University School of Medicine, Hangzhou 310009, China
*   Correspondence: mujjun@mail.xjtu.edu.cn

Abstract: This study aimed to develop a noninvasive, economical and effective subclinical renal damage (SRD) risk assessment tool to identify high-risk asymptomatic people from a large-scale population and improve current clinical SRD screening strategies. Based on the Hanzhong Adolescent Hypertension Cohort, SRD-associated variables were identified and the SRD risk assessment score model was established and further validated with machine learning algorithms. Longitudinal follow-up data were used to identify child-to-adult SRD risk score trajectories and to investigate the relationship between different trajectory groups and the incidence of SRD in middle age. Systolic blood pressure, diastolic blood pressure and body mass index were identified as SRD-associated variables. Based on these three variables, an SRD risk assessment score was developed, with excellent classification ability (AUC value of ROC curve: 0.778 for SRD estimation, 0.729 for 4-year SRD risk prediction), calibration (Hosmer—Lemeshow goodness-of-fit test $p = 0.62$ for SRD estimation, $p = 0.34$ for 4-year SRD risk prediction) and more potential clinical benefits. In addition, three child-to-adult SRD risk assessment score trajectories were identified: increasing, increasing-stable and stable. Further difference analysis and logistic regression analysis showed that these SRD risk assessment score trajectories were highly associated with the incidence of SRD in middle age. In brief, we constructed a novel and noninvasive SRD risk assessment tool with excellent performance to help identify high-risk asymptomatic people from a large-scale population and assist in SRD screening.

Keywords: subclinical renal damage; machine learning; risk assessment tool; group-based trajectory modeling; screening strategy

Citation: Chen, C.; Liu, G.; Chu, C.; Zheng, W.; Ma, Q.; Liao, Y.; Yan, Y.; Sun, Y.; Wang, D.; Mu, J. A Novel and Noninvasive Risk Assessment Score and Its Child-to-Adult Trajectories to Screen Subclinical Renal Damage in Middle Age. *Bioengineering* 2023, 10, 257. https://doi.org/10.3390/bioengineering10020257

Academic Editors: Pedro Miguel Rodrigues, João Alexandre Lobo Marques, João Paulo do Vale Madeiro and Peter Hauser

Received: 13 January 2023
Revised: 10 February 2023
Accepted: 13 February 2023
Published: 15 February 2023

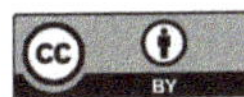

1. Introduction

Chronic kidney disease (CKD) is defined as abnormalities in kidney structure or function for at least 3 months with implications for health [1]. CKD has become a major public health concern due to its high prevalence and all-cause mortality [2,3]. The Global Burden of Disease Study reported that 697.5 million individuals suffered from CKD in 2017, with an overall prevalence of 9.1% [4]. A systematic review on the regional prevalence of CKD in Asia showed a substantial variation in CKD prevalence ranging from 7.0% in South Korea to 34.3% in Singapore, while China and India had the highest absolute number of people with CKD (159.8 million and 140.2 million, respectively) [5]. CKD is associated with a high risk of hospitalization, cardiovascular events, cognitive dysfunction, morbidity and all-cause mortality [6–8]. In addition, CKD may be accompanied by several other complications, including anemia, secondary hyperparathyroidism and electrolyte disturbances, creating substantial health care costs [9–11] and indicating the urgent need to prevent and manage renal damage progression at an early stage. Subclinical renal damage (SRD) is an early, asymptomatic renal abnormality characterized by a moderate increase in urinary albumin excretion or a moderate reduction in the glomerular filtration rate [12]. SRD can be defined by an estimated glomerular filtration rate (eGFR) between 30 and 60 mL/min/1.73 m^2 or an elevated urinary albumin-to-creatinine ratio (uACR) more than 2.5 mg/mmol in men and 3.5 mg/mmol in women. The Hanzhong Adolescent Hypertension Cohort showed that the incidence of SRD in northern China was 13.1% [13]. Individuals with SRD tend to also have hypertension and diabetes mellitus [14], which further worsen renal function [1]. Early SRD detection and screening are essential to slow disease progression and reduce the risk of complications, morbidity and mortality, because the SRD condition can correspond to the stages of CKD (G3a stage, G3b stage in GFR Category and A2 stage, A3 stage in persistent albuminuria category) according to the 2012 KDIGO Clinical Practice Guideline for the Evaluation and Management of CKD [1]. Patients in these stages are mainly assessed as having moderately increased risk or high risk for concurrent complications and future outcomes; these are also the critical periods for early diagnosis and intervention for CKD. Currently, the detection and screening of renal function rely on biochemical assays with blood or urine samples. Serum creatinine can be used to evaluate eGFR and urine microalbumin, and creatinine can be used to evaluate uACR [15]. Biochemical analysis is the gold standard but is costly for long-term follow-up or large-scale population screening [16,17]. In addition, SRD is clinically asymptomatic and despite that renal function can be estimated by the measurement of serum creatinine concentration, urine protein or albumin concentration, it is still difficult to apply routine large-scale SRD screening, especially for asymptomatic adults, due to the lack of more economical and effective noninvasive risk assessment tools for SRD [1,18]. Hence, a simple and noninvasive risk assessment tool is urgently needed for SRD screening.

It has been reported that diabetes, hypertension, older age, obesity and smoking are independent risk factors for the development and progression of renal dysfunction [6,19–21]. Some studies have established prediction models for CKD risk based on these factors [22–24]. However, little attention has been given to the establishment of SRD risk assessment tools and the longitudinal observation of these tools. Recently, tracking trajectory patterns over time has accounted for dynamic changes and provided an important dimension for consideration. Group-based trajectory modeling is one of the approaches that considers variations in time [25]. Previous studies have suggested that long-term BP trajectories and long-term BMI trajectories are associated with the incidence of SRD [13,15,26]. However, single-variable trajectory practices are generally far from making full use of multivariate longitudinal data and the interrelationship of different variables.

In this study, we used data from Hanzhong Adolescent Hypertension Cohort to develop a noninvasive, economical and effective SRD risk assessment tool to identify high-risk asymptomatic people from a large-scale population and improve current clinical SRD screening strategies.

2. Materials and Methods

2.1. Cohorts and Participants

This study included participants from the Hanzhong Adolescent Hypertension Cohort, an ongoing prospective study initiated in 1987 that is focused on cardiovascular risk factor development. The Hanzhong Adolescent Hypertension Cohort recruited a total of 4623 schoolchildren from 26 rural sites of three towns in Hanzhong, Shaanxi, China in 1987, and several follow-ups were conducted in the following 30 years [27]. The inclusion criteria of the present study were as follows: aged 6–15 years in 1987, able to speak Mandarin to ensure effective communication, participated in the latest follow-up and had laboratory test data in 2017. For further trajectory analysis, complete blood pressure and BMI data during the 30-year follow-up were required. During the selection, individuals who had a history of myocardial infarction, heart failure, stroke, renal failure, or peripheral artery disease were excluded from the analysis. We conducted data collection in 1989, 1992, 1995, 2005, 2013 and 2017. In the 30 years of follow-up time, migration, death, mental illness and military service mainly contributed to the loss of follow-up. This study was clinically registered (NCT02734472) and approved by the Ethics Committee of First Affiliated Hospital of Xi'an Jiaotong University (Ethical Approval number: XJTU1AF2015LSL-047). All subjects gave written informed consent in advance. In addition, we obtained the consent of a parent/guardian for participants <18 years of age.

2.2. Anthropometric Measurements

Baseline clinical information, including demographic characteristics, histories of hypertension, hyperlipidemia, stroke and diabetes, history of cigarette smoking and alcohol consumption and cardiovascular complications, was collected using a standardized self-questionnaire. Body weight, height, waist circumference and hip circumference were measured by trained staff via standardized procedures. Body mass index (BMI) was calculated as weight in kilograms divided by height in meters squared (kilograms per meter squared). The average values of replicate measurements were used for further analysis.

2.3. Blood Pressure Measurements

Systolic and diastolic blood pressure were measured three times by trained and certified staff via WHO recommended procedures (in a seated position in a quiet and comfortable environment, 5-min rest before measurement, 2-min interval between examinations). Mean values of blood pressure were used for further analysis.

2.4. Biochemical Parameter Measurements

In this study, biochemical parameters, including total cholesterol (TC), triglyceride (TG), LDL cholesterol (LDL-C), HDL cholesterol (HDL-C), total bilirubin, serum creatinine, urinary uric acid (UA), creatinine and albumin levels, were measured according to standardized procedures. uACR (milligrams per millimole) was evaluated as urine albumin (in milligrams) divided by urine creatinine (in millimoles). eGFR was estimated by the Modification of Diet in Renal Disease (MDRD) calculation formula for Chinese patients with chronic kidney disease: eGFR = 175 × serum creatinine (in milligrams per deciliter) $^{-1.234}$ × age (in years) $^{-0.179}$ (×0.79 for females) [28].

2.5. Definitions

In this study, subclinical renal damage was defined as an eGFR between 30 and 60 mL/min/1.73 m^2 or a uACR more than 2.5 mg/mmol in men and 3.5 mg/mmol in women [15]. Cigarette smokers were defined as subjects with >six months of smoking history during their lifetime (continuous or cumulative) [29]. Participants who reported that they drank alcohol (liquor, beer or wine) every day and that their alcohol consumption lasted for more than 6 months were defined as drinkers [30].

2.6. Statistical Analysis

To identify effective and reliable clinical parameters with high screening or early diagnostic value for SRD, we analyzed the cross-sectional data in 2017 (n = 2303) and provided a novel feature selection strategy by combining three machine learning methods (complete-case analyses), including LASSO regression, random forest and the SVM-REF algorithm. LASSO regression was performed via the R package "glmnet" [31], the random forest method was carried out by the R package "randomForest" and the SVM-REF approach was achieved by the R packages "sigFeature" and "e1071". A logistic regression model was constructed based on the R package "rms". The 2303 participants were randomly assigned to the training set (70%, n = 1611) and the internal validation set (30%, n = 692). The R package "pROC" was used to calculate the area under the curve (AUC) value of the receiver operating characteristic (ROC) curve [32]. In addition, calibration curve analysis and the Hosmer—Lemeshow goodness-of-fit test were performed using the R packages "rms" and "ResourceSelection". Decision curve analysis was conducted by the R package "rmda" to evaluate the potential clinical application value and net benefit.

Next, group-based trajectory modeling was achieved by the "traj" package [33] in R software to identify the optimal number of subgroups with similar SRD risk score trajectories among those with complete blood pressure and BMI data during the 30-year follow-up in this cohort (n = 1048, complete-case analysis). Categorical data are summarized as frequencies and percentages. Continuous variables are reported as the mean ± standard deviation (if normally distributed) or the median (25th and 75th percentile ranges). Independent sample *t*-tests, one-way ANOVA, Mann—Whitney U tests and Kruskal—Wallis tests were performed for the difference analysis of continuous variables according to their group, distribution and variance. Logistic regression analysis was carried out by SPSS software (SPSS Inc., Chicago, IL, USA). Statistical significance was considered at a two-sided *p* value <0.05 for all analyses.

3. Results

3.1. Study Population

The flow chart of the present study was shown in Figure 1. Overall, the latest follow-up data (the 7th follow-up, in 2017) of 2303 participants were included in the cross-sectional analysis to perform the machine learning feature selection and identify variables highly associated with SRD. Then, these 2303 participants were randomly assigned to the training set (70%, n = 1611) and the internal validation set (30%, n = 692). The training set was used to construct the SRD risk score model and the validation set was used to evaluate the SRD estimation performance. The data in 2013 (the 6th follow-up) were also included to evaluate the 4-year SRD risk prediction performance. The characteristics included in the model construction and validation of the participants in the training and internal validation sets are shown in Table 1. All variables have no significant differences between the training and internal validation sets, which suggested the data consistency and reasonableness of grouping. In addition, participants with complete blood pressure and BMI data during the 30-year follow-up were included in further group-based trajectory modeling analysis to identify the SRD risk score trajectories (n = 1048).

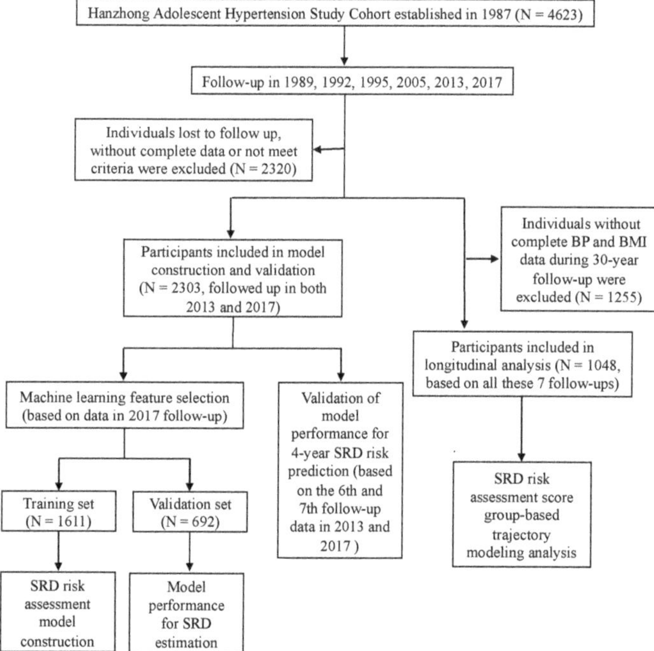

Figure 1. Flow chart of research design.

Table 1. Characteristics of the participants in the training and internal validation sets.

Characteristics	Total	Training Set	Internal Validation Set	*p* Value
SBP (mmHg)	121.3 (112.7–131.3)	121.7 (113.0–131.3)	120.8 (112.0–131.3)	0.363
DBP (mmHg)	76.0 (69.3–84.3)	76.3 (70.0–84.3)	75.3 (68.3–84.7)	0.096
BMI (kg/cm^2)	23.8 (21.9–26.0)	23.8 (21.9–26.2)	23.8 (21.9–25.6)	0.397
eGFR (mL/min per 1.73 m^2)	96.9 (87.1–106.1)	96.5 (86.8–105.8)	98.2 (88.0–106.6)	0.096
uACR (mg/mmol)	0.95 (0.62–1.68)	0.95 (0.62–1.69)	0.96 (0.63–1.65)	0.939
SRD (n, %)	276 (13.2)	203 (13.9)	73 (11.7)	0.177

SBP, systolic blood pressure; DBP, diastolic blood pressure; BMI, body mass index; eGFR, estimated glomerular filtration rate; uACR, urinary albumin-to-creatinine ratio; SRD, subclinical renal damage.

3.2. Feature Selection

A heatmap (Figure S1 in Supplementary Materials) showed the correlation among SRD and other 25 SRD-associated variables (anthropometric parameters, blood pressure level, biochemical parameters, diabetes history, etc.). Considering the data multicollinearity, it is necessary to conduct feature selection to identify the most important variables and then construct SRD risk models. In this study, we combined three machine learning algorithms to achieve accurate feature selection, including LASSO regression analysis, the random forest algorithm and the SVM-RFE algorithm. In LASSO regression analysis, 10-fold cross-validation was performed to detect the optimal AUC value and minimal parameters. Finally, we selected six features among 25 variables: systolic blood pressure, diastolic blood pressure, BMI, triglyceride, heart rate and diabetes (Figure 2A). The SVM-RFE algorithm was also used to achieve feature selection according to the optimal classification accuracy. Four variables were identified as key features: diastolic blood pressure, systolic blood pressure, BMI and body weight (Figure 2B). In addition, the random forest algorithm suggested six features (diastolic blood pressure, systolic blood pressure, BMI, triglyceride, serum chloride and serum potassium) to reach the minimum cross-validation error (Figure 2C). Meanwhile, based on the mean decrease in the Gini coefficient, the importance of variables in the random forest model were calculated (Figure 2D). Finally, by combining these three machine learning feature selection algorithms, we selected diastolic blood pressure, systolic blood pressure and BMI as hub variables for further analysis and model construction.

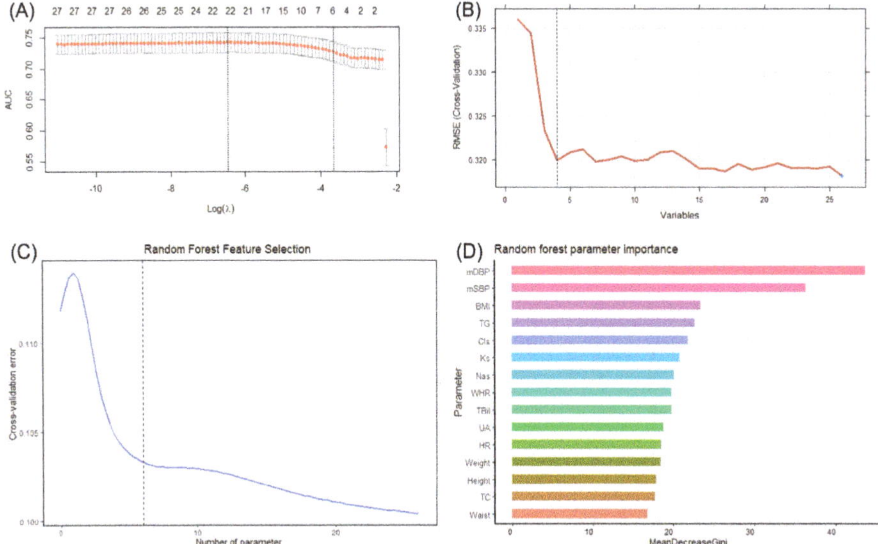

Figure 2. Machine learning feature selection strategies in this study. (**A**) LASSO regression analysis. Six features were identified including SBP, DBP, BMI, triglyceride, heart rate and diabetes. (**B**) SVM-RFE

algorithm feature selection. Four features were identified: DBP, SBP, BMI and body weight. (**C**) Random forest algorithm feature selection. Six features were selected: DBP, SBP, BMI, triglyceride, serum chloride and serum potassium. (**D**) Importance of the parameters was assessed by a random forest algorithm. AUC, area under the curve; RMSE, root mean square error; mDBP, mean diastolic blood pressure; mSBP, mean systolic blood pressure; BMI, body mass index; TG, triglyceride; Cls, serum chloride iion; Ks, serum potassium; Nas, serum sodium; WHR, weight-to-height ratio; TBil, total bilirubin; UA, uric acid; HR, heart rate; TC, total cholesterol.

3.3. Construction and Validation of the SRD Risk Assessment Model

Logistic regression analysis was performed to establish an SRD risk assessment model based on data from the training set: SRD index = 0.020143 × SBP + 0.039718 × DBP + 0.063076 × BMI − 9.211994, SRD risk score = $1/(1 + e^{-\text{SRD index}})$. Meanwhile, a corresponding nomogram was constructed to achieve more efficient clinical application (Figure 3A). In detail, according to SBP, DBP and BMI data, total points can be calculated to evaluate the diagnostic possibility of SRD. High possibility indicates the need for further blood or urine testing to determine renal function, while low possibility indicates little need to take further tests, so as to achieve large-scale screening or self-monitoring. Next, we validated the classification ability of the model, and the AUC value of the ROC curve reached 0.778 (for SRD real-time estimation) and 0.729 (for 4-year SRD risk prediction) in the internal validation set (Figure 3B,C). The optimal cutoff value for SRD real-time estimation is 0.153, which leads to a sensitivity of 0.685 and specificity of 0.779. Meanwhile, the optimal cutoff value for 4-year SRD risk prediction is 0.117 which leads to a sensitivity of 0.767 and a specificity of 0.598. The calibration curve analysis and the Hosmer—Lemeshow goodness-of-fit test ($p = 0.62$ for SRD real-time estimation, $p = 0.34$ for SRD 4-year risk prediction) indicated that this model had good calibration in both SRD real-time estimation and SRD 4-year risk prediction (Figure 3D,E). In addition, as the SRD estimation decision curve analysis (DCA) showed, compared to the SRD screening decision strategies currently used in clinical practice, which mainly focus on the specific higher-risk conditions, such as hypertension, obesity and diabetes, more potential net benefit can be obtained in all ranges of risk thresholds using this SRD assessment model to assist in SRD screening decision making (Figure 3F,G). The results of the SRD 4-year risk prediction DCA also supported this conclusion. In fact, SBP, DBP and BMI data are easy to collect in clinical practice by noninvasive examination, which indicates that it is possible for our models to evaluate or predict the SRD risk and identify high-risk asymptomatic people from a large-scale population, which can improve existing SRD screening strategies.

(A)

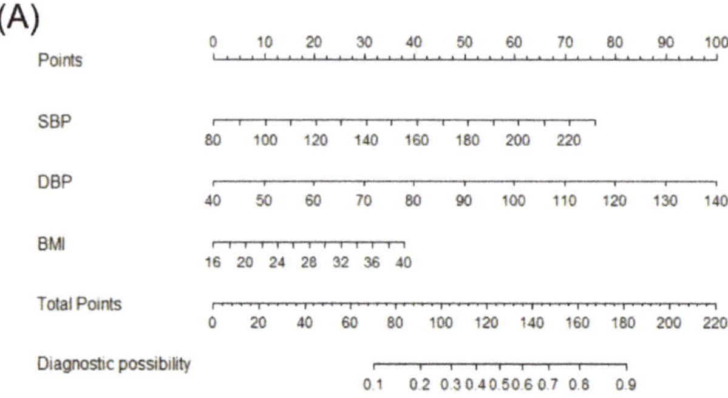

Figure 3. *Cont.*

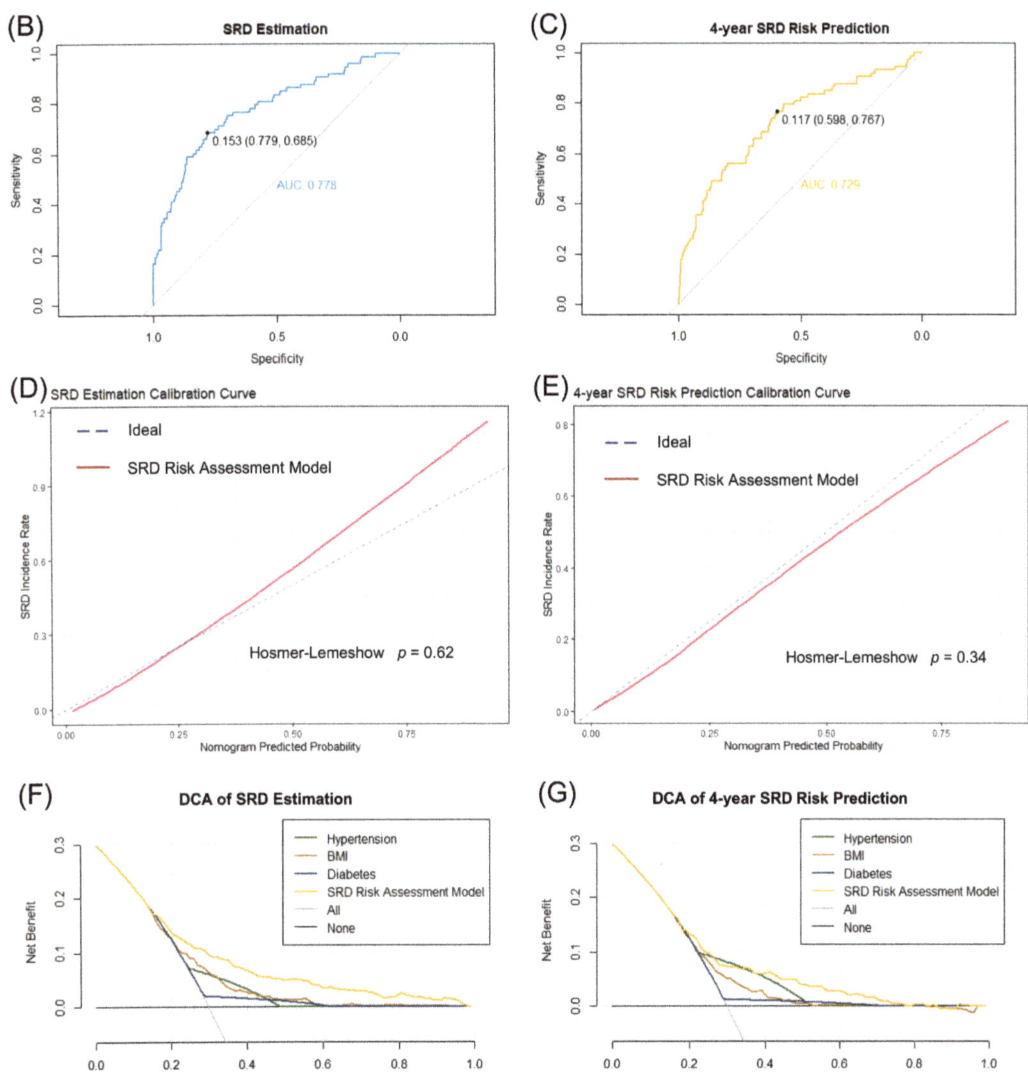

Figure 3. SRD risk assessment model construction and validation. (**A**) Nomogram for SRD risk. Diagnostic possibility can be calculated based on SBP, DBP and BMI. (**B,C**) AUC value of the ROC curve in the internal validation set. The SRD estimation AUC value can reach 0.778 and the 4-year SRD risk prediction AUC value can reach 0.729. (**D,E**) Calibration analysis for this SRD risk assessment model. (**F,G**) Decision curve analysis for hypertension, diabetes, BMI and this SRD risk assessment model, which showed this model had greater potential clinical benefits than each individual variable used to assess SRD risk in current clinical practice such as hypertension, diabetes and BMI. SRD, subclinical renal damage; SBP, systolic blood pressure; DBP, diastolic blood pressure; BMI, body mass index; AUC, area under the curve; DCA, decision curve analysis.

3.4. SRD Risk Score Trajectory

SRD risk scores during the 30-year follow-up were calculated based on the diastolic blood pressure, systolic blood pressure and BMI data. Then, we performed group-based trajectory modeling analysis and identified three SRD risk score trajectory groups: stable, increasing-stable and increasing (Figure 4). The SRD risk scores of all three groups have trends of increasing with age from childhood to middle age and have similar slope increases before about 25 years old. After this age, the stable group (n = 376; 35.9%) endured relatively lower SRD risk score levels and SRD risk scores compared to the other two group, which continued to increase. The increasing-stable group (n = 404; 38.5%) was characterized by SRD risk scores increasing to a relatively higher level and then holding steady after about 40 years old. Meanwhile, the increasing group (n = 268; 25.6%) was characterized by a sustained increase from childhood to middle age and reached a higher level than both the stable group and increasing-stable group.

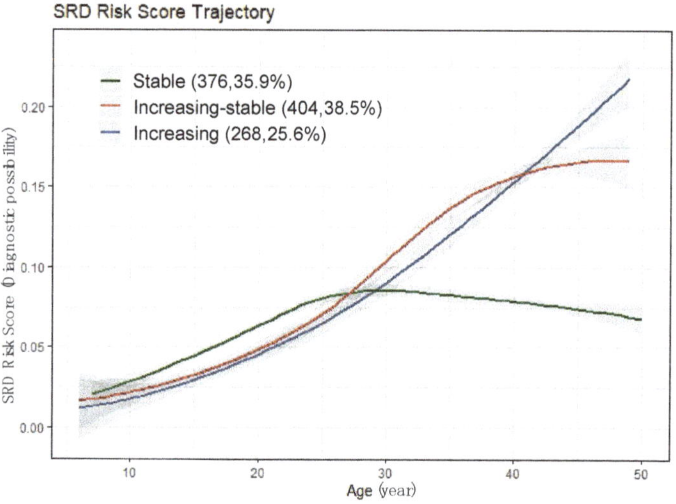

Figure 4. Three SRD risk score trajectory groups identified in this study using group-based trajectory modeling analysis: stable group, increasing-stable group and increasing group. SRD, subclinical renal damage.

3.5. Cardiovascular Risk Factors for SRD Risk Score Trajectory Groups

Table 2 shows the data of partial anthropometry and biochemical indicator tests in 1987 and 2017 according to these three SRD risk score groups. Among these 1048 participants, 583 (55.6%) were males and 465 (44.4%) were females. The median age in 2017 was 43 years old. Differences in the proportion of males, age, incidence of hyperlipidemia, incidence of hypertension, current smoking, alcohol consumption, waist circumference, hip circumference, TC, TG, LDL-C, HDL-C, serum uric acid, serum creatinine, urine albumin and uACR were statistically significant (p <0.05). Occupation, education, marital status, incidence of carotid atherosclerosis, heart rate (both in 1987 and in 2007), urine uric acid (uUA) and eGFR were not significantly different. Individuals in the SRD risk score stable group were more likely to be females, and more likely to have a lower waist circumference, hip circumference, TC, TG, LDL-C and serum UA. In addition, the SRD risk score increasing group a higher incidence of hyperlipidemia and hypertension, as well as higher rate of current smoking and alcohol consumption.

Table 2. Demographic characteristics and cardiovascular risk factors by the SRD risk score trajectory groups.

	Total	Stable	Increasing-Stable	Increasing	*p* Value
Male (%)	583	169 (45.1)	258 (63.7)	156 (58.2)	<0.001
Age (years)	43.0 (41.0–46.0)	43.0 (41.0–46.0)	43.0 (40.0–45.0)	43.0 (41.0–45.0)	0.049
Occupation (%)	1011				0.383
Farmer	408	146 (40.1)	157 (40.3)	105 (40.9)	
Worker	194	63 (17.3)	82 (21.0)	49 (19.1)	
Business	81	35 (9.6)	30 (7.7)	16 (6.2)	
Governor	21	5 (1.4)	13 (3.4)	3 (1.2)	
Other	307	115 (31.6)	108 (27.7)	84 (32.7)	
Marital status (%)	1041				0.064
Unmarried or other	15	4 (1.1)	8 (2.1)	3 (1.2)	
Married	1015	365 (97.1)	387 (97.0)	263 (98.9)	
Divorced	11	7 (1.9)	4 (1.0)	0 (0.0)	
Education (%)	1016				0.553
Primary school or less	73	24 (6.6)	27 (6.9)	22 (18.7)	
Middle school	628	221 (60.5)	240 (61.2)	167 (64.5)	
High school	226	82 (22.5)	92 (23.5)	52 (20.1)	
College or more	89	38 (10.4)	33 (8.4)	18 (6.9)	
Current smoking (%)	450	126 (34.8)	200 (51.9)	124 (49.2)	<0.001
Alcohol consumption (%)	321	96 (26.5)	141 (36.6)	84 (33.3)	0.011
SRD (%)	138	33 (8.8)	54 (13.4)	51 (19.0)	0.001
AS (%)	139	48 (12.9)	55 (13.9)	36 (13.7)	0.922
Hyperlipidemia	424	119 (31.6)	170 (42.1)	135 (50.4)	<0.001
Hypertension	172	10 (2.7)	65 (16.1)	97 (36.2)	<0.001
Heart rate 1987 (beats/min)	78.0 (72.0–84.0)	78.0 (72.0–84.0)	78.0 (72.0–84.0)	78.0 (72.0–84.0)	0.983
Heart rate 2017 (beats/min)	73.0 (66.0–80.0)	72.5 (66.0–79.0)	73.0 (66.0–80.0)	75.0 (69.0–82.0)	0.072
Waist (cm)	84.8 (78.2–92.2)	80.8 (75.5–87.2)	87.0 (79.7–94.3)	89.4 (82.4–95.5)	<0.001
Hips (cm)	92.2 (88.8–95.9)	90.7 (87.7–93.4)	93.4 (89.5–97.0)	93.7 (90.4–97.0)	<0.001
TC (mmol/L)	4.48 (4.03–5.00)	4.40 (3.92–4.87)	4.49 (4.02–5.08)	4.58 (4.17–5.18)	0.001
TG (mmol/L)	1.39 (1.01–2.01)	1.20 (0.89–1.66)	1.44 (1.08–2.03)	1.64 (1.13–2.44)	<0.001
LDL–C (mmol/L)	2.49 (2.11–2.88)	2.44 (2.05–2.78)	2.48 (2.13–2.95)	2.55 (2.22–3.00)	0.006
HDL-C (mmol/L)	1.13 (0.99–1.33)	1.20 (1.02–1.42)	1.12 (0.98–1.29)	1.09 (0.95–1.29)	<0.001
Serum uric acid (µmol/L)	283.2 (226.2–338.8)	264.9 (212.5–316.8)	300.7 (239.7–352.6)	293.8 (243.3–352.2)	<0.001
Urine uric acid (µmol/L)	1298.5 (914.8–1984.5)	1291.5 (897.5–1994.5)	1317.0 (981.5–1951.0)	1283.0 (889.0–2090.0)	0.268
Serum creatinine (µmol/L)	76.3 (66.7–86.8)	73.7 (65.3–82.9)	78.8 (68.6–88.8)	77.0 (69.7–88.0)	<0.001
Urine albumin (mg/L)	8.0 (4.1–13.7)	6.4 (3.1–11.1)	9.0 (4.8–14.2)	9.2 (5.2–22.5)	<0.001
eGFR (mL/min per 1.73 m^2)	97.2 (87.0–106.3)	97.2 (86.2–107.0)	97.7 (87.1–106.3)	94.3 (85.9–106.0)	0.260
uACR (mg/mmol)	0.98 (0.64–1.72)	0.85 (0.57–1.33)	0.99 (0.64–1.96)	1.25 (0.74–2.34)	<0.001

AS, atherosclerosis; TC, total cholesterol; TG, triglycerides; LDL-C, low density lipoprotein cholesterol; HDL-C, high density lipoprotein cholesterol.

3.6. Association between Novel SRD Risk Score Trajectories and Subclinical Renal Damage

SRD incidence was significantly different among the three SRD risk score groups ($p < 0.05$). Figure 5A shows that the SRD risk score increasing group had a higher SRD incidence rate in middle age (19%) compared to stable group (8.8%) and stable-increasing group (13.4%). We found that the uACR was significantly different among the three SRD risk score groups ($p < 0.05$), whereas the GFR was not significantly different ($p = 0.26$). The increasing group had a significantly higher uACR level (1.25 (0.74–2.34)) than the increasing-stable group (0.99 (0.64–1.96)) and the stable group (0.85 (0.57–1.33)). Additionally, the uACR levels between the stable, stable-increasing and increasing group were also significantly different ($p = 0.002$ for stable group compared to stable-increasing group, $p < 0.001$ for stable group compared to increasing group, $p = 0.011$ for stable-increasing group compared to increasing group). Moreover, the increasing group had a lower eGFR (94.3 (85.9–106.0)) compared to stable group (97.2 (86.2–107.0)) and stable-increasing group (97.7 (87.1–106.3)). The scatter diagrams of uACR levels and eGFR levels among these three groups are shown in Figure 5B,C. Next, logistic regression was performed to investigate the association between the SRD risk score trajectory groups and SRD incidence. The trajectory groups were defined as dummy independent variables, and the stable group was the control group in the logistic regression. Our results showed that the increasing group and increasing-stable group had significantly greater odds of SRD incidence in middle age than the stable group. The increasing-stable group had an OR of 1.6 (95% CI, 1.01 to 2.54), and the increasing group had an OR of 2.44 (95% CI, 1.53 to 3.91). The adjusted logistic regression model showed that ORs were slightly attenuated after adjustment for gender and age. The increasing-stable group had an OR of 1.53 (95% CI, 0.96 to 2.43), and the increasing group had an OR of 2.39 (95% CI, 1.49 to 3.84). Additional adjustment for waist circumference, hip circumference, TC, TG, LDL-C and HDL-C also attenuated the ORs. The increasing-stable group had an OR of 1.25 (95% CI, 0.77 to 2.05), and the increasing group had an OR of 1.75 (95% CI, 1.05 to 2.91). Finally, after further adjusting for the incidence of current smoking and alcohol consumption, the ORs of the increasing-stable group were 1.24 (95% CI, 0.76 to 2.03) and the ORs of the increasing group were 1.73 (95% CI, 1.04 to 2.89). These results indicated that these SRD risk score trajectories can serve as a strong predictor for the SRD incidence risk in middle age (Table 3). In addition, through long-term trajectory analysis, we can also demonstrate the good performance and reliability of this SRD risk assessment score in longitudinal observation.

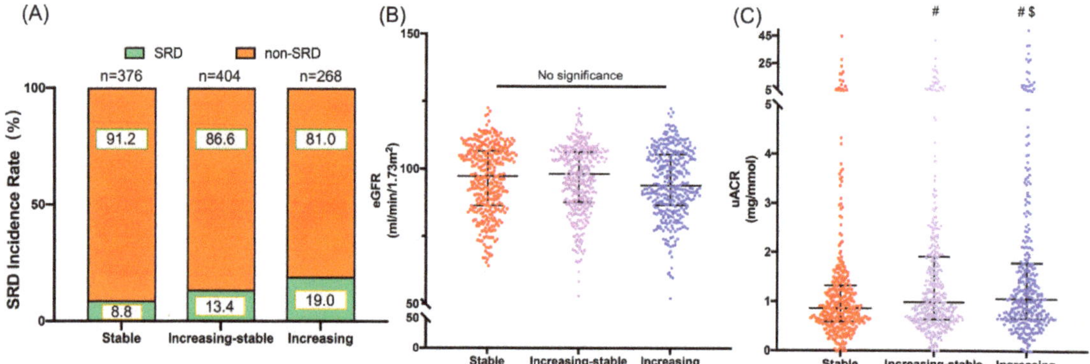

Figure 5. Renal damage of different trajectories groups. (**A**) SRD incidence rate among the three SRD risk score trajectory groups. (**B,C**) Scatter diagrams of eGFR levels and uACR levels among these three SRD risk score trajectory groups. SRD, subclinical renal damage; eGFR, estimated glomerular filtration rate; uACR, urinary albumin-to-creatinine ratio. [#] $p < 0.05$ vs. stable group and [$] $p < 0.05$ vs. increasing-stable group.

Table 3. Adjusted odds ratios and 95% confidence intervals of the association of SRD risk score trajectory groups with subclinical kidney damage.

Trajectory Groups	No. of Subjects with SRD in 2017	Unadjusted	Model 1	Model 2	Model 3
Stable	33 (8.8)	1.00	1.00	1.00	1.00
Increasing-stable	54 (13.4)	1.60 (1.01–2.54)	1.53 (0.96–2.43)	1.25 (0.77–2.05)	1.24 (0.76–2.03)
Increasing	51 (19.0)	2.44 (1.53–3.91)	2.39 (1.49–3.84)	1.75 (1.05–2.91)	1.73 (1.04–2.89)

Model 1 = gender, age in 2017. Model 2 = Model 1 + waist circumference, hip circumference, TC, TG, LDL-C and HDL-C in 2017. Model 3 = Model 2 + current smoking and alcohol consumption in 2017.

4. Discussion

4.1. Main Findings

Three predictive factors (SBP, DBP and BMI) for SRD in middle age were identified using an integrated feature selection strategy. Based on these three predictive factors, a novel noninvasive SRD risk assessment model was established that showed excellent classification ability, calibration and potential clinical benefits for SRD estimation and SRD 4-year risk prediction. These results indicated that it is possible for our models to identify high-risk asymptomatic people from a large-scale population and help the clinical SRD early screening decision in middle age. Additionally, through subsequent cohort analysis, we identified three trajectory groups for this novel SRD risk assessment score using 30-year follow-up data. We found that the incidence of SRD in middle age and uACR levels were highly associated with these risk score trajectories. Further logistic regression analysis indicated that these SRD risk score trajectories can serve as a strong predictor for the SRD incidence risk in middle age. Therefore, longitudinal observation further confirmed the value of this risk score to generate individualized risk estimates and further participate in clinical screening decisions for SRD in middle age. In summary, we constructed a novel, simple and low-cost risk assessment tool for SRD screening, which presented good performance in predicting SRD risk in middle age. The convenience of this model makes it possible to assess the SRD risk of asymptomatic people and then carry out further SRD screening.

4.2. Prior Studies and the Focus of our Investigation

The detection and screening for SRD is critical because it can correspond to the CKD stages (G3a stage, G3b stage in GFR Category and A2 stage, A3 stage in persistent albuminuria category) which are associated with moderately increased risk (yellow risk) or high risk (orange risk) for the concurrent complications and future outcomes; these are also are the most critical periods for early diagnosis and intervention for CKD. However, SRD is usually asymptomatic until an advanced disease stage, and estimation methods of renal function, such as the measurement of serum creatinine concentration, urine protein or albumin concentration are costly for long-term follow-up or large-scale screening [34,35]. In current clinical practice, only patients with specific higher-risk conditions, such as hypertension, obesity and diabetes are recommended to be screened for renal function conditions or SRD. It is still difficult to apply routine SRD screening in a large-scale general population, especially for asymptomatic adults, due to the lack of a more economical and effective noninvasive risk assessment tool for SRD [1,36]. Therefore, a simple and noninvasive SRD risk assessment tool is urgently needed to assist in the SRD screening decision and improve large-scale SRD screening strategies. SRD is attributed to several risk factors, such as hypertension, diabetes, older age and obesity [37–39]. There have been numerous efforts to construct prediction models for the risk of decreasing eGFR in CKD [22,24]. However, the estimation or prediction of SRD can be more useful than only predicting a decrease in eGFR from the perspective of identifying the prognostic risk of CKD. In addition, too many variables and biochemical examination results were included in existing models, which complicated their translation to clinical practice for large-scale screening. Hence, in this study, we provided a novel feature-selection strategy by combining three machine learning methods, and first established an SRD risk assessment model calculated only by SBP, DBP and BMI data, which may have greater utility in clinical application. Additionally, our risk assessment model had better performance than those in previous studies: excellent classification ability (AUC value of the ROC curve: 0.778 for SRD estimation, 0.729 for 4-year SRD risk prediction in the validation set), calibration (Hosmer—Lemeshow goodness-of-fit test $p = 0.62$ for SRD estimation, $p = 0.34$ for 4-year SRD risk prediction) and potential clinical benefits.

In addition, most existing prediction models lack a longitudinal cohort analysis, such as group-based trajectory modeling analysis, which could reflect the relationship between model trajectory and SRD incidence [40,41]. Therefore, in the current study, we combined SBP, DBP and BMI data to calculate a novel SRD risk assessment score and then performed a trajectory analysis. Ultimately, three trajectory groups (increasing, increasing-stable, and stable) were identified based on 30-year follow-up data, and the incidence of SRD in middle age and uACR levels were highly associated with these risk score trajectories. Compared with the stable group, the increasing group and increasing-stable group had a significantly higher uACR. In addition, the results of the logistic regression showed that these three SRD risk assessment score trajectories could serve as ideal predictors of the incidence of SRD in middle age. Several other studies and some of our previous works have tried to investigate the relationship between SRD incidence and its risk-factor trajectories, such as SBP trajectory, DBP trajectory, MAP trajectory and BMI trajectory [13,15]. However, single-variable trajectory analyses have limitations because they ignore the interaction among multiple factors [42]. Hence, the group-based trajectory analysis for the SRD risk assessment score in the current work, which gives full consideration to the characteristics of SBP, DBP and BMI, is also a breakthrough for SRD-associated trajectory modeling analysis strategies.

4.3. Limitations and Future Directions

The present study used a community-based cohort followed for 30 years, which represents a large population. It is prospective in nature and consists of representative data from the general population. However, it should be noted that this study has the following limitations. First, our study used a racially-homogenous cohort from multiple rural areas in northern China, which limited the generalizability of our results, and validation using other cohorts with different backgrounds of ethnicities and populations will be performed in our further studies. Second, this work was not externally validated, which may also have limited the generalizability of our results. Notwithstanding this limitation, our study provided a novel SRD risk assessment tool that has both good performance in cross-sectional analysis and longitudinal analysis as well as the convenience of clinical application. In addition, to our knowledge, this is the first study to perform a group-based trajectory modeling longitudinal analysis for an SRD risk assessment tool, which revealed that realistic SRD outcomes in middle age correspond to the development trend of the risk score suggested by the SRD risk assessment model.

5. Conclusions

In conclusion, we used a large community-based cohort followed for 30 years to establish a novel, simple and low-cost SRD risk assessment tool and performed longitudinal group-based trajectory analysis for this tool. Internal validation suggested that our risk assessment model has excellent classification ability (AUC value of the ROC curve: 0.778 for SRD estimation, 0.729 for 4-year SRD risk prediction), calibration (Hosmer—Lemeshow goodness-of-fit test $p = 0.62$ for SRD estimation, $p = 0.34$ for 4-year SRD risk prediction) and potential clinical benefits. Further longitudinal trajectory analysis also confirmed the reliability of this SRD risk assessment score. Considering the good clinical utility, simplicity and convenience as well as the excellent performance of our model, it can identify high-risk asymptomatic people from a large-scale population and improve current clinical SRD screening strategies.

Supplementary Materials: The following supporting information can be downloaded at: https://www.mdpi.com/article/10.3390/bioengineering10020257/s1, Figure S1: Heat map for the correlation between SRD-associated variables.

Author Contributions: Conceptualization, C.C. (Chen Chen), G.L. and J.M.; Data curation, C.C. (Chao Chu), W.Z., Q.M., Y.L., Y.Y., Y.S. and D.W.; Formal analysis, C.C. (Chen Chen) and G.L.; Writing—Original Draft Preparation, C.C. (Chen Chen) and G.L.; Writing—Review & Editing, C.C. (Chen Chen) and J.M. All authors have read and agreed to the published version of the manuscript.

Funding: This research was funded by the National Natural Science Foundation of China No. 82070437 (J.M.) and No. 82200472 (W.Z.), the Clinical Research Award of the First Affiliated Hospital of Xi'an Jiaotong University (XJTU1AF–CRF–2019–004), the Key Project of the Ministry of Science and Technology of China(2017YFC0211703), the Chinese Academy of Medical Sciences & Peking Union Medical College (2017–CXGC03–2) and International Joint Research Center for Cardiovascular Precision Medicine of Shaanxi Province (2020GHJD–14).

Institutional Review Board Statement: This study was clinically registered (NCT02734472) and approved by the Ethics Committee of First Affiliated Hospital of Xi'an Jiaotong University (Ethical Approval number: XJTU1AF2015LSL–047).

Informed Consent Statement: Informed consent was obtained from all subjects involved in the study. Written informed consent has been obtained from the patients to publish this paper.

Data Availability Statement: Not applicable.

Conflicts of Interest: The authors declare no conflict of interest.

References

1. Inker, L.A.; Astor, B.C.; Fox, C.H.; Isakova, T.; Lash, J.P.; Peralta, C.A.; Kurella Tamura, M.; Feldman, H.I. KDOQI US Commentary on the 2012 KDIGO Clinical Practice Guideline for the Evaluation and Management of CKD. *Am. J. Kidney Dis.* **2014**, *63*, 713–735. [CrossRef] [PubMed]
2. Levey, A.S.; de Jong, P.E.; Coresh, J.; El Nahas, M.; Astor, B.C.; Matsushita, K.; Gansevoort, R.T.; Kasiske, B.L.; Eckardt, K.-U. The definition, classification, and prognosis of chronic kidney disease: A KDIGO Controversies Conference report. *Kidney Int.* **2011**, *80*, 17–28. [CrossRef] [PubMed]
3. Couser, W.G.; Remuzzi, G.; Mendis, S.; Tonelli, M. The contribution of chronic kidney disease to the global burden of major noncommunicable diseases. *Kidney Int.* **2011**, *80*, 1258–1270. [CrossRef]
4. GBD 2017 Disease and Injury Incidence and Prevalence Collaborators. Global, regional, and national incidence, prevalence, and years lived with disability for 354 diseases and injuries for 195 countries and territories, 1990–2017: A systematic analysis for the Global Burden of Disease Study 2017. *Lancet* **2018**, *392*, 1789–1858. [CrossRef] [PubMed]
5. Liyanage, T.; Toyama, T.; Hockham, C.; Ninomiya, T.; Perkovic, V.; Woodward, M.; Fukagawa, M.; Matsushita, K.; Praditpornsilpa, K.; Hooi, L.S.; et al. Prevalence of chronic kidney disease in Asia: A systematic review and analysis. *BMJ Glob. Health* **2022**, *7*, e007525. [CrossRef]
6. Webster, A.C.; Nagler, E.V.; Morton, R.L.; Masson, P. Chronic Kidney Disease. *Lancet* **2017**, *389*, 1238–1252. [CrossRef]
7. Reiss, A.B.; Miyawaki, N.; Moon, J.; Kasselman, L.J.; Voloshyna, I.; D'Avino, R., Jr.; De Leon, J. CKD, arterial calcification, atherosclerosis and bone health: Inter–relationships and controversies. *Atherosclerosis* **2018**, *278*, 49–59. [CrossRef]
8. Obrador, G.T.; Levin, A. CKD Hotspots: Challenges and Areas of Opportunity. *Semin. Nephrol.* **2019**, *39*, 308–314. [CrossRef]
9. Drawz, P.; Rahman, M. Chronic kidney disease. *Ann. Intern. Med.* **2015**, *162*, ITC1-16. [CrossRef]
10. Ballew, S.; Matsushita, K. Cardiovascular Risk Prediction in CKD. *Semin. Nephrol.* **2018**, *38*, 208–216. [CrossRef]
11. Gaitonde, D.Y.; Cook, D.L.; Rivera, I.M. Chronic Kidney Disease: Detection and Evaluation. *Am. Fam. Physician* **2017**, *96*, 776–783.
12. Mulè, G.; Calcaterra, I.; Costanzo, M.; Geraci, G.; Guarino, L.; Foraci, A.C.; Vario, M.G.; Cerasola, G.; Cottone, S. Relationship Between Short-Term Blood Pressure Variability and Subclinical Renal Damage in Essential Hypertensive Patients. *J. Clin. Hypertens.* **2015**, *17*, 473–480. [CrossRef]
13. Yan, Y.; Zheng, W.; Ma, Q.; Chu, C.; Hu, J.; Wang, K.; Liao, Y.; Chen, C.; Yuan, Y.; Lv, Y.; et al. Child-to-adult body mass index trajectories and the risk of subclinical renal damage in middle age. *Int. J. Obes.* **2021**, *45*, 1095–1104. [CrossRef]
14. Wang, Y.; Du, M.-F.; Gao, W.-H.; Fu, B.-W.; Ma, Q.; Yan, Y.; Yuan, Y.; Chu, C.; Chen, C.; Liao, Y.-Y.; et al. Risk factors for subclinical renal damage and its progression: Hanzhong Adolescent Hypertension Study. *Eur. J. Clin. Nutr.* **2020**, *75*, 531–538. [CrossRef]
15. Zheng, W.; Mu, J.; Chu, C.; Hu, J.; Yan, Y.; Ma, Q.; Lv, Y.; Xu, X.; Wang, K.; Wang, Y.; et al. Association of Blood Pressure Trajectories in Early Life with Subclinical Renal Damage in Middle Age. *J. Am. Soc. Nephrol.* **2018**, *29*, 2835–2846. [CrossRef]
16. Moyer, V.A. Screening for chronic kidney disease: U.S. Preventive Services Task Force recommendation statement. *Ann. Intern. Med.* **2012**, *157*, 567–570. [CrossRef]

17. Levin, A.; Stevens, P.E. Early detection of CKD: The benefits, limitations and effects on prognosis. *Nat. Rev. Nephrol.* **2011**, *7*, 446–457. [CrossRef]
18. Stevens, P.E.; Levin, A. Evaluation and management of chronic kidney disease: Synopsis of the kidney disease: Improving global outcomes 2012 clinical practice guideline. *Ann. Intern. Med.* **2013**, *158*, 825–830. [CrossRef]
19. Xie, X.; Atkins, E.; Lv, J.; Bennett, A.; Neal, B.; Ninomiya, T.; Woodward, M.; MacMahon, S.; Turnbull, F.; Hillis, G.S.; et al. Effects of intensive blood pressure lowering on cardiovascular and renal outcomes: Updated systematic review and meta-analysis. *Lancet* **2016**, *387*, 435–443. [CrossRef]
20. Kramer, H.; Luke, A.; Bidani, A.; Cao, G.; Cooper, R.; McGee, D. Obesity and Prevalent and Incident CKD: The Hypertension Detection and Follow-Up Program. *Am. J. Kidney Dis.* **2005**, *46*, 587–594. [CrossRef]
21. Vivante, A.; Golan, E.; Tzur, D.; Leiba, A.; Tirosh, A.; Skorecki, K.; Calderon-Margalit, R. Body mass index in 1.2 million adolescents and risk for end–stage renal disease. *Arch. Intern. Med.* **2012**, *172*, 1644–1650. [CrossRef] [PubMed]
22. Nelson, R.G.; Grams, M.E.; Ballew, S.H.; Sang, Y.; Azizi, F.; Chadban, S.J.; Chaker, L.; Dunning, S.C.; Fox, C.; Hirakawa, Y.; et al. Development of Risk Prediction Equations for Incident Chronic Kidney Disease. *JAMA* **2019**, *322*, 2104–2114. [CrossRef] [PubMed]
23. Chien, K.-L.; Lin, H.-J.; Lee, B.-C.; Hsu, H.-C.; Lee, Y.-T.; Chen, M.-F. A Prediction Model for the Risk of Incident Chronic Kidney Disease. *Am. J. Med.* **2010**, *123*, 836–846. [CrossRef] [PubMed]
24. Lerner, B.; Desrochers, S.; Tangri, N. Risk Prediction Models in CKD. *Semin. Nephrol.* **2017**, *37*, 144–150. [CrossRef]
25. Nagin, D.S.; Jones, B.L.; Passos, V.L.; Tremblay, R.E. Group–based multi–trajectory modeling. *Stat. Methods Med. Res.* **2018**, *27*, 2015–2023. [CrossRef]
26. Yan, Y.; Ma, Q.; Liao, Y.; Chen, C.; Hu, J.; Zheng, W.; Chu, C.; Wang, K.; Sun, Y.; Zou, T.; et al. Blood pressure and long-term subclinical cardiovascular outcomes in low-risk young adults: Insights from Hanzhong adolescent hypertension cohort. *J. Clin. Hypertens.* **2021**, *23*, 1020–1029. [CrossRef]
27. Chu, C.; Dai, Y.; Mu, J.; Yang, R.; Wang, M.; Yang, J.; Ren, Y.; Xie, B.; Dong, Z.; Yang, F.; et al. Associations of risk factors in childhood with arterial stiffness 26 years later: The Hanzhong adolescent hypertension cohort. *J. Hypertens.* **2017**, *35* (Suppl. 1), S10–S15. [CrossRef]
28. Ma, Y.-C.; Zuo, L.; Chen, J.-H.; Luo, Q.; Yu, X.-Q.; Li, Y.; Xu, J.-S.; Huang, S.-M.; Wang, L.-N.; Huang, W.; et al. Modified Glomerular Filtration Rate Estimating Equation for Chinese Patients with Chronic Kidney Disease. *J. Am. Soc. Nephrol.* **2006**, *17*, 2937–2944. [CrossRef]
29. Shiffman, S.; Tindle, H.; Li, X.; Scholl, S.; Dunbar, M.; Mitchell-Miland, C. Characteristics and smoking patterns of intermittent smokers. *Exp. Clin. Psychopharmacol.* **2012**, *20*, 264–277. [CrossRef]
30. Li, X.X.; Zhao, Y.; Huang, L.X.; Xu, H.X.; Liu, X.Y.; Yang, J.J.; Zhang, P.J.; Zhang, Y.H. Effects of smoking and alcohol consumption on lipid profile in male adults in northwest rural China. *Public Health* **2018**, *157*, 7–13. [CrossRef]
31. Friedman, J.H.; Hastie, T.; Tibshirani, R. Regularization Paths for Generalized Linear Models via Coordinate Descent. *J. Stat. Softw.* **2010**, *33*, 1–22. [CrossRef]
32. Robin, X.; Turck, N.; Hainard, A.; Tiberti, N.; Lisacek, F.; Sanchez, J.-C.; Müller, M. pROC: An open-source package for R and S+ to analyze and compare ROC curves. *BMC Bioinform.* **2011**, *12*, 77. [CrossRef]
33. Trinh, M.H.; Sundaram, R.; Robinson, S.L.; Lin, T.C.; Bell, E.M.; Ghassabian, A.; Yeung, E.H. Association of Trajectory and Covariates of Children's Screen Media Time. *JAMA Pediatr.* **2020**, *174*, 71–78. [CrossRef]
34. Chen, T.K.; Knicely, D.H.; Grams, M.E. Chronic Kidney Disease Diagnosis and Management: A Review. *JAMA* **2019**, *322*, 1294–1304. [CrossRef]
35. Teasdale, E.J.; Leydon, G.; Fraser, S.; Roderick, P.; Taal, M.W.; Tonkin-Crine, S. Patients' Experiences After CKD Diagnosis: A Meta-ethnographic Study and Systematic Review. *Am. J. Kidney Dis.* **2017**, *70*, 656–665. [CrossRef]
36. McClellan, W.M.; Ramirez, S.P.B.; Jurkovitz, C. Screening for Chronic Kidney Disease: Unresolved Issues. *J. Am. Soc. Nephrol.* **2003**, *14*, S81–S87. [CrossRef]
37. Bruce, M.A.; Griffith, D.M.; Thorpe, R.J.J. Stress and the kidney. *Adv. Chronic Kidney Dis.* **2015**, *22*, 46–53. [CrossRef]
38. Kronenberg, F. Emerging risk factors and markers of chronic kidney disease progression. *Nat. Rev. Nephrol.* **2009**, *5*, 677–689. [CrossRef]
39. Hallan, S.; de Mutsert, R.; Carlsen, S.; Dekker, F.W.; Aasarød, K.; Holmen, J. Obesity, smoking, and physical inactivity as risk factors for CKD: Are men more vulnerable? *Am. J. Kidney Dis.* **2006**, *47*, 396–405. [CrossRef]
40. Mattsson, M.; Maher, G.; Boland, F.; Fitzgerald, A.P.; Murray, D.M.; Biesma, R. Group-based trajectory modelling for BMI trajectories in childhood: A systematic review. *Obes. Rev.* **2019**, *20*, 998–1015. [CrossRef]
41. Nagin, D.S.; Odgers, C.L. Group-Based Trajectory Modeling in Clinical Research. *Annu. Rev. Clin. Psychol.* **2010**, *6*, 109–138. [CrossRef] [PubMed]
42. Kagura, J.; Adair, L.S.; Munthali, R.J.; Pettifor, J.M.; Norris, S. Association Between Early Life Growth and Blood Pressure Trajectories in Black South African Children. *Hypertension* **2016**, *68*, 1123–1131. [CrossRef] [PubMed]

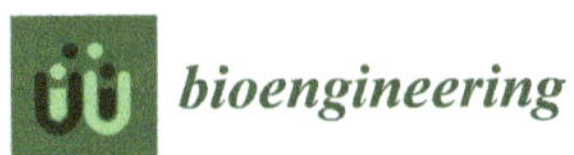 *bioengineering*

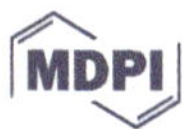

Review

COVID-19 Detection by Means of ECG, Voice, and X-ray Computerized Systems: A Review

Pedro Ribeiro [1], João Alexandre Lobo Marques [2] and Pedro Miguel Rodrigues [1,*]

[1]   CBQF—Centro de Biotecnologia e Química Fina—Laboratório Associado, Escola Superior de Biotecnologia, Universidade Católica Portuguesa, Rua de Diogo Botelho 1327, 4169-005 Porto, Portugal
[2]   Laboratory of Applied Neurosciences, University of Saint Joseph, Macao SAR 999078, China
*   Correspondence: pmrodrigues@ucp.pt

Abstract: Since the beginning of 2020, Coronavirus Disease 19 (COVID-19) has attracted the attention of the World Health Organization (WHO). This paper looks into the infection mechanism, patient symptoms, and laboratory diagnosis, followed by an extensive assessment of different technologies and computerized models (based on Electrocardiographic signals (ECG), Voice, and X-ray techniques) proposed as a diagnostic tool for the accurate detection of COVID-19. The found papers showed high accuracy rate results, ranging between 85.70% and 100%, and F1-Scores from 89.52% to 100%. With this state-of-the-art, we concluded that the models proposed for the detection of COVID-19 already have significant results, but the area still has room for improvement, given the vast symptomatology and the better comprehension of individuals' evolution of the disease.

Keywords: COVID-19; artificial intelligence; signal processing; image processing; computerized diagnostic systems

Citation: Ribeiro, P.; Marques, J.A.L.; Rodrigues, P.M. COVID-19 Detection by Means of ECG, Voice, and X-ray Computerized Systems: A Review. *Bioengineering* **2023**, *10*, 198. https://doi.org/10.3390/bioengineering10020198

Academic Editors: Yunfeng Wu and Larbi Boubchir

Received: 13 December 2022
Revised: 31 January 2023
Accepted: 1 February 2023
Published: 3 February 2023

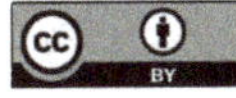

1. Introduction

The World Health Organization (WHO) has been on alert since early 2020 regarding the Coronavirus Disease 19 (COVID-19). Nowadays, with well over 6 million deaths worldwide [1], the scientific community is developing new ways to detect the disease.

1.1. Mechanism

COVID-19 is a disease caused by a Severe Acute Respiratory Syndrome-Coronavirus-2 (SARS-CoV-2) [2], which is a single, positive-strand Ribonucleic acid (RNA) virus that causes severe respiratory syndrome in humans. SARS-CoV-2 belongs to the family Coronaviridae and is divided into alpha (α-CoV), beta (β-CoV), gamma (γ-CoV), and delta (δ-CoV) coronaviruses. It was initially detected in bats, and the first cases of the disease were detected in a market in China. For this particular case, SARS-CoV-2 is a coronavirus genetically similar to β-CoV which, similar to α-CoV, can infect mammals [3–5].

SARS-CoV-2 uses Angiotensin Converting Enzyme 2 (ACE2), which is a receptor in the cell surface, to start the infection. After the binding of the spike protein with the ACE2 receptor, the invasion process is triggered by host cell proteases. The virus releases the RNA into the host cell, then the RNA is translated into viral replicase polyproteins. The negative RNA copies of the viral genome are produced by the enzyme replicase using the positive RNA genome. During transcription, RNA polymerase produces a series of subgenomic mRNAs and translates them into viral proteins. The RNA genome is assembled into virions in Golgi and Endoplasmic Reticulum (ER), which bud into the ERGIC (ER–Golgi intermediate compartment) and are released out of the cell [3–5].

SARS-CoV-2 uses ACE2 to initiate the infection process. This receptor is present in the kidney, blood vessels, heart, and the lungs, which means it can cause respiratory, cardiovascular, gastrointestinal, and central nervous system diseases [3–5].

In the next section, the most frequent symptoms identified in COVID-19 patients, as well as eventual complications, are briefly presented.

1.2. Symptoms

COVID-19 patients may present mild to severe symptoms, with a substantial portion of the population not demonstrating any type of symptoms. The reported symptoms include fever, cough, and shortness of breath. A small segment of the population presented some gastrointestinal symptoms such as vomiting, diarrhea, and pain in the abdominal area [4,5].

Cardiovascular complications have been reported in COVID-19 patients as well. The reports have described acute cardiac injury, cardiogenic shock, electrocardiographic (ECG) changes, right ventricular dysfunction, thromboembolic complications, and tachyarrhythmias [6].

1.3. Laboratory Diagnostic

Diagnosing active cases of COVID-19 is one of the most important tasks for controlling the pandemic. Laboratory testing techniques have been developed to obtain an accurate diagnosis of COVID-19. The most common techniques are Nucleic Acid Amplification Test (NAAT) and Antigen detection [4,7].

NAAT is a technology used to diagnose an active COVID-19 infection by the use of Real-Time Polymerase Chain Reaction (RT-PCR) assay to detect SARS-CoV-2 RNA from the upper respiratory tract [4,7].

Antigen detection tests are tests used to detect the presence of SARS-CoV-2 viral proteins. Most of the available antigen kits require samples taken from the nasal cavity or nasopharynx, with some kits allowing samples from saliva as well [7].

1.4. Rational for the Review

To determine the most suitable computerized resources to detect COVID-19, we investigated the scientific literature available up to November 2022. A research study was conducted in the Cochrane reviews database and in the PubMed/MEDLINE database to find the most up to date pieces of evidence and guidelines. We have read and analyzed the results based on the most popular indicators for evaluating classifiers algorithms, such as Accuracy, F1-Score, Sensitivity, and Specificity. With these metrics, it is possible to compare the proposed models in the literature and how they could possibly distinguish COVID-19 patients from other types of diseases or healthy control groups.

1.5. Objectives/Questions for the Review to Address

This review will analyze and compare a variety of computerized systems that detect COVID-19, with the main goal of determining if it is possible to accurately detect COVID-19 without the need for an RT-PCR test, preferably considering noninvasive methods.

2. Methods

2.1. Document Search

The document search was done using Google Scholar as the electronic search engine and was based on available literature from the databases Elsevier, Wiley, Knowledge E, Frontiers Media, SBMU Journals, Jaypee Brothers Medical Publishing, Springer Science and Business Media, MDPI, IEEE, Cold Spring Harbor Laboratory, Tech Science Press, and arXiv. The articles were accepted if they had at least two participant groups: COVID-19 patients and a Control group, and provided at least the metric Accuracy of their model.

The document search was performed between April 2022 and November 2022. The search keywords used were "COVID-19 AI Detection", "COVID-19", "COVID-19 Detection", "COVID-19 detection ECG", "COVID-19 detection X-ray", "COVID-19 detection Voice", "COVID-19 detection ECG Accuracy", "COVID-19 detection X-ray Accuracy", "COVID-19 detection Voice Accuracy", "COVID-19 WHO", "COVID-19 Heart Variable

Rate", "COVID-19 Image processing", "COVID-19 Voice analyzes", "COVID-19 cough detection", "COVID-19 signal processing", "COVID-19 Accuracy", "COVID-19 computerized system", and "COVID-19 breathing detection".

2.2. Search Strategy

The article search process was initialized by searching the Keyword "COVID-19" on Google Scholar. Due to the recent appearance of COVID-19 we limited the search between the years 2020 and 2022, resulting in 483,000 papers. Later, we searched for the keywords "COVID-19 Detection", resulting in 12,000 papers.

For the next step of our search, we took into consideration which parts of the body are the most affected by the disease and searched for the most common biomedical signals/images. We selected X-ray, Voice, and ECG as the biomedical signal/image sources and searched for the keywords "COVID-19 detection ECG" (950 papers), "COVID-19 detection Voice" (2100 papers), and "COVID-19 detection X-ray" (6300 papers).

As the inclusion criterion, we required that the articles must at least use Accuracy as a classification metric. For that we added the keyword "Accuracy" to the previous search, resulting in 855 papers with keywords "COVID-19 detection ECG Accuracy", 1750 papers for the search "COVID-19 detection Voice Accuracy" and 6020 papers for the search "COVID-19 detection X-ray Accuracy".

The exclusion criteria used were to discard state-of-the-art, reviews, systematic reviews, duplicate paper, and irrelevant abstracts, giving us a total of 550 papers.

Of the 550 papers for full-text analysis, 1 paper was removed because it was retracted and 249 papers were rejected because they did not allow public access to the database, did not give an exact number of samples present in the database, or did not indicate the number of samples used for training/testing.

In the final step of our search, 280 papers were removed because they did not provide a code or the applied process was not explained well enough for us to reproduce the proposed methodology. In the end, 20 papers were included in this review.

2.3. Limitations

Our review presents some limitations on the methods applied to obtain the references. For example, the use of Google Scholar as a search engine, although being capable of indicating papers from a variety of different publishers or even being capably of analyzing a full paper, its searching proprieties can present some limitations, e.g., the way we can apply the exclusion criteria, if we ask the search engine to discard state-of-the-art, reviews, and systematic reviews, it may exclude some original research articles because, e.g., "state-of-art" is included in those papers and it is an exclusion keyword. This type of limitation can remove several papers from the search that may present some interesting findings.

Due to the purpose of the present review being concerned with COVID-19 detection by using computerized systems, the code used and classification model are the most important information to provide. With that in mind, another limitation was the lack of documentation or even the sharing of algorithms to make the proposed methodology reproducible, which led to the exclusion of papers that did not provide any way for us to reproduce and fully understand the methodology.

Figure 1 shows the number of papers per publisher obtained for this review.

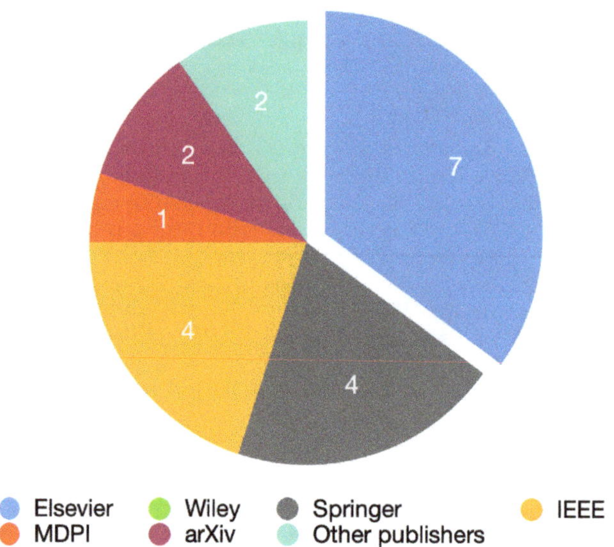

Figure 1. Pie chart with all the publishers used.

2.4. Year of Publication Present in the Review

The publication interval considered papers published between 2020 and 2022. Figure 2 shows the number of selected papers for each year.

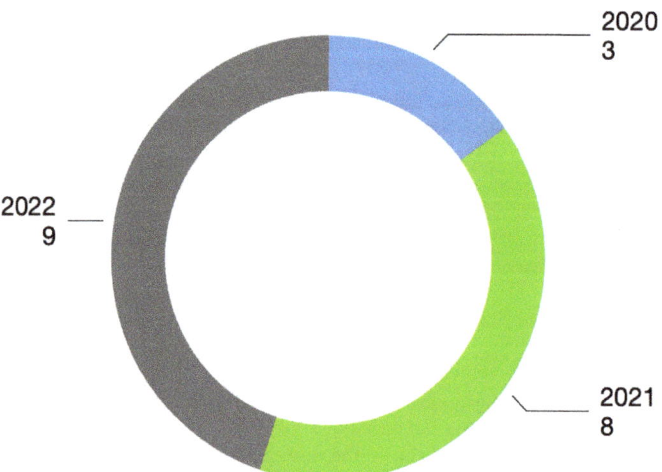

Figure 2. Year of publication.

The papers used in this review investigated the use of three different computerized systems: Voice processing, cardiovascular analysis based on Electrocardiogram (ECG) signal, and pulmonary assessment based on X-ray images.

3. Results

3.1. COVID-19 Detection Based on ECG Processing

Most of the impact of COVID-19 is focused on the respiratory system, but the virus can also cause a variety of cardiac complications, including myocardial injury, heart failure, cardiogenic shock, and cardiac arrhythmias, which shows the importance of ECG [8,9].

ECG is an exam that can monitor the electrical activity of the heart. In the early cases of COVID-19, myocardial Injury was found in patients that were infected with the virus [10].

As one of the most used clinical examination methods, it is of great importance to study the changes in the electrocardiographic activity, as well as to understand the ECG features related to COVID-19 [11].

In a study done in 2020 by Bergamaschi et al. [10], 269 patients were admitted with COVID-19. The ECGs were made at the admission date and after 1 week from hospitalization. The authors evaluated the correlation between ECGs findings and major adverse events (MAE). The study concluded that abnormal ECG at hospitalization and elevated baseline Troponin values were more common in patients who developed MAE. Other studies [11–15] concluded that Troponin is a good indicator to access the severity of the infection and the ECG might be an easy tool for risk stratification in such patients. In the same year, another study done by Angeli et al. [16] concluded that the evolution of ECG abnormalities is independent of the severity of pulmonary tract infection and reflects a wide spectrum of cardiovascular complications.

Looking into the ECG abnormalities, several studies found that the S-T segment alteration was the most frequent ECG finding and signs of left ventricular hypertrophy were associated with a worse prognosis [2,11,14,15], concluding that abnormal T wave or the presence of S-T segment elevation/depression can have a good prognostic in predicting the mortality of COVID-19 patients [11,14,15].

A study carried out by Bassiouni et al. [17] created several deep learning models and classifiers to distinguish COVID-19 from other cardiovascular diseases (CVDs) and Control, having the best Accuracy result of 99.74% with the ECGConvnet being used as a classifier. The ECGConvnet was the proposed system used in this study and it demonstrated that it is possible to develop an automatic diagnosis system for COVID-19 based on deep learning using ECG images.

A study [18] done in 2022 aimed to automatically utilize ECG signals to detect COVID-19. The ECG signal was obtained from ECG paper records, then the electrocardiographic signal was entered as input into a one-dimensional convolutional neural network (1D-CNN), and the authors tried to correctly diagnose the pathologies present in the database. The investigators separated the database into three different classes: COVID-19, Normal, and Other. The Other class contained the diseases myocardial infarction (MI), abnormal heartbeats, and recovered myocardial infarction (RMI). The investigation obtained an Accuracy of 83.17%, an F1-score of 85.38%, a Sensitivity of 84.81%, and a Specificity of 86.28% when using the three classes at the same time as the target.

Another study [19] submitted in 2022 approached the automatic detection of COVID-19 by utilizing models of Convolutional Neural Networks (CNN). The investigators tested the CNN pre-trained models ResNet50, DenseNet-201, VGG16, VGG19, Inceptionv3, and Inceptionresnetv2. ECG pre-processing was performed to eliminate undesirable distortions. Then, a data augmentation technique was implemented as a way to artificially inflate the dataset before entering the CNN models, and from all the models tested in this study, the VGG16 model had the best result of Accuracy with 81.39% for a target containing Normal ECGs and COVID-19 patients.

Attallah [20] investigated the use of Bi-Layers of deep features integration to diagnose COVID-19 based on ECG images. The paper used a methodology with four stages: preprocessing, feature extraction and integration, feature selection, and classification. The features were extracted from the last average pooling layer and the last fully connected layer from some pre-trained CNNs, which were the ResNet-50, the DenseNet-201, the Inception-V3, Xception, and the Inception-ResNet. The study concluded with 98.80% Accuracy, 98.8%

Specificity, and a Sensitivity of 98.8% when doing a Binary classification between Normal ECGs and COVID-19 ECGs. The Multi-class Classification, which was the same class as the Binary plus Abnormal ECGs, had 91.73% Accuracy, 91.80% F1-Score, 95.9% Specificity, and 91.7% Sensitivity.

Sobahi et al. [21] published an article in 2022 that demonstrated an ECG-based COVID-19 detection. The investigators approached the situation with the use of an attention-based 3D CNN model with residual connections (RC). The database that was used contained 12-lead ECG printouts and was distributed between three classes: normal subjects, COVID-19 patients, and patients with abnormal heartbeat (AHB). The CNN model was comprised of 19 layers: 1 image 3D input, 3 3D convolution layers, 3 batch normalization layers, 3 rectified linear unit (ReLu) layers, 2 dropout layers, 2 additional layers, 1 Sigmoid layer, 1 Elementwise Multiplication layer, a fully connected layer, a softmax and classification layers. The study concluded with a Binary Classification (COVID-19 patients vs. Normal subjects) Accuracy of 99% and a Multiclass Classification (Covid patients vs. Normal subjects vs. Abnormal Heartbeat patients) Accuracy of 92%.

An investigation [22] published in 2022 considered a public dataset containing ECG images to diagnose COVID-19. Inside the database, there were five distinct categories, such as normal, COVID-19, MI, AHB, and RMI. They tested six different CNN models as a way to distinguish COVID-19 from the other types of classes. The models were ResNet18, ResNet50, ResNet101, InceptionV3, DenseNet201, and MobileNetv2. The investigators used six different classes: normal, COVID-19, MI, AHB, RMI, and CVDs. They also visualized three different classification schemes: a Binary classification between the normal class and the COVID-19 class, a three-class classification between the normal class, the COVID-19 class, and the CVDs class, and a five-class classification between the normal class, the COVID-19 class, the MI class, the AHB class, and the RMI class. For the Binary classification, the best result was 99.1% Accuracy, for the three-class classification the best Accuracy result was 97.36%, and for the five-class classification the best Accuracy was 97.83%.

Even though COVID-19 is, for the most part, a respiratory or lung disease, the cardiac system can also suffer significant damage. One common complaint of COVID-19 patients is the appearance of palpitations or even the rise of symptoms similar to a heart attack, which includes chest pain, shortness of breath, and Echocardiogram changes [23].

A non-invasive method such as the biomarker Heart Rate Variability (HRV) is a way to assess the Autonomic Nervous System (ANS) activity as an interaction between the respiratory, cardiovascular, and nervous systems, which means that it can be another possible way of studying the difference between COVID-19 and non-COVID-19 patients [24].

A study done by Mishra et al. [25], in 2020 took advantage of the heart rate sensors present on wearable devices. The authors found that elevated resting heart rates and outlying HR/steps measurements were altered, usually in advance of the symptoms.

A study [26] published in 2021 used a methodology in which the data was collected through a smartphone camera using photoplethysmography technology, wrist-worn smartwatches, and wrist-worn bands synchronized with a smartphone app. The investigators used three different classes: Before COVID-19, during COVID-19, and after COVID-19 for patients that used the smartphone app and were positive for the disease. They concluded that there was no statistically significant interaction between the HRV indicators before, during, and after COVID-19 illness. However, they found statistical differences in the standard deviation of normal-to-normal intervals (SDNN) and root mean square of successive normal-to-normal interval differences (RMSSD) for some patients.

Another study done by Hasty et al. [27] compared the levels of C-reactive protein (CRP), which is a marker of systemic inflammation, associated with severe disease in bacterial or viral infections [28], with the SDNN. In this experiment, they used patients that presented hypoxic respiratory failure requiring high-flow nasal cannula or mechanical ventilation, and the experiment was done for seven days. The study concluded that there was a drop of more than 40% in the standard deviation of the interval between heartbeats (SDNN) followed by more than a tripling of CRP in the 72 h that followed.

3.2. COVID-19 Detection Based on Voice Processing

Voice can be diagnosed and analyzed to determine the presence of a respiratory disease [29].

Let us take a look at the use of speech for disease detection. Speech is a complex process that requires the coordination of the brain, muscles, and respiratory system. The smallest changes in a person's speech may be the early signs of a disease, for example, a disease such as Parkinson's, which can be associated with tremors of the vocal cords [30].

One of the focal areas for COVID-19 is the lungs. The virus can cause lung complications such as pneumonia or even acute respiratory distress syndrome. For example, the use of systems to detect the slight changes in our voices that we humans are unable to hear is extremely important to detect a pathology that can provoke breathing difficulties [31].

Voice signal as a way to detect COVID-19 might be used not only with speech but also with coughing. Cough detection can be used to differentiate coughing sounds, and the coughing produced by COVID-19 is possibly one of the ways to go for the detection of the pathology [32–34].

An article [35] published in 2022 demonstrated the possibility of detecting COVID-19 through coughing. In this study, the researchers used four different classes: COVID-19 positive, COVID-19 negative, non-COVID-19 subjects, and non-COVID subjects with pertussis cough. The study demonstrated the feasibility of the automatic diagnosis of COVID-19 from coughs with an Accuracy, F1-Score, Specificity, and Sensitivity close to 90%, using Random Forest as the classifier.

Another study [36] from 2021 investigated the use of symbolic recurrence quantification measures with MFCC features for the automatic detection of COVID-19 in cough sounds of healthy and sick individuals. The investigators used the XGBoost as the classifier and the results obtained by the created model achieved an Accuracy of 99% with an F1-Score of 69%, for sustained vowels.

A study carried out by Dash et al. [37] developed a new feature that they called COVID-19 Coefficient (C-19CC). In speech recognition, the normal frequency scale to the perceptual frequency scale and the frequency range of the filter values are fixed. The characteristics of speech signals vary from disease to disease. In the case of the detection of COVID-19, mainly the coughing sounds, the bandwidth, and properties are quite different from the complete speech signal. The Accuracy result for C-19CC was 85.70% while using SVM to classify coughing sounds.

Atmaja et al. [38] submitted a paper in 2022 related to COVID-19 detection through coughing. The investigators proposed a transfer learning approach as a way to improve the performance of COVID-19 detection by incorporating cough detection, cough segmentation, and data augmentation. Cough detection was used to remove non-cough signals. Cough segmentation was used to segregate several coughs in a waveform into individual coughs and data augmentation was used to increase the number of samples used for deep learning. The investigators used three different datasets, Coswara, COUGHVID, and ComParE-CCS, having a total of 2026 samples, after cough detection and cough segmentation. The study used the Mel spectrogram to get the feature of the acoustic signal. The study concluded with an Accuracy of 88.19% using the CNN14 as a classifier, which is a Convolutional Neural Network that has 14 layers between the input layer and the output layer.

In 2020, a study done by Imran et al. [39] compared different types of cough and used artificial intelligence to distinguish patients with COVID-19 and patients without COVID-19. The study concluded that it is possible to create an app that can accurately distinguish COVID-19 and non COVID-19 patients by using Deep Transfer Learning-based Multi Class classifier, having an Accuracy of 92.64%.

Verde et al. [40] compared the performance of some machine learning techniques to correctly detect COVID-19 by analyzing the voice. The study, published in 2021, used a crowd-sourced database named Coswara, which is a database present on the GitHub platform and contains samples of coughing, breathing, and voice sounds from each subject. The investigators evaluated the sustained phonation of the vowels "a", "e", and "o", because it avoided any linguistic artifacts due to the different languages present in the database. The features that were extracted from the voice samples were Fundamental Frequency (F^0), Jitter and Shimmer, Harmonic to Noise Ratio (HNR), Mel-Frequency Cepstral Coefficients (MFCC), First and second derivatives of cepstral coefficient, Spectral Centroid (SC), and Spectral Roll-off (SR). The Machine Learning techniques used were divided into several groups, which were Bayes, Functions, Lazy, Meta, Rules, and Trees. The investigation concluded with the SVM Algorithm, present in the Machine Learning Functions, having the best overall result, obtaining an Accuracy of 97.07%, an F1-score of 82.35%, and a Specificity of 97.37%.

Silva et al. [41] used the Coswara dataset to extract features, such as Energy, Entropies, Correlation Dimension, Detrended Fluctuation Analysis, Lyapunov Exponent, and Fractal Dimensions, in a multi-band analysis done by Wavelet Transform. After the extraction, a feature selection was made and the selected features served as entries for an ensemble machine learning model (XGBoost). The classification results presented accuracies higher than 83%, obtained for all Binary pairs, with a special mention to the pair Healthy control vs. all stages of COVID-19, which had been discriminated with an Accuracy of 98.46%.

3.3. COVID-19 Detection Based on Image Processing

Image processing is the process of obtaining visible images of the inner body structure. The goal of this process is its use for scientific and medicinal purposes, as well as, tissue visual representation [42].

The use of Image processing is an interesting way to approach the diagnosis of COVID-19 because of the virus nature. The pathology can cause damage to the lungs and with the use of equipment such as Computed Tomography (CT) Scanners that can create an image of the affected organ, it can be used to complement the already existing diagnosis exams [43].

A research done by Salman et al. [44] aimed to construct a model by using deep learning tools for detecting COVID-19 pneumonia on high-resolution X-rays. The investigators used a CNN InceptionV3 as the classifier and obtained an Accuracy of 100%, which is a comparable performance against expert radiologists.

In another study conducted by DeGrave et al. [45], the researchers used Artificial intelligence (AI) to demonstrate that deep learning systems can detect COVID-19 from chest radiographs. They concluded that the deep learning models rely on confounding factors rather than medical pathology, which means that the systems appear accurate with the used dataset but failed when tested with new data.

In 2021, an investigation was conducted using AI and X-rays images. Öztaş et al. [46] compared the detection of COVID-19 between X-ray images and Blood test data. The study used ResNet-18 and squeezenet as training models to classify the images and a multi-layer neural network to diagnose the blood test. The researchers concluded that the ResNet-18 performs slightly better than squeezenet even though both have obtained almost 98% Accuracy. When comparing the X-ray methodology to the blood test methodology, The radio-graphic images performed better, having an Accuracy of almost 98%, compared to the 72% Accuracy obtained using the multi-layer neural network for the blood test.

Wu et al. [47] published an article about the use of deep Convolutional Neural Networks (CNNs) to diagnose positive COVID-19 cases, using X-ray images as their input. The proposed architectures for the CNN followed a simple LeNet-5, where the two structures were *in_6c_2p_12c_2p* and *in_8c_2p_16c_2p*. Each structure had the number of input nodes and c or p for the type of layers, which in this case were the convolution and pooling layers, respectively. This article obtained a final Accuracy of 98.83%, demonstrating that this can be another possible research direction.

Another study [48], also done with X-ray images, illustrated an automated diagnosis model from a dataset of X-ray images of patients with severe bacterial pneumonia, reported COVID-19 disease, and normal cases. The findings in this article indicate that deep learning with X-ray imagery could retrieve important biomarkers relevant for COVID-19 disease detection, obtaining a 96.73% of Accuracy on a modified ResNet-18.

Using the same type of images as the previously referred articles related to Image Processing, a paper [49] was done where the researchers used a methodology based on the deep feature plus support vector machine (SVM). The dataset was separated into three categories: COVID-19, pneumonia, and normal. The highest Accuracy was 98.66%, achieved by a combination of ResNet50 plus SVM.

Fang et al. [50] investigated the use of classifiers to identify positive cases of COVID-19. The article that was published in 2021, used chest x-ray images as input for the classifiers and they proposed a multi-stage residual network, named MSRCovXNet, for effective detection of the pathology. The investigators also used ResNet-18 as the feature extractor. The proposed network was optimized by fusing two feature enhancement modules, one containing local information and the other containing semantic information. The network obtained a precision of 98.90% for the detection of COVID-19 and, when using the COVIDGR dataset as the input, an average Accuracy of 82.20% was achieved.

An article [51] published in 2020 proposed an alternative method to determine the COVID-19 cases from normal or abnormal cases by using X-ray images. The investigators proposed the use of an enhanced cuckoo search optimization algorithm (CS) using fractional-order calculus (FO) and four different heavy-tailed distributions: the Mittag-Leffler distribution, Cauchy distribution, Pareto distribution, and Weibull distribution. The classification, done by using a KNN model, contained three classes: normal patients, COVID-19-infected patients, and pneumonia patients. The experiment used 18 different datasets and the best Accuracy result was 100%.

Table 1 indicates the strategy used in state-of-the-art methods to diagnose COVID-19 and Table 2 presents the discrimination rates of the previously presented methods.

Table 1. State-of-the-art methods of the present review.

Ref.	Dataset	Data Augmentation	Source	Features	Machine Learning Classifier	Cross-Validation
[17]	ECG images dataset of cardiac and COVID-19 patients (1937 records)	Yes	ECG	Feature extraction from ECGConvnet (transfer learning)	ECGConvnet	Yes
[18]	ECG images dataset of cardiac and COVID-19 patients (1937 records)	No	ECG	Feature extraction from SERes-Net18 (transfer learning)	SEResNet18	Yes
[19]	ECG images dataset of cardiac and COVID-19 patients (1937 records)	Yes	ECG	Feature extraction with VGG16 pre-trained (transfer learning)	CNN VGG16	Yes
[20]	ECG images dataset of cardiac and COVID-19 patients (1937 records)	Yes	ECG	ResNet-50, Inception V3, Xception, InceptionResNet and DenseNet-201 pre-tained feature extraction (transfer learning)	ECG-BiCoNet (CNN)	Yes
[21]	ECG images dataset of cardiac and COVID-19 patients (1937 records)	Yes	ECG	Feature extraction from 3D CNN (transfer learning)	3D CNN	Yes
[22]	ECG images dataset of cardiac and COVID-19 patients (1937 records)	Yes	ECG	Feature extraction from InceptionV3 pre-trained (transfer learning)	CNN	Yes
[35]	UdL+UC+Coswara+Virufy+Pertussis (813 samples)	Yes	Voice	Energy, instantaneous frequency, instantaneous frequency peak, Shannon entropy, instantaneous entropy, spectral information entropy, spectral information, and kurtosis	Random Forest	Yes
[36]	Corona Voice Detect project with Voca.ai (3415 samples)	Yes	Voice	Mel frequency cepstral coefficients	XGBoost	Yes
[37]	Crowd-sourced Respiratory Sound Data	Yes	Voice	C-19CC	SVM	Yes
[38]	Coswara + COUGHVID + ComPare-CCS (2026 samples)	Yes	Voice	Log Mel Spectrogram	CNN14	No
[39]	ESC-50 (5435 samples)	No	Voice	Mel frequency cepstral coefficients	Deep Transfer Learning-based Multi Class classifier	Yes

Table 1. *Cont.*

Ref.	Dataset	Data Augmentation	Source	Features	Machine Learning Classifier	Cross-Validation
[40]	Coswara database (1027 samples)	No	Voice	Fundamental frequency, jitter and shimmer, harmonic to noise ratio, mel-frequency cepstral coefficients, first and second derivatives of cepstral coefficient, spectral centroid and spectral Roll-off	SVM	No
[41]	Coswara database (909 samples)	No	Voice	Energy, entropies, correlation dimension, detrended fluctuation analysis, Lyapunov Exponent and fractal dimensions	XGBoost	Yes
[46]	Covid chestxray dataset + Chex Pert dataset (5370 samples)	No	X-ray	Feature extraction from Resnet18 pre-trained (transfer learning)	Resnet18	Yes
[47]	Covid chestxray dataset + Chex Pert dataset (5184 samples)	Yes	X-ray	Feature extraction from LetNet-5 (transfer learning)	Extreme Learning Machine	No
[44]	Covid chestxray dataset + Kaggle repository + Open-i repository (160 samples)	Yes	X-ray	Deep feature extraction based on VGG16, ResNet50 and InceptionV3 (transfer learning)	CNN Inceptionv3	No
[48]	Covid chestxray dataset + Labeled Optical Coherence Tomography + Chest X-ray Images for Classification	Yes	X-ray	Feature extraction from CNN (transfer learning)	Modified ResNet-18	No
[49]	Covid chestxray dataset + Kaggle repository (50 samples)	Yes	X-ray	Feature extracted by CNN ResNet50 (transfer learning)	SVM	No
[50]	Covidx Dataset (14,003 samples)	Yes	X-ray	Feature extracted by ResNet-18 (transfer learning)	MSRCovXNet (multi-stage residual network)	Yes
[51]	COVID-19 CHEST X-RAY DATABASE+ COVID-19 Database + COVID-Chestxray Database + ChestX-ray8 + chest-xray-pneumonia (1560 samples)	No	X-ray	Contrast, correlation, energy, entropy, homogeneity, Mittag-Leffler distribution, Pareto distribution, and Cauchy distribution	KNN	No

Table 2. State-of-the-art methods that fit on the present review - discrimination rates (N/A: not applicable).

Ref.	Accuracy	F1-Score	Sensitivity	Specificity
[17]	99.74%	99.70%	99.70%	≈100%
[18]	83.17%	85.38%	84.81%	86.28%
[19]	81.39%	N/A	N/A	N/A
[20]	91.73%	91.80%	91.70%	95.90%
[21]	92.00%	92.03%	95.99%	92.00%
[22]	97.83%	97.82%	97.83%	98.86%
[35]	85.53%	85.58%	85.96%	85.09%
[36]	99.00%	69.00%	70.00%	N/A
[37]	85.70%	N/A	N/A	N/A
[38]	88.19%	N/A	N/A	N/A
[39]	92.64%	92.66%	92.64%	97.55%
[40]	97.07%	82.35%	93.33%	97.37%
[41]	98.46%	N/A	N/A	N/A
[46]	≈98%	N/A	N/A	N/A
[47]	98.83%	N/A	N/A	N/A
[44]	100%	100%	100%	100%
[48]	96.73%	N/A	N/A	N/A
[49]	95.38%	95.52%	97.29%	93.47%
[50]	82.20%	N/A	N/A	N/A
[51]	100%	N/A	N/A	N/A

4. Discussion

The main objective of this review was to answer the following research question: is it possible to accurately detect COVID-19 without the need for an RT-PCR test, preferably considering noninvasive methods?

4.1. ECG Processing

Looking into Table 2, in the articles related to the ECG [17–22], we can see high Accuracy results on all articles, with the lowest percentage being 81.39% and the highest percentage being 99.74%. The majority of the articles presented four discrimination metrics and just one provided Accuracy as the only metric.

Refs. [17,18,20–22] presented the metric F1-score. In these articles, we saw values ranging from 85.38% to 99.70%, which means that some models could correctly predict all the classes or had slight difficulty detecting some classes.

Of all the articles that had four metrics, the article by Nguyen et al. had the least favorable results, with Accuracy presenting 83.17% as the lowest percentage and Specificity obtained 86.28% as the highest result. These results demonstrated that some classes were not classified correctly.

4.2. Voice Processing

Looking into Table 2, in the articles related to the Voice signal [35–41], three articles presented Accuracy as the only metric. In those articles, the results of Accuracy were 85.70% and 98.46%, demonstrating that they have high Accuracy but are not able to correctly detect all the predicted classes.

The other three articles presented the Accuracy and the F1-score. The first article presented an Accuracy of 99.00% and an F1-score of 69.00%. The second article showed an Accuracy of 92.64% and an F1-score of 92.66%. The third article presented an Accuracy of 97.07% and an F1-score of 82.35%. The three articles presented high Accuracy percentage results but the first article demonstrated the lowest F1-Score result, indicating a low recall and precision, which is confirmed by the Sensitivity of 70.00%.

Three articles presented the four metrics, 85.53% Accuracy, 85.58% F1-score, 85.96% Sensitivity, 85.09% Specificity, 92.64% of Accuracy, 92.66% F1-score, 92.64% Sensitivity and 97.55% Specificity and 97.07% Accuracy, 82.35% F1-score, 93.33% Sensitivity and 97.37% Specificity, respectively. By looking into the four metrics at the same time, we can see high results for all the metrics but the articles done by Tena et al. had an overall higher difficulty to classify some tests.

4.3. X-ray Processing

Regarding the articles related to X-ray [44,46–51] presented in Table 2, five articles showed Accuracy as the only metric to evaluate the models. The Accuracy results ranged between 82.2% and 100%, which shows, in some models, difficulty in correctly predicting the classes.

The article by Sethy et al. showed three additional metrics apart from Accuracy. The results showed 95.38% Accuracy, 95.52% F1-score, 97.29% Sensitivity, and 93.47% Specificity. With this high percentage, we can see the false positive having a greater impact, making the F1-Score and the Specificity have a lower percentage when compared to the Accuracy.

Salman et al. used a model that gave us four metrics: Accuracy, F1-Score, Sensitivity, and Specificity. The results were 100% in all metrics, which shows that the model can predict all classes without difficulties. However, by combining training, validation, and testing there was a total of 160 X-ray images. Despite the nice methodology flow, conclusions about the results (100% Accuracy) should be carefully done, as the relatively small dataset is not good enough for being split it into testing, training, and validation groups for drawing conclusions.

4.4. Critical Analysis for the Selected Papers

The performance results presented in Table 2 show some interesting values. However, we note that there is a good portion of the paper that needed to perform data augmentation as a way to artificially increase the number of samples, especially for the COVID-19 classes. This type of process can lead to an overfitting set of results, meaning that the same samples can be used for the training and testing stages, which leads to an increase in the discrimination rates.

A direct comparison between papers was not possible, even though there are a couple of articles that share the same database. This is due to the use of data augmentation, which was referred to in the previous paragraph, the use of different features, as some were extracted from the pre-trained classifier, and the use of a smaller sample size for the training/testing, making it impossible to know if the same sample was used between papers that used the same database.

5. Conclusions

Even though COVID-19 already has different types of vaccines, the quick and accurate detection of the pathology is extremely important for the prevention of worst-case scenarios.

In this paper, we have reviewed a few articles related to three different types of computerized diagnostic support systems: ECG (including Heart Rate Variability), Voice, and X-ray.

We conclude that the computerized detection of COVID-19 already has promising results in the literature, showing that it might be possible to detect the disease without the need for an RT-PCR test. However, there is still room for improvement, given the vast symptomatology and better comprehension of an individual's evolution of the disease.

Future Directions

The goals defined for this review were accomplished, however for future directions, it would be interesting to combine a variety of research engines and analyze the existing methodologies for the COVID-19 prognosis.

Another contribution that we believe will bring a huge benefit is the increase of the number of public databases available and that the sample size of those databases should be enlarged, especially for the COVID-19 positive groups. This would make the algorithms already developed more robust, paving the way for their implementation in clinical settings.

Author Contributions: Conceptualization, P.R., J.A.L.M. and P.M.R.; methodology, P.R.; validation, P.M.R. and J.A.L.M.; writing—original, P.R.; writing—review and editing, P.M.R. and J.A.L.M.; supervision, J.A.L.M. and P.M.R.; funding acquisition, P.M.R. All authors have read and agreed to the published version of the manuscript.

Funding: This research was funded by National Funds from FCT—Fundação para a Ciência e a Tecnologia through projects UIDB/50016/2020.

Institutional Review Board Statement: Not applicable.

Informed Consent Statement: Not applicable.

Data Availability Statement: Not applicable.

Conflicts of Interest: The authors declare no conflict of interest.

References

1. WHO Coronavirus (COVID-19) Dashboard. Available online: https://covid19.who.int/ (accessed on 22 August 2022).
2. Mehraeen, E.; Alinaghi, S.; Nowroozi, A.; Dadras, O.; Alilou, S.; Shobeiri, P.; Behnezhad, F.; Karimi, A. A systematic review of ECG findings in patients with COVID-19. *Indian Heart J.* **2020**, *72*, 500–507. [CrossRef]
3. Yesudhas, D.; Srivastava, A.; Gromiha, M. COVID-19 outbreak: history, mechanism, transmission, structural studies and therapeutics. *Infection* **2020**, *49*, 199–213. [CrossRef] [PubMed]

4. Hosseini, E.; Kashani, N.; Nikzad, H.; Azadbakht, J.; Bafrani, H.; Kashani, H. The novel coronavirus Disease-2019 (COVID-19): Mechanism of action, detection and recent therapeutic strategies. *Virology* **2020**, *551*, 1–9. [CrossRef]

5. Ciotti, M.; Ciccozzi, M.; Terrinoni, A.; Jiang, W.; Wang, C.; Bernardini, S. The COVID-19 pandemic. *Crit. Rev. Clin. Lab. Sci.* **2020**, *57*, 365–388. [CrossRef] [PubMed]

6. Chinitz, J.; Goyal, R.; Harding, M.; Veseli, G.; Gruberg, L.; Jadonath, R.; Maccaro, P.; Gandotra, P.; Ong, L.; Epstein, L. Bradyarrhythmias in patients with COVID-19: Marker of poor prognosis? *Pacing Clin. Electrophysiol.* **2020**, *43*, 1199–1204. [CrossRef] [PubMed]

7. Lai, C.; Lam, W. Laboratory testing for the diagnosis of COVID-19. *Biochem. Biophys. Res. Commun.* **2021**, *538*, 226–230. [CrossRef]

8. Long, B.; Brady, W.; Bridwell, R.; Ramzy, M.; Montrief, T.; Singh, M.; Gottlieb, M. Electrocardiographic manifestations of COVID-19. *Am. J. Emerg. Med.* **2021**, *538*, 96–103. [CrossRef]

9. COVID-19: Cardiac Manifestations in Adults. Available online: https://www.uptodate.com/contents/covid-19-cardiac-manifestations-in-adults (accessed on 31 October 2022).

10. Bergamaschi, L.; D'Angelo, E.; Paolisso, P.; Toniolo, S.; Fabrizio, M.; Angeli, F.; Donati, F.; Magnani, I.; Rinaldi, A.; Bartoli, L.; et al. The value of ECG changes in risk stratification of COVID-19 patients. *Ann. Noninvasive Electrocardiol.* **2021**, *26*, e12815. [CrossRef] [PubMed]

11. Wang, Y.; Chen, L.; Wang, J.; He, X.; Huang, F.; Chen, J.; Yang, X. Electrocardiogram analysis of patients with different types of COVID-19. *Ann. Noninvasive Electrocardiol.* **2020**, *25*, e12806. [CrossRef]

12. Chorin, E.; Dai, M.; Kogan, E.; Wadhwani, L.; Shulman, E.; Nadeau-Routhier, C.; Knotts, R.; Bar-Cohen, R.; Barbhaiya, C.; Aizer, A.; et al. Electrocardiographic risk stratification in COVID-19 patients. *Front. Cardiovasc. Med.* **2021**, *8*, 636073. [CrossRef]

13. Yang, D.; Li, J.; Gao, P.; Chen, T.; Cheng, Z.; Cheng, K.; Deng, H.; Fang, Q.; Yi, C.; Fan, H.; et al. The prognostic significance of electrocardiography findings in patients with coronavirus disease 2019: A retrospective study. *Clin. Cardiol.* **2021**, *44*, 963–970. [CrossRef]

14. Aghajani, M.; Toloui, A.; Aghamohammadi, M.; Pourhoseingholi, A.; Taherpour, N.; Sistanizad, M.; Neishaboori, A.; Asadpoordezaki, Zi.; Miri, R. Electrocardiographic findings and in-hospital mortality of COVID-19 patients; a retrospective cohort study. *Arch. Acad. Emerg. Med.* **2021**, *9*, e45.

15. Kaliyaperumal, D.; Bhargavi, K.; Ramaraju, K.; Nair, K.; Ramalingam, S.; Alagesan, M. Electrocardiographic Changes in COVID-19 Patients: A Hospital-based Descriptive Study. *Indian J. Crit. Care Med.* **2022**, *26*, 43–48. [CrossRef] [PubMed]

16. Angeli, F.; Spanevello, A.; Ponti, R.; Visca, D.; Marazzato, J.; Palmiotto, G.; Feci, D.; Reboldi, G.; Fabbri, L.; Verdecchia, P. Electrocardiographic features of patients with COVID-19 pneumonia. *Eur. J. Intern. Med.* **2020**, *78*, 101–106. [CrossRef]

17. Bassiouni, M.; Hegazy, I.; Rizk, N.; El-Dahshan, E.; Salem, A. Automated Detection of COVID-19 Using Deep Learning Approaches with Paper-Based ECG Reports. *Circuits Syst. Signal Process.* **2022**, *41*, 5535–5577. [CrossRef] [PubMed]

18. Nguyen, T.; Pham, H.; Le, H.; Nguyen, A.; Thanh, N.; Do, C. Detecting COVID-19 from digitized ECG printouts using 1D convolutional neural networks. *PLoS ONE* **2022**, *17*, e0277081. [CrossRef]

19. Shahin, I.; Nassif, A.; Alsabek, M. COVID-19 Electrocardiograms Classification using CNN Models. In Proceedings of the 2021 14th International Conference on Developments in eSystems Engineering (DeSE), Sharjah, United Arab Emirates, 7–10 December 2021.

20. Attallah, O. ECG-BiCoNet: An ECG-based pipeline for COVID-19 diagnosis using Bi-Layers of deep features integration. *Comput. Biol. Med.* **2022**, *142*, 105210. [CrossRef]

21. Sobahi, N. Attention-based 3D CNN with residual connections for efficient ECG-based COVID-19 detection. *Comput. Biol. Med.* **2022**, *143*, 105335. [CrossRef]

22. Rahman, T. COV-ECGNET: COVID-19 detection using ECG trace images with deep convolutional neural network. *Health Inf. Sci. Syst.* **2022**, *10*, 1. [CrossRef]

23. Heart Problems after COVID-19. Available online: https://www.hopkinsmedicine.org/health/conditions-and-diseases/coronavirus/heart-problems-after-covid19 (accessed on 25 October 2022).

24. Heart Rate Variability Disturbances and Biofeedback Treatment in COVID-19 Survivors. Available online: https://www.escardio.org/Journals/E-Journal-of-Cardiology-Practice/Volume-21/heart-rate-variability-disturbances-and-biofeedback-treatment-in-covid-19-surviv (accessed on 25 October 2022).

25. Mishra, T.; Wang, M.; Metwally, A.; Bogu, G.; Brooks, A.; Bahmani, A.; Alavi, A.; Celli, A.; Higgs, E.; Dagan-Rosenfeld, O.; et al. Early detection of COVID-19 using a smartwatch. *medRxiv* **2020**, *in press*.

26. Ponomarev, A.; Tyapochkin, K.; Surkova, E.; Smorodnikova, E.; Pravdin, P. Heart Rate Variability as a Prospective Predictor of Early COVID-19 Symptoms. *medRxiv* **2021**, *in press*.

27. Hasty, F.; Garcia, G.; Dávila, H.; Wittels, S.; Hendricks, S.; Chong, S. Heart Rate Variability as a Possible Predictive Marker for Acute Inflammatory Response in COVID-19 Patients. *Mil. Med.* **2021**, *186*, e34–e38. [CrossRef] [PubMed]

28. Smilowitz, N.; Kunichoff, D.; Garshick, M.; Shah, B.; Pillinger, M.; Hochman, J.; Berger, J. C-reactive protein and clinical outcomes in patients with COVID-19. *Eur. Heart J.* **2021**, *42*, 2270—2279. [CrossRef]

29. Hassan, A.; Shahin, I.; Alsabek, M. COVID-19 Detection System using Recurrent Neural Networks. In Proceedings of the 2020 International Conference on Communications, Computing, Cybersecurity, and Informatics (CCCI), Sharjah, United Arab Emirates, 3–5 November 2020; pp. 1–5.

30. Diagnosing Disease by Voice. Available online: https://www.pfizer.com/news/articles/diagnosing_disease_by_voice (accessed on 24 October 2022).

31. COVID-19 Lung Damage. Available online: https://www.hopkinsmedicine.org/health/conditions-and-diseases/coronavirus/what-coronavirus-does-to-the-lungs (accessed on 24 October 2022).

32. Deshpande, G.; Schuller, B. An overview on audio, signal, speech, & language processing for COVID-19. *arXiv* **2020**, arXiv:2005.08579.

33. Feng, K.; He, F.; Steinmann, J.; Demirkiran, I. Deep-learning Based Approach to Identify COVID-19. In Proceedings of the SoutheastCon 2021, Atlanta, GA, USA, 10–13 March 2021; pp. 1–4.

34. Despotovic, V. Detection of COVID-19 from voice, cough and breathing patterns: Dataset and preliminary results. *Comput. Biol. Med.* **2021**, *138*, 104944. [CrossRef]

35. Tena, A.; Clarià, F.; Solsona, F. Automated detection of COVID-19 cough. *Biomed. Signal Process. Control* **2022**, *71*, 103175. [CrossRef]

36. Mouawad, P.; Dubnov, T.; Dubnov, S. Robust detection of COVID-19 in cough sounds. *SN Comput. Sci.* **2021**, *2*, 34. [CrossRef] [PubMed]

37. Dash, T.; Mishra, S.; Panda, G.; Satapathy, S. Detection of COVID-19 from speech signal using bio-inspired based cepstral features. *Pattern Recognit.* **2021**, *117*, 107999. [CrossRef]

38. Atmaja, B.; Zanjabila, S.; Sasou, A. Cross-dataset COVID-19 Transfer Learning with Cough Detection, Cough Segmentation, and Data Augmentation. *arXiv* **2022**, arXiv:2210.05843.

39. Imran, A.; Posokhova, I.; Qureshi, H.; Masood, U.; Riaz, M.; Ali, K.; John, C.; Hussain, M.; Nabeel, M. AI4COVID-19: AI enabled preliminary diagnosis for COVID-19 from cough samples via an app. *Inform. Med. Unlocked* **2020**, *20*, 100378. [CrossRef]

40. Verde, L.; Pietro, G.; Ghoneim, A.; Alrashoud, M.; Al-Mutib, K.; Sannino, G. Exploring the Use of Artificial Intelligence Techniques to Detect the Presence of Coronavirus COVID-19 Through Speech and Voice Analysis. *IEEE Access* **2021**, *9*, 65750–65757. [CrossRef]

41. Silva, G.; Batista, P.; Rodrigues, P.M. COVID-19 activity screening by a smart-data-driven multi-band voice analysis. *J. Voice* **2022**, *in press*. [CrossRef]

42. Abdallah, Y.; Alqahtani, T. Research in Medical Imaging Using Image Processing Techniques. In *Medical Imaging—Principles and Applications*; IntechOpen: London, UK, 2019.

43. Tello-Mijares, S.; Woo, L. Computed Tomography Image Processing Analysis in COVID-19 Patient Follow-Up Assessment. *J. Healthc. Eng.* **2021**, *2021*, 8869372. [CrossRef] [PubMed]

44. Salman, F.; Abu-Naser, S.; Alajrami, E.; Abu-Nasser, B.; Alashqar, B. COVID-19 detection using artificial intelligence. *Int. J. Acad. Eng. Res.* **2020**, *4*, 18–25.

45. DeGrave, A.; Janizek, J.; Lee, S. AI for radiographic COVID-19 detection selects shortcuts over signal. *Nat. Mach. Intell.* **2021**, *3*, 610–619. [CrossRef]

46. Öztaş, A.; Boncukcu, D.; Ozteke, E.; Demir, M.; Mirici, A.; Mutlu, P. Covid19 Diagnosis: Comparative Approach Between Chest X-ray and Blood Test Data. In Proceedings of the 2021 6th International Conference on Computer Science and Engineering (UBMK), Ankara, Turkey, 15–17 September 2021; Volume 6, pp. 472–477.

47. Wu, C.; Khishe, M.; Mohammadi, M.; Karim, S.; Rashid, T. Evolving deep convolutional neutral network by hybrid sine–cosine and extreme learning machine for real-time COVID19 diagnosis from X-ray images. *Soft Comput* **2021**, *25*, 1–20. [CrossRef]

48. Al-Falluji, R.; Katheeth, Z.; Alathari, B. Automatic detection of COVID-19 using chest X-ray images and modified ResNet18-based convolutional neural networks. *Comput. Mater. Contin.* **2021**, *66*, 1301–1313.

49. Sethy, P.; Behera, S. Detection of coronavirus disease (COVID-19) based on deep features. *IJMEMS* **2020**, *5*, 643–651.

50. Fang, Z.; Ren, J.; MacLellan, C.; Li, H.; Zhao, H.; Hussain, A.; Fortino, G. A Novel Multi-Stage Residual Feature Fusion Network for Detection of COVID-19 in Chest X-ray Images. *IEEE Trans. Mol. Biol. Multi-Scale Commun.* **2022**, *8*, 17–27. [CrossRef]

51. Yousri, D.; Elaziz, M.; Abualigah, L.; Oliva, D.; Al-qaness, M.; Ewees, A. COVID-19 X-ray images classification based on enhanced fractional-order cuckoo search optimizer using heavy-tailed distributions . *Appl. Soft Comput.* **2020**, *101*, 107052. [CrossRef] [PubMed]

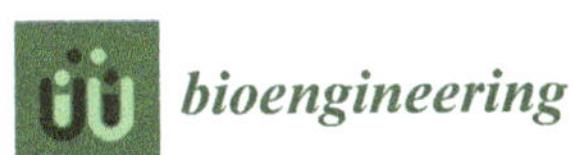 *bioengineering*

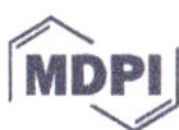

Article

ECG Measurement Uncertainty Based on Monte Carlo Approach: An Effective Analysis for a Successful Cardiac Health Monitoring System

Jackson Henrique Braga da Silva [1], Paulo Cesar Cortez [1], Senthil K. Jagatheesaperumal [2] and Victor Hugo C. de Albuquerque [1,*]

[1]   Department of Teleinformatics Engineering, Federal University of Ceará, Fortaleza 60455-970, Brazil
[2]   Department of Electronics and Communication Engineering, Mepco Schlenk Engineering College, Sivakasi 626005, India
*   Correspondence: victor.albuquerque@ieee.org; Tel.: +55-85-985-246-835

Abstract: Measurement uncertainty is one of the widespread concepts applied in scientific works, particularly to estimate the accuracy of measurement results and to evaluate the conformity of products and processes. In this work, we propose a methodology to analyze the performance of measurement systems existing in the design phases, based on a probabilistic approach, by applying the Monte Carlo method (MCM). With this approach, it is feasible to identify the dominant contributing factors of imprecision in the evaluated system. In the design phase, this information can be used to identify where the most effective attention is required to improve the performance of equipment. This methodology was applied over a simulated electrocardiogram (ECG), for which a measurement uncertainty of the order of 3.54% of the measured value was estimated, with a confidence level of 95%. For this simulation, the ECG computational model was categorized into two modules: the preamplifier and the final stage. The outcomes of the analysis show that the preamplifier module had a greater influence on the measurement results over the final stage module, which indicates that interventions in the first module would promote more significant performance improvements in the system. Finally, it was identified that the main source of ECG measurement uncertainty is related to the measurand, focused towards the objective of better characterization of the metrological behavior of the measurements in the ECG.

Keywords: Measurement uncertainty; Monte Carlo method; ECG; Cardiac health

Citation: Silva, J.H.B.d.; Cortez, P.C.; Jagatheesaperumal, S.K.; de Albuquerque, V.H.C. ECG Measurement Uncertainty Based on Monte Carlo Approach: An Effective Analysis for a Successful Cardiac Health Monitoring System. *Bioengineering* **2023**, *10*, 115. https://doi.org/10.3390/bioengineering10010115

Academic Editors: Pedro Miguel Rodrigues, João Alexandre Lobo Marques and João Paulo do Vale Madeiro

Received: 7 December 2022
Revised: 7 January 2023
Accepted: 11 January 2023
Published: 13 January 2023

1. Introduction

The field of medicine has considerably evolved with the help of engineering and the development of systems capable of monitoring patients and measuring their vital signs so that decisions can be made by a specialist regarding the care of that patient. In this context, the instruments used to measure and monitor a patient's vital signs play a critical role, which requires great reliability in their measurement results. Small variations or ranges of uncertainties related to the measurement results of these instruments can lead to catastrophic effects [1]. Thus, focusing on the bioengineering perspective, measurement devices must be reliable and robust to manage such uncertainties [2].

With the current issues in the context of the analysis and development of measurement systems, one of the ways to assess the quality of measurement results is through the evaluation of the uncertainty related to the obtained results [3]. The analysis of measurement uncertainty is a task that can be applied in research and development, with several domains of knowledge acquired through theoretical, empirical, or hybrid studies [4].

Several recent works, such as [5–7], performed measurement uncertainty analyses to validate measurement systems and/or methods. In these works, uncertainty was used with the objective of evaluating the confidence level of the results or with the objective of comparing results obtained from different methods. In works such as [8,9], measurement uncertainty was used as a basis for decision making and conformity assessment. It is noteworthy that the work in [9] proposed a method for which the measurement uncertainty analysis showed the need to improve the metrological performance of the method with a target value for the measurement uncertainty, which is one of the recommendations in [4].

On the other hand, in many recent works such as [10,11], how the uncertainty analysis was performed or even the uncertainty of the presented results was not indicated. These works addressed various measurement methods in which, not necessarily, the measurement system was the focus. However, much attention is drawn to the fact that many other recent works, such as [12–14], proposed a new sensor or a new measurement system, none of which showed how the measurement uncertainty was analyzed.

Approaching it in a more specific way, the state of the art of uncertainty analysis of ECG measurement, which will be the object of study of this work, is highlighted in works such as [15], which identifies the main sources of the uncertainty in the results of ECG measurement and evaluates its influence on the QRS, SST, and QRST curves, as well as on the interpretation of these results. The work by [16] evaluates the accuracy of its results only by the repeatability and reproducibility of an algorithm implemented to identify diseases from the digitized images of ECG curves such as the QRS, which already bring with them the uncertainties identified in works such as that of [15]. It can be stated that in these cases, repeatability and reproducibility characterize only the uncertainty related to the process of scanning and classifying the ECG images, which must be taken into account along with all other sources of uncertainty that are present during the process of measurement and the generation of these images. In [17], the authors quantified the sources of uncertainty, using statistical techniques based on Monte Carlo, to more accurately classify cardiac arrhythmias with AI. It should be noted that in works where the uncertainty was quantified, the classification method used data that already included other uncertainties, inherited from the process of measuring the ECG signal. Several other works such as [18–20] used uncertainty as a parameter to evaluate the performance of the methods proposed in their respective works.

Measurement uncertainty is a parameter that makes it possible to confidently state how good a measurement method or system is or how much better it is compared with others. In works such as [21,22], the measurement uncertainty was experimentally analyzed, after interfacing the sensors with the system. However, these analyses can be carried out theoretically [3,4] and can be analyzed before designing or implementing a measurement system. Measurement uncertainty analysis can be used to show how well the behavior of a measurement system is known in the design phase and how much the performance of this system can be improved. Few works were reported on using least-square analysis for the measurement of observational uncertainties [23] and unequally spaced non-stationary time series signals [24].

In this context, this work proposes a methodology that uses measurement uncertainty as a parameter to evaluate performance and guide actions to improve projects and the development of measurement systems. In this methodology, the Monte Carlo method (MCM) is used, the essence of which is to perform numerical simulations from a large number of repetitions and reach conclusions from the statistical analysis of the obtained responses. The proposed methodology is based on the acquired knowledge, which has been developed over time and published by the International Bureau of Weights and Measures (BIPM) in their guides. Based on such standards, MCM strategies are widely used in the literature for transmission line resistance computation [25], the assessment of truth uncertainties based on error feeds [4], and the propagation of distribution uncertainty measurement [3] applications. Furthermore, MCM was used for measuring compressive concrete strength in [26], which facilitated the analysis of robustness and sensitivity factors. In [27], MCM was used for invariance measurement for assessing the capabilities of conventional and recent measurement strategies. Additionally, the authors in [28] used MCM simulation for performing more realistic measurements in the modeling of additive manufacturing applications. It highlights the impact of the MCM approach for assessing the measurements of the lattice structures manufactured through additive techniques.

This work differs from the previous ones precisely because it uses systematic numerical simulations and uncertainty as a performance parameter during the analysis of measurement system design. The articles cited in the characterization of the state-of-the-art research on the evaluation of the uncertainties in the measurements performed with an ECG, in general, used this parameter for the interpretation and/or classification of measurement results and subsequent decision making related to the diagnosis of diseases. The detailed description of the proposed methodology of this work is elaborated in Section 2.2, which is then applied to evaluate the performance of electrocardiogram (ECG) signals. Simply put, the contribution of this work is twofold:

- Contribute to filling a small gap in the state of the art of evaluating the uncertainty of measurements performed with an ECG;
- Present a methodology capable of identifying opportunities for improvement in measurement system projects, using measurement uncertainty as a parameter.

Very recently, in [16], the authors developed a conversion algorithm to transform image-based ECGs into digital signals. Further, in [17], an uncertainty-aware deep-learning-based predictive framework was developed for assessing the uncertainties of the model. However, none of these studies focused on uncertainty measurement in ECG signals.

Earlier, more prominent works on ECG signals were performed by authors, particularly to classify heart arrhythmia using deep learning [29], automated cardiac arrhythmia detection [30], and arrhythmia classification [31]. Further, with the support of Internet of Things (IoT) platforms, related works were reported on the classification optimization of short ECG segments [32] and atrial fibrillation recognition and detection using Artificial Intelligence of Things (AIoT).

2. Materials and Methods

2.1. Datasets

The ECG is an essential means of monitoring the cardiac activities of patients. Using standardized electrodes, carefully placed at specific points on the patient's body, it is possible to record the heart's electrical signals. A standard ECG uses 3, 5, or 12 electrodes [33]. With more electrodes placed over the patient's body, more information could be acquired from the setup.

The ECG basically measures the electrical activities generated from the flow of blood in the heart [34]. By monitoring the heart's electrical signals, it is possible to assess the conditions and health status of the patient. The response curves of the measured signals shown in Figure 1 indicate the normal conditions of the patients, which are obtained after the iterated processing of the signals captured from the electrodes.

In Figure 2, a sample is presented of the four classes of typical ECG signals, which are postoperative telemetry data acquired from 418 patients who underwent various types of cardiac surgery [35]. These data were used to train the classification algorithm, which identifies cardiac problems based on the ECG waveform.

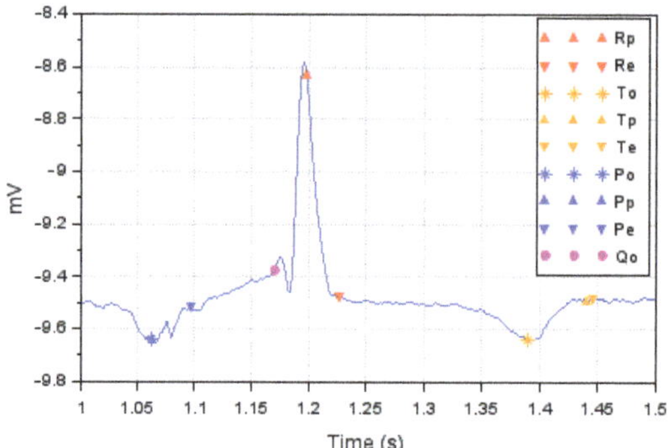

Figure 1. A normal ECG waveform for one cardiac cycle representing positive and negative deflection from baseline.

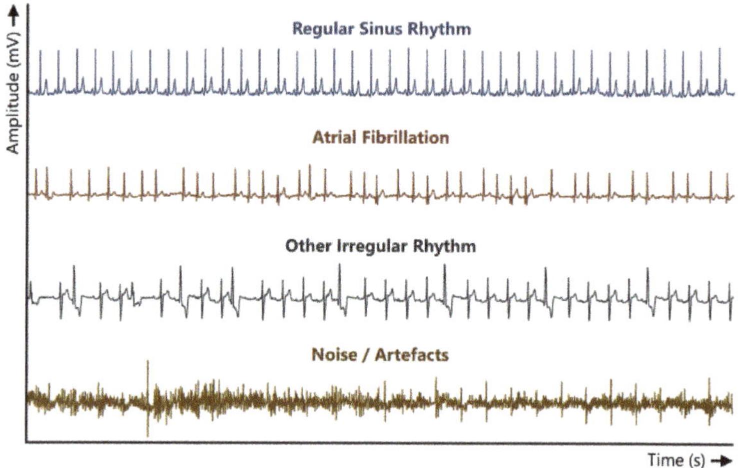

Figure 2. Typical ECG segments of the four different classes [35].

The noise/artifacts class, shown in Figure 2, represents those signals that cannot be interpreted by a specialist due to noise or other associated factors, e.g., patient movements or pacemaker activity [35]. There are certain crucial factors that must be taken into account when designing and using an ECG, such as frequency distortion, saturation or clipping distortion, ground loops, artifacts from large electrical transients, and interference from other electrical devices [36]. These factors are important not only for biomedical engineers but also for healthcare professionals who use this instrument in their decision making.

All sources of interference in the values indicated by an ECG generate uncertainties that may affect the interpretation of these results and, consequently, the diagnosis of diseases. Few recent works, such as [37–40], showed ways to ensure reliability when analyzing the parameters acquired by considering the ECG signals, taking into account the uncertainty of these values.

As ECG monitoring devices are widely used as a diagnostic tool, and there are several manufacturers for this instrument, performance requirements have been established by international standards over the years in order to guarantee the reliability of the values indicated by these instruments. Table 1 provides a summary of the most recent performance requirements established in the standard developed in [41].

In addition to the requirements shown in Table 1, the standard in [41] establishes the requirements for evaluating the performance of such equipment, based on the overall system error and frequency response. Input signals should be limited in amplitude and rate of slew to ±5 mV and 125 mV/s, respectively, and should be reproduced on the output recording medium with a maximum instantaneous deviation of ±5% or ±40 microvolts (μV), whichever is greater [41].

In addition to the standard [41], which establishes minimum safety and performance requirements for ECG monitoring equipment, the International Organization of Legal Metrology (OIML) has published the international recommendation [41], which establishes requirements for the calibration and verification of the ECG monitoring system. These standards provide guidelines that can be used to identify and quantify sources of uncertainty in the measurement of ECG signals.

Table 1. Requirement of ECG monitoring devices and their description [41].

Requirement Description	Min/Max	Units	Value
Operating conditions:			
Line voltage	Range	V RMS	104 to 1127
Frequency	Range	Hz	60 ± 1
Temperature	Range	°C	25 ± 10
Relative humidity	Range	%	50 ± 20
Atmospheric pressure	Range	kPa	70 to 106
Input Dynamic Range:			
Range of linear operations of input signal	Min	mV	±5
Allowed variation of amplitude with dc offset	Max	%	±5
Gain control, accuracy, and stability:			
Gain error	Max	%	5
Gain change rate/min	Max	%/min	±0.33
Total gain change/h	Max	%	±3
Time base selection and accuracy:			
Time base error	Max	%	±5
Output display:			
Error of rulings	Max	%	±2
Time marker error	Max	%	±2
Accuracy of input signal reproduction:			
Overall error for signals	Max	%	±5
Error in lead weighting factors	Max	%	5
Hysteresis after 15 mm deflection from baseline	Max	mm	0.5
Standardizing voltage:			
Amplitude error	Max	%	±5
System noise:			
Multichannel crosstalk	Max	%	2
Baseline stability:			
Baseline drift rate RTI	Max	μV/s	10
Total baseline drift RTI (2 min period)	Max	μV	500

2.2. Methods

The methodology proposed in this work involves the performance evaluation of a measurement system and can be applied even in the design phase. The methodology basically consists of a form of synthesis and analysis, taking into account the measurement uncertainty of the system under development. The application of this methodology is schematically presented in Figure 3.

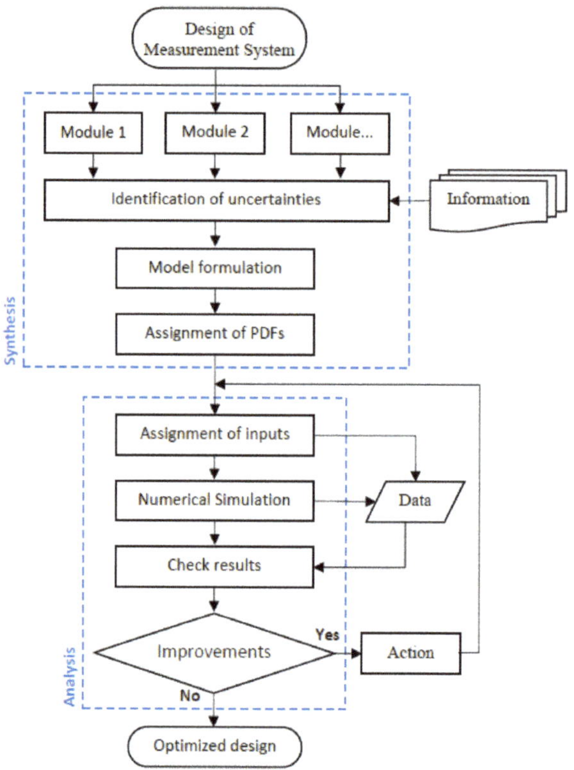

Figure 3. The sequence of stages involved in the synthesis and analysis phases of the proposed methodology.

For the performance evaluation of a measurement system, with its pre-project or initial project already elaborated, this measurement system must initially be divided into modules and, with the information gathered in the project synthesis, the input quantities and primary sources of measurement uncertainty must be identified.

It is necessary to know how these modules are interconnected, and how they behave individually and together. With this knowledge, it is possible to determine a mathematical model for the system, capable of characterizing the metrological behavior of the complete system, as well as the behavior of each module individually. Guidelines for the mathematical modeling of a measurement system can be found in [4].

As the analysis is performed using statistical tools, it is necessary to assign each of the sources of uncertainty a probability density function (PDF) that characterizes its random behavior [25].

The analysis phase highlighted in Figure 3 presents the iterative process where the various ranges and other necessary parameters are assigned to the input quantities. Following this process, the MCM is applied through the numerical simulation of the previously defined mathematical model, and the outputs are analyzed in comparison with the desired performance of the system.

In addition to this methodology, proposing the use of measurement uncertainty as a parameter to evaluate the performance of a measurement system, the application of the MCM also stands out for numerical simulations using a probabilistic approach, which can be implemented in software for mathematical computation, as shown in Algorithm 1.

Algorithm 1 MCM implementation.

$X[x_1, x_2, x_3, \ldots, x_n]; U[u_1, u_2, u_3, \ldots, u_n]$

$M \leftarrow c_1$ //Initialize M (number of iterations)
$A[n : M]$ // The array A is declared
$A(1, 1 : M) \leftarrow f(M, x_1, u_1, pdf)$ //Assigns random number with proper PDF
$A(2, 1 : M) \leftarrow f(M, x_2, u_2, pdf)$
$A(3, 1 : M) \leftarrow f(M, x_3, u_3, pdf)$

$\vdots$

$A(n, 1 : M) \leftarrow f(M, x_n, u_n, pdf)$
$Y[n + 1 : M + 2]$ //The array Y is declared

$Y(n + 1, 1 : M) \leftarrow g(A)$ //Function g defines the mathematical model
$Y(n + 1, M + 1) \leftarrow average(Y(n + 1, 1 : M))$
$A(n + 1, M + 2) \leftarrow standardDeviation(Y(n + 1, 1 : M))$
$B[n : M] \leftarrow h(n, X)$ //The array B is declared with n lines constants

$for\ i = 1\ to\ n$

$Z[1 : M] \leftarrow B(i : M)$
$B(i : M) \leftarrow A(i : M)$
$Y(i, 1 : M) \leftarrow g(B)$
$Y(i, M + 1) \leftarrow average(Y(i, 1 : M))$
$Y(i, M + 2) \leftarrow standardDeviation(Y(i, 1 : M))$
$B(i : M) \leftarrow Z$

This algorithm requires coherent values as input variables for the quantities under analysis and estimates the measurement uncertainties associated with each of the input parameters. Its output is a data vector containing the values of the output quantity considering the influence of each measurement uncertainty source individually, as well as considering the influence of all uncertainty sources acting concurrently.

The M parameter is the minimum number of simulations recommended for the MCM application. This number depends on the desired confidence level p (or coverage probability) for the application so the higher the desired confidence level, the greater the M should be and, consequently, the greater the computational effort required for simulation. M can be determined by Equation (1).

$$M = \frac{1}{(1 - p)} \cdot 10^4 \tag{1}$$

The number of input variables is represented by n, and function f, in Algorithm 1, is used to generate random numbers according to the PDF suitable for the behavior of the measurement uncertainty associated with the input variable. The measurement uncertainty expression guide [25] provides valid recommendations for PDF assignments.

The looping statement in Algorithm 1 is implemented to evaluate the influence on the output, based on the uncertainty source acting individually. However, these looping statements can be modified to assess the influence of a group of uncertainty sources, which would characterize the behavior of a system module.

It is worth noting that the mathematical model implemented through numerical simulation helps to gain awareness of the metrological behavior of the system as a whole, as well as of each module individually. Through this analysis, the relative performance of each module against the performance of the complete system could be evaluated. This analysis is very convenient to identify which action will promote a significant improvement in the performance of the system, as well as to evaluate the costs for such improvement. Thus, an optimized design can be achieved by considering the best cost–benefit ratio.

The methodology proposed in this work was applied to evaluate the performance of ECG signal measurement. In Section 2.1, the formation of the knowledge/information base is presented, which basically comprises the description of the measurement process through the parameters and metrological requirements that are necessary to characterize and delimit the system under development. The synthesis and analysis phases of the proposed methodology are presented in Section 3.

3. Results

The application of the proposed methodology began with the collection of information and the clear definition of the measurement system, with the identification of modules and other fundamental parts for its proper functioning. In this application, the high input impedance electrical circuit module is presented in Figure 4, which was divided into two modules. The first half was the preamplifier phase, where the first stage of amplification of the input signal occurred. In the second half of the module, the signal was filtered and passed through the second amplification stage.

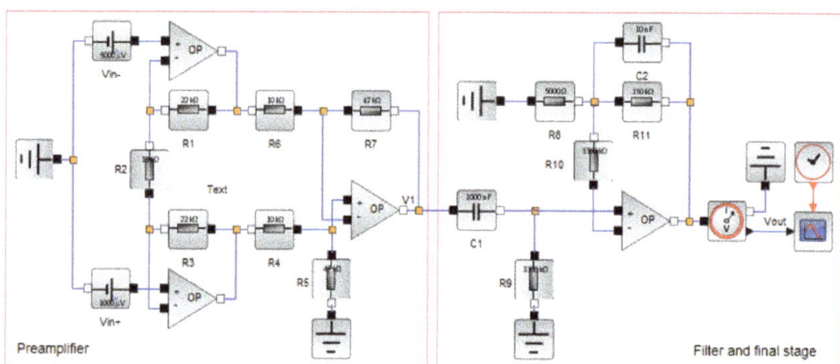

Figure 4. A simplified ECG system with preamplification and filter stages.

3.1. Formulation of the Model

The ECG monitoring system design, shown in Figure 4, was modeled using the Xcos tool from Scilab version 6.1.1, a free open-source cross-platform numerical computational tool. Considering the few idealizations for the circuit represented in Figure 4, we have $R_1 = R_3$; $R_4 = R_6$; $R_5 = R_7$, and $R_9 = R_{10}$, for which the transfer function can be formulated as shown in Equation (2), for the preamplifier, and in Equation (3), for the final stage:

$$v_1 = \left(1 + \frac{2R_1}{R_2}\right)\frac{R_5}{R_4}(v_{in+} - v_{in-}) \tag{2}$$

$$v_{out} = \left(1 + \frac{R_{11}}{R_8}\right)(v_1) \tag{3}$$

From Equations (4) and (5), we could estimate the cut-off frequencies of the first and second modules, respectively, which are responsible for attenuating the effect of noise in the input signal.

$$f_1 = \frac{1}{2\pi C_1 R_9} \tag{4}$$

$$f_2 = \frac{1}{2\pi C_2 R_{11}} \tag{5}$$

With these equations, it is possible to evaluate the behavior of each module, in isolation and of the system as a whole. It is also possible to evaluate the contribution of each element of this circuit to estimate the accuracy of the system. Moreover, it guarantees the possibility to identify exactly where to act, substituting an element or improving the performance of a specific module and, consequently, of the measurement system under development.

3.2. PDF Assignment

For each of the uncertainty sources, which were considered to be significant in the previous analysis, quantities were assigned, their average value was determined (μ), and their range of variation was characterized by the standard deviation (σ) or between an interval of (a, b). In addition to the quantities, the assigned PDFs characterized their random behavior. Table 2 presents the quantities and the PDF of the uncertainty sources considered for analysis in this article.

The parameters presented in Table 2 were categorized into three groups of factors, with the aim of better organizing the knowledge about the metrological behavior of ECG signals. The first group gathered the factors related to the measurement, that is, the electrical signals, which were the factors not completely under the control of whoever develops the measurement system. The second group brought together the factors related to the measurement system, which were factors internal to the system that could be analyzed to identify opportunities for improvement in the system. Finally, the third group gathered the external factors, which were the factors related to the environment, where the measurements were carried out. The factors related to the environment were not the focus of the application but must be treated with due attention.

Table 2. The input quantities and their PDFs assigned on the basis of available information.

Quantity	PDF	Parameters				
		μ	σ	a	b	Unit
Measurand:						
v_{in+}	$N(\mu,\sigma)$	0.30	0.04			mV
v_{in-}	$N(\mu,\sigma)$	0.00	0.04			mV
Baseline	$N(\mu,\sigma)$	3.00	0.01			mV
Measuring system:						
R_1	$R(a,b)$	22.00		21.78	22.22	kΩ
R_2	$R(a,b)$	10.00		9.90	10.10	kΩ
R_4	$R(a,b)$	10.00		9.90	10.10	kΩ
R_5	$R(a,b)$	47.00		46.53	47.47	kΩ
R_8	$R(a,b)$	5.00		4.95	5.05	kΩ
R_9	$R(a,b)$	3.30		2.27	3.33	MΩ
R_{11}	$R(a,b)$	150.00		148.50	151.50	kΩ
C_1	$U(a,b)$	1.00		0.99	1.01	μF
C_2	$U(a,b)$	10.00		9.90	10.10	nF
Environment:						
Noise	$N(\mu,\sigma)$	0.00	0.01			mV

In this work, all external interference was considered for analysis in the form of noise inputs pertaining to the measurement signal. The analysis was carried out through the Cardiovascular Wave Analysis module of the Scilab software. This module provides ECG data files (open-access databases) that were used in the simulations performed in this work. In Figure 5, the signal generated by this tool is depicted, from which the parameters related to the baseline and noise of the signal were obtained.

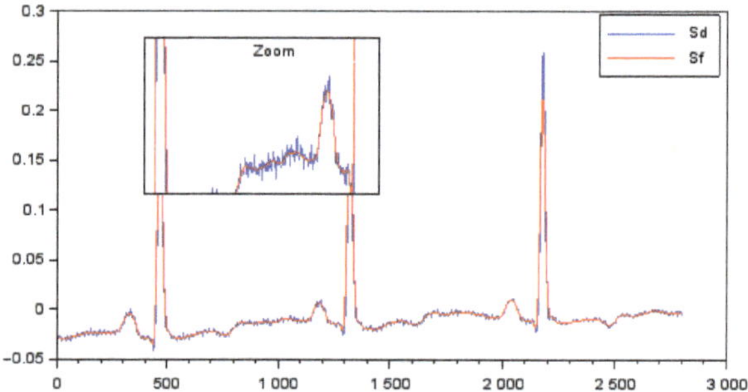

Figure 5. Detrended signal (Sd) and filtered signal (Sf).

In the proposed methodology, the MCM was used to analyze the sources of uncertainty, for which inferences were estimated through numerical iterations. Moreover, the method is also recommended for situations in which the linearization of the mathematical model of measurement provides an inadequate representation, or the PDF of the output quantity significantly deviates from a Gaussian distribution or a t-distribution [25].

The essence of MCM is to perform numerical simulations from a large number of repetitions and to obtain conclusions about the phenomenon under study from the statistical analysis of the responses obtained. The MCM in this work was carried out with Algorithm 1, following the prescribed measurement guidelines [25].

For the implementation of the MCM, normal, rectangular, and U-shaped PDFs were often used to achieve the desired characteristics of the system under test. The PDFs used to generate the sample values were implemented in the Scilab software tool. For this implementation, $M = 2 \times 10^5$ samples were used in order to obtain results, with a confidence level of 95%.

As an initial response, output data were obtained with a normal probability distribution, providing a mean of 2596 mV, and a standard deviation of 57 mV, as shown in Figure 6. The measurement uncertainty, calculated for a coverage probability of 95%, was ±112 mV, which corresponded to 4.32% of the mean value.

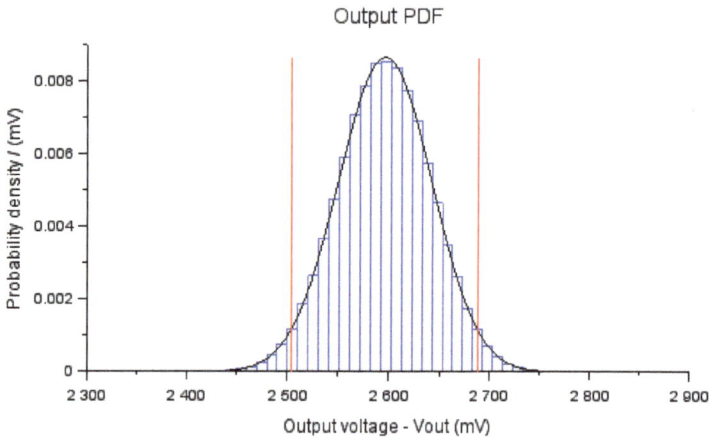

Figure 6. PDF for V_{out} obtained using the MCM for the approximate model (3) using the information summarized in Table 2.

The previous results refer to the simulation in which all uncertainty sources acted simultaneously. However, this simulation strategy can also be applied by varying only one or a set of uncertainty sources at a time, to assess their level of influence on the results.

Figure 7 shows the PDFs obtained with the application of the MCM for the two modules of the measurement system under study, and they were analyzed separately. It is noteworthy that the probability function of the first module followed a normal curve, and the second module formed a triangular curve. This fact highlights the importance of using MCM in this methodology since traditional analytical methods, as observed in [3], assume that the outputs are characterized by a normal probability distribution curve.

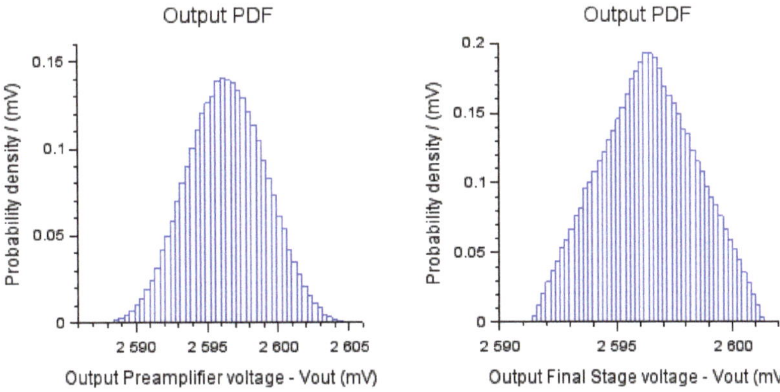

Figure 7. PDF for preamplifier and final stage.

The use of MCM guarantees greater assurance in the results obtained with the application of the methodology proposed in this work, since this method allows the propagation of uncertainty in modules, in addition to the propagation of the PDFs [25].

In Table 3, the results of the simulation of the sources of uncertainty considered significant in this work are tabulated based on the analysis performed individually as well as in blocks.

Table 3. Individual or block simulation of uncertainty sources.

Source of Uncertainty	Vout (mV)			U_{95} (%)
	μ	σ	U_{95}	
Measurand:				
v_{in}	2596	44	87	3.36
Baseline	2596	8	15	0.59
Measuring system:				
Preamplifier	2596	27	54	2.07
Final stage	2596	20	39	1.55
Environment:				
Noise	2596	8	15	0.59

In the initial analysis, the use of precision resistors of 1% was considered in the electrical circuit of the setup (Table 2). By considering the use of high-precision resistors of 0.1% of the nominal value only in the preamplifier module, an output with a mean of 2596 mV, a standard deviation of 50 mV, and an uncertainty of 99 mV was obtained, which corresponded to 3.80% of the average value. It is evident from this observation that, in terms of the average value, the contribution of the preamplifier module dropped from 2.07% to 0.21%.

Considering the use of resistors with an accuracy of 0.1% in the entire experimental setup shown in Figure 4, an uncertainty of 90 mV was achieved, which corresponded to

3.47% of the average value. This indicated a 0.85% improvement in the accuracy of the ECG signal under analysis. In Table 4, the simulation results are presented considering the implementation, with the suggested improvement actions.

Table 4. Individual or block simulation of uncertainty sources after design improvements.

Source of Uncertainty	Vout (mV)			U_{95} (%)
	μ	σ	U_{95}	
Measurand:				
v_{in}	2596	45	87	3.36
Baseline	2596	8	15	0.59
Measuring system:				
Preamplifier	2596	3	5	0.21
Final stage	2596	2	4	0.15
Environment:				
Noise	2596	8	15	0.59

A comparison of the quantitative results of Table 4 with the results presented in Table 3 highlights the potential of the methodology proposed in this work to identify and direct improvement actions in measurement system projects, which, in turn, can be analyzed through computer simulations before their respective implementations.

3.3. Validation and Comparisons with the Literature

In terms of evaluating measurement uncertainty, the most widespread method in the literature is the analytical method published in ISO-GUM, cited in works such as [3,4,25]. In these studies, basically, a combined standard uncertainty is calculated at approximately 68% confidence level, using the expression:

$$u(Y) = \sqrt{\left(\frac{\partial y}{\partial X_1} u(X_1)\right)^2 + \left(\frac{\partial y}{\partial X_2} u(X_2)\right)^2 + \ldots + \left(\frac{\partial y}{\partial X_n} u(X_n)\right)^2} \tag{6}$$

where $u(Y)$ is the combined standard uncertainty of the output quantity, and $u(X_i)$ is the standard uncertainty assigned to the i-th input quantity being combined. To calculate the expanded uncertainty for a confidence level of 95%, Equation (7) is used:

$$U_{95} = k \cdot u(Y) \tag{7}$$

where $k = 1.96$ for a confidence level of 95%, considering the effective degrees of freedom tending to infinity.

Applying this method to the problem in question and taking the data from Table 2 as inputs, an uncertainty of ± 161 mV was found, which corresponded to 6.21% of the measured value. It is noteworthy that, for the same parameters and input values, the value found with the methodology proposed in this work was 4.32% of the measured value.

Comparing the result obtained by applying the methodology presented in this work with the result of applying the methodology used in the literature on the evaluation of measurement uncertainty, it is highlighted that the methodology proposed in this work presented more precise results.

4. Discussion

As shown in Table 3, baseline variations and noise interference had a negligible influence on the obtained results. From these results, it is evident that the most significant uncertainty was associated with variations in the input signal.

There are several causes for input signal variations as the most significant source of uncertainty, such as the placement of sensors on the patient's body, patient movements during measurements, electromagnetic interference from other equipment, and other sources of uncertainty that are not under the control of who designs the measurement system.

It is noteworthy that the second most significant source of uncertainty was associated with the preamplifier module. From the estimated observations on the uncertainty information, the designer can assess how much the measurement system uncertainty can be reduced by acting on a specific module in the system.

As previously stated in the aforementioned discussion, the source with the greatest contribution of uncertainty was related to the input signal, which in turn was related to the measurand. However, it is noteworthy that the identified improvement actions promoted significant reductions in the contributions of the analyzed modules. To promote further improvements, it would be recommended to act smartly on system parameters to improve the stability of the baseline or reduce the effect of noise on the measured signal.

In Figure 8, the power spectrum of the noisy signal is plotted centered at the zero frequency before and after noise removal. The power amplitude is represented as the squared magnitude of a signal's Fourier transform, normalized by the number of frequency samples. If the input signal noise, as well as the signal itself, is of low frequency (below 50 Hz before the filter), it would be challenging to remove the noise without significantly affecting the signal of interest. With the chosen filter applied in this work, it was possible to remove noise with a frequency above 30 Hz, as can be observed in Figure 8.

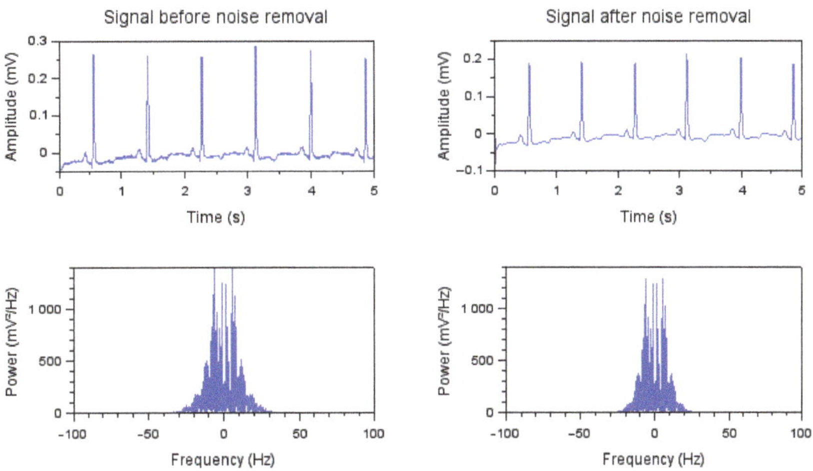

Figure 8. ECG signals power as a function of frequency before and after noise removal.

In the spectrogram of the filtered signal, shown in Figure 9, which covers the time interval of 1 to 2 s, it is possible to notice that the remaining noise and a good part of the signal of interest were of low power and practically constant over the measurement period. The analysis of Figures 8 and 9 reveals that particular attention must be paid when applying filters so that the significant data of the ECG signal of interest are not lost.

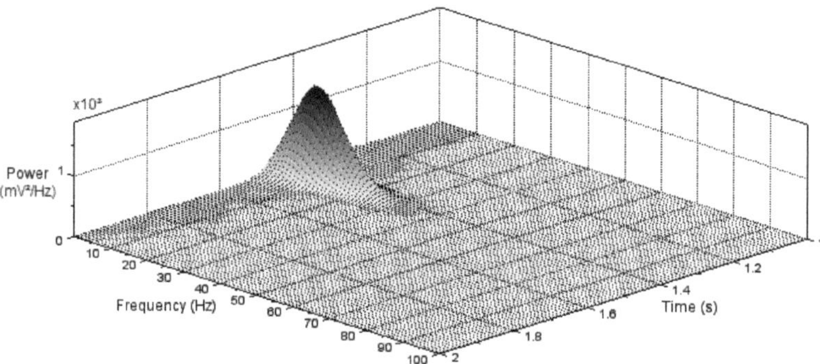

Figure 9. Time–frequency spectrogram after noise removal.

In order to improve the performance of the ECG acting on the source of uncertainty related to the input signal, in addition to the use of signal-processing techniques and noise filtering, it is necessary to carry out investigations taking into account the measurement procedure and the functioning mode of the used sensor. In future works, procedures that can measure the electrical activity of the heart, or even other signals, can be investigated so that the results are not so influenced by the positioning of the sensors and the movement of the patients. Likewise, future investigations can be carried out with the aim of identifying sensors that are not as susceptible to noise from the environment.

As regards the limitations of the methodology proposed in this work, it should be noted that it was tested with problems in the time domain; therefore, for applications in the frequency domain, adjustments in the proposed algorithm are necessary. It should also be noted that the successful implementation of this methodology is strongly limited by the ability of the mathematical model to describe the metrological behavior of the elements and/or modules that constitute the measurement system under analysis.

5. Conclusions

The methodology presented in this work demonstrates the probabilistic uncertainty from the measurement system, with the measurements and analysis performed on an ECG monitoring system. The methodology uses a probabilistic approach for the evaluation of measurement uncertainty, through the application of the MCM, to evaluate the performance of signals measured from an ECG monitoring system. With the performed analysis, it was possible to reach the desired situation, for which the ECG measurement uncertainty would be 3.47% in relation to the measurement result, subjected to a confidence level of 95%. With this analysis, it was also possible to identify strategic points where actions can be taken to further improve the accuracy of the measurement system, such as actions to improve baseline stability or actions to reduce the effect of noise. It is noteworthy that the application of this methodology revealed that the sources of uncertainty related to the input signal, directly related to the measurand, was 3.36% of the measured value, which was almost the measurement uncertainty of the ECG itself. Thus, studies can be carried out with the objective of better investigating the behavior of the measurement system and, consequently, improving the measurement process, as well as increasing the reliability of the results. It is concluded that a more detailed and reliable understanding of the behavior of a measurement system, as well as the individual behavior of an element or a module of that system, makes it possible to act more efficiently to improve the method's performance.

Author Contributions: Conceptualization, P.C.C., S.K.J. and V.H.C.d.A.; methodology, P.C.C., J.H.B.d.S. and V.H.C.d.A.; software, J.H.B.d.S. and P.C.C.; validation, S.K.J. and V.H.C.d.A.; formal analysis, P.C.C. and V.H.C.d.A.; investigation, J.H.B.d.S. and S.K.J.; writing—original draft preparation, J.H.B.d.S. and S.K.J.; writing—review and editing, P.C.C. and V.H.C.d.A.; visualization, J.H.B.d.S. and P.C.C.; supervision, P.C.C., S.K.J. and V.H.C.d.A.; project administration, P.C.C. and V.H.C.d.A. All authors have read and agreed to the published version of the manuscript.

Funding: This work has been supported by the National Council for Scientific and Technological Development (CNPq) via grant n° 305517/2022-8, and 313599/2019-0.

Institutional Review Board Statement: Not applicable.

Informed Consent Statement: Not applicable.

Data Availability Statement: Not applicable.

Conflicts of Interest: The authors declare no conflict of interest.

References

1. Wu, D.; Tang, Y. An improved failure mode and effects analysis method based on uncertainty measure in the evidence theory. *Qual. Reliab. Eng. Int.* **2020**, *36*, 1786–1807. [CrossRef]
2. Bennett, K.J.; Pizzolato, C.; Martelli, S.; Bahl, J.S.; Sivakumar, A.; Atkins, G.J.; Solomon, L.B.; Thewlis, D. EMG-informed neuromusculoskeletal models accurately predict knee loading measured using instrumented implants. *IEEE Trans. Biomed. Eng.* **2022**, *69*, 2268–2275. [CrossRef] [PubMed]
3. Cox, M.; Harris, P.; Siebert, B.L. Evaluation of measurement uncertainty based on the propagation of distributions using Monte Carlo simulation. *Meas. Tech.* **2003**, *46*, 824–833. [CrossRef]
4. Von Clarmann, T.; Compernolle, S.; Hase, F. Truth and Uncertainty. A critical discussion of the error concept versus the uncertainty concept. *Atmos. Meas. Tech.* **2022**, *15*, 1145–1157. [CrossRef]
5. Gitelson, A.; Viña, A.; Inoue, Y.; Arkebauer, T.; Schlemmer, M.; Schepers, J. Uncertainty in the evaluation of photosynthetic canopy traits using the green leaf area index. *Agric. For. Meteorol.* **2022**, *320*, 108955. [CrossRef]
6. Separovic, L.; Lourenço, F.R. Measurement uncertainty evaluation of an analytical procedure for determination of terbinafine hydrochloride in creams by HPLC and optimization strategies using Analytical Quality by Design. *Microchem. J.* **2022**, *178*, 107386. [CrossRef]
7. da Silva, R.J.B.; Saame, J.; Anes, B.; Heering, A.; Leito, I.; Näykki, T.; Stoica, D.; Deleebeeck, L.; Bastkowski, F.; Snedden, A.; et al. Evaluation and validation of detailed and simplified models of the uncertainty of unified pHabsH2O measurements in aqueous solutions. *Anal. Chim. Acta* **2021**, *1182*, 338923. [CrossRef]
8. Petri, D.; Carbone, P.; Mari, L. Quality of measurement information in decision-making. *IEEE Trans. Instrum. Meas.* **2020**, *70*, 1003816. [CrossRef]
9. Yang, H.; Cai, Y.; Zhu, B.; Xuan, G.; Li, X.; Sun, L.; Cheng, L. A Universal Measurement Method for Nanoparticle Number Concentration Based On Atomic Force Microscope. *IEEE Trans. Nanotechnol.* **2021**, *20*, 852–859. [CrossRef]
10. Galli, A.; Giorgi, G.; Narduzzi, C. Standardized Gaussian Dictionary for ECG Analysis a Metrological Approach. *IEEE Open J. Instrum. Meas.* **2022**, *1*, 4000209. [CrossRef]
11. Li, N.; Wang, L.; Jia, J.; Yang, Y. A novel method for the image quality improvement of ultrasonic tomography. *IEEE Trans. Instrum. Meas.* **2020**, *70*, 5000810. [CrossRef]
12. Uguz, D.U.; Canbaz, Z.T.; Antink, C.H.; Lüken, M.; Leonhardt, S. A Novel Sensor Design for Amplitude Modulated Measurement of Capacitive ECG. *IEEE Trans. Instrum. Meas.* **2022**, *71*, 4000710. [CrossRef]
13. Wang, Q.; Zhao, L.; Yang, T.; Liao, Z.; Xue, X.; Wu, B.; Zhang, W.; Zang, J.; Cui, D.; Zhang, Z.; et al. A mathematical model of a piezoelectric micro-machined hydrophone with simulation and experimental validation. *IEEE Sens. J.* **2021**, *21*, 13364–13372. [CrossRef]
14. Lim, A.; Schonewille, A.; Forbrigger, C.; Looi, T.; Drake, J.; Diller, E. Design and Comparison of Magnetically-Actuated Dexterous Forceps Instruments for Neuroendoscopy. *IEEE Trans. Biomed. Eng.* **2020**, *68*, 846–856. [CrossRef] [PubMed]
15. Lux, R.L. Uncertainty of the electrocardiogram: Old and new ideas for assessment and interpretation. *J. Electrocardiol.* **2000**, *33*, 203–208. [CrossRef]
16. Randazzo, V.; Puleo, E.; Paviglianiti, A.; Vallan, A.; Pasero, E. Development and Validation of an Algorithm for the Digitization of ECG Paper Images. *Sensors* **2022**, *22*, 7138. [CrossRef]
17. Aseeri, A.O. Uncertainty-Aware Deep Learning-Based Cardiac Arrhythmias Classification Model of Electrocardiogram Signals. *Computers* **2021**, *10*, 82. [CrossRef]
18. Jahmunah, V.; Ng, E.; Tan, R.S.; Oh, S.L.; Acharya, U.R. Uncertainty quantification in DenseNet model using myocardial infarction ECG signals. *Comput. Methods Programs Biomed.* **2023**, *229*, 107308. [CrossRef]
19. Sadda, P.; Ghebermicael, D.; Emerenini, U. Uncertainty modeling can identify erroneous computer ECG reads. *Heart Rhythm* **2021**, *18*, 1. [CrossRef]

20. Honarvar, H.; Agarwal, C.; Somani, S.; Vaid, A.; Lampert, J.; Wanyan, T.; Reddy, V.Y.; Nadkarni, G.N.; Miotto, R.; Zitnik, M.; et al. Enhancing convolutional neural network predictions of electrocardiograms with left ventricular dysfunction using a novel sub-waveform representation. *Cardiovasc. Digit. Health J.* **2022**, *3*, 220–231. [CrossRef]

21. Al-Obaidi, K.; Valyrakis, M. A sensory instrumented particle for environmental monitoring applications: Development and calibration. *IEEE Sens. J.* **2021**, *21*, 10153–10166. [CrossRef]

22. Luo, X.; Shi, C.; Zeng, H.Q.; Ewurum, H.C.; Wan, Y.; Guo, Y.; Pagnha, S.; Zhang, X.B.; Du, Y.P.; He, X. Evolutionarily Optimized Electromagnetic Sensor Measurements for Robust Surgical Navigation. *IEEE Sens. J.* **2019**, *19*, 10859–10868. [CrossRef]

23. Ghaderpour, E.; Ghaderpour, S. Least-squares spectral and wavelet analyses of V455 Andromedae time series: The life after the super-outburst. *Publ. Astron. Soc. Pac.* **2020**, *132*, 114504. [CrossRef]

24. Ghaderpour, E.; Pagiatakis, S.D. Least-squares wavelet analysis of unequally spaced and non-stationary time series and its applications. *Math. Geosci.* **2017**, *49*, 819–844. [CrossRef]

25. Tolić, I.; Milićević, K.; Tokić, A. Measurement uncertainty of transmission line resistance calculation using 'Guide to the Expression of Uncertainty in Measurement' and adaptive Monte–Carlo method. *IET Sci. Meas. Technol.* **2017**, *11*, 339–345. [CrossRef]

26. Dao, D.V.; Adeli, H.; Ly, H.B.; Le, L.M.; Le, V.M.; Le, T.T.; Pham, B.T. A sensitivity and robustness analysis of GPR and ANN for high-performance concrete compressive strength prediction using a Monte Carlo simulation. *Sustainability* **2020**, *12*, 830. [CrossRef]

27. Pokropek, A.; Davidov, E.; Schmidt, P. A Monte Carlo simulation study to assess the appropriateness of traditional and newer approaches to test for measurement invariance. *Struct. Equ. Model. Multidiscip. J.* **2019**, *26*, 724–744. [CrossRef]

28. Lozanovski, B.; Downing, D.; Tran, P.; Shidid, D.; Qian, M.; Choong, P.; Brandt, M.; Leary, M. A Monte Carlo simulation-based approach to realistic modelling of additively manufactured lattice structures. *Addit. Manuf.* **2020**, *32*, 101092. [CrossRef]

29. Cui, J.; Wang, L.; He, X.; De Albuquerque, V.H.C.; AlQahtani, S.A.; Hassan, M.M. Deep learning-based multidimensional feature fusion for classification of ECG arrhythmia. *Neural Comput. Appl.* **2021**, 1–15. [CrossRef]

30. de Albuquerque, V.H.C.; Nunes, T.M.; Pereira, D.R.; Luz, E.J.d.S.; Menotti, D.; Papa, J.P.; Tavares, J.M.R. Robust automated cardiac arrhythmia detection in ECG beat signals. *Neural Comput. Appl.* **2018**, *29*, 679–693. [CrossRef]

31. Luz, E.J.d.S.; Nunes, T.M.; De Albuquerque, V.H.C.; Papa, J.P.; Menotti, D. ECG arrhythmia classification based on optimum-path forest. *Expert Syst. Appl.* **2013**, *40*, 3561–3573. [CrossRef]

32. Zhang, X.; Jiang, M.; Wu, W.; de Albuquerque, V.H.C. Hybrid feature fusion for classification optimization of short ECG segment in IoT based intelligent healthcare system. *Neural Comput. Appl.* **2021**, 1–15. [CrossRef]

33. Betts, J.G.; Young, K.A.; Wise, J.A.; Johnson, E.; Poe, B.; Kruse, D.H.; Korol, O.; Johnson, J.E.; Womble, M.; DeSaix, P. *Anatomy and Physiology*; Jordan University of Science and Technology: Ar-Ramtha, Jordan, 2013 .

34. Berkaya, S.K.; Uysal, A.K.; Gunal, E.S.; Ergin, S.; Gunal, S.; Gulmezoglu, M.B. A survey on ECG analysis. *Biomed. Signal Process. Control* **2018**, *43*, 216–235. [CrossRef]

35. Wesselius, F.J.; van Schie, M.S.; De Groot, N.M.; Hendriks, R.C. An accurate and efficient method to train classifiers for atrial fibrillation detection in ECGs: Learning by asking better questions. *Comput. Biol. Med.* **2022**, *143*, 105331. [CrossRef] [PubMed]

36. Webster, J.G. *Medical Instrumentation: Application and Design*; John Wiley & Sons: Hoboken, NJ, USA, 2009.

37. Bond, R.R.; Novotny, T.; Andrsova, I.; Koc, L.; Sisakova, M.; Finlay, D.; Guldenring, D.; McLaughlin, J.; Peace, A.; McGilligan, V.; et al. Automation bias in medicine: The influence of automated diagnoses on interpreter accuracy and uncertainty when reading electrocardiograms. *J. Electrocardiol.* **2018**, *51*, S6–S11. [CrossRef] [PubMed]

38. Perez, Y.; Tobert, K.E.; Saunders, M.J.; Sorensen, K.B.; Bos, J.M.; Ackerman, M.J. Diagnostic accuracy of the 12-lead electrocardiogram in the first 48 hours of life for newborns of a parent with congenital long QT syndrome. *Heart Rhythm* **2022**, *19*, 969–974. [CrossRef] [PubMed]

39. Monedero, I. A novel ECG diagnostic system for the detection of 13 different diseases. *Eng. Appl. Artif. Intell.* **2022**, *107*, 104536. [CrossRef]

40. Merdjanovska, E.; Rashkovska, A. Comprehensive survey of computational ECG analysis: Databases, methods and applications. *Expert Syst. Appl.* **2022**, *203*, 117206. [CrossRef]

41. Wong, K.C.; Klimis, H.; Lowres, N.; von Huben, A.; Marschner, S.; Chow, C.K. Diagnostic accuracy of handheld electrocardiogram devices in detecting atrial fibrillation in adults in community versus hospital settings: A systematic review and meta-analysis. *Heart* **2020**, *106*, 1211–1217. [CrossRef]

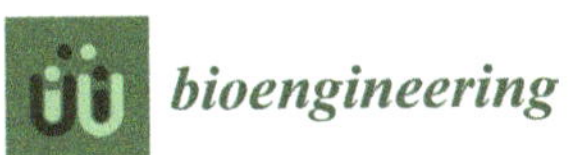 *bioengineering*

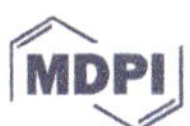

Communication

Distinction of Different Colony Types by a Smart-Data-Driven Tool

Pedro Miguel Rodrigues *, Pedro Ribeiro and Freni Kekhasharú Tavaria

CBQF—Centro de Biotecnologia e Química Fina–Laboratório Associado, Escola Superior de Biotecnologia, Universidade Católica Portuguesa, Rua de Diogo Botelho 1327, 4169-005 Porto, Portugal
* Correspondence: pmrodrigues@ucp.pt

Abstract: Background: Colony morphology (size, color, edge, elevation, and texture), as observed on culture media, can be used to visually discriminate different microorganisms. Methods: This work introduces a hybrid method that combines standard pre-trained CNN keras models and classical machine-learning models for supporting colonies discrimination, developed in Petri-plates. In order to test and validate the system, images of three bacterial species (*Escherichia coli*, *Pseudomonas aeruginosa*, and *Staphylococcus aureus*) cultured in Petri plates were used. Results: The system demonstrated the following *Accuracy* discrimination rates between pairs of study groups: 92% for *Pseudomonas aeruginosa* vs. *Staphylococcus aureus*, 91% for *Escherichia coli* vs. *Staphylococcus aureus* and 84% *Escherichia coli* vs. *Pseudomonas aeruginosa*. Conclusions: These results show that combining deep-learning models with classical machine-learning models can help to discriminate bacteria colonies with good *accuracy* ratios.

Keywords: petri-plates; colonies; machine-learning models; discrimination

1. Introduction

Evaluation of the number of viable microorganisms in a sample is a commonly used method in most microbiology laboratories. The method consists of counting visible colonies on agar plates and calculating the number of colony-forming units per mL (or gram) of the sample. For example, it is widely used for food, clinical, environmental, and drug safety testing. The counting of bacteria is usually carried out manually, and is, therefore, subjective and error-prone [1]. At present, automatic digital counters are common in laboratories and some have highly efficient automatic counting methods, which have replaced manual counting methods.

Although the counting of visible colonies on agar plates is the most commonly used method to assess bacterial populations, with the advantage of only considering the counts of viable cells [2], it is time-consuming, laborious and requires at least 24 h or more for visible colonies to form. This can be a considerable limitation in some situations, such as quality control of certain foods and in clinical settings, where fast results are required so that actions can rapidly be implemented.

One important factor in cell counting is the analyst's ability to see colonies distinctly. Colony morphology is used to select bacteria as phenotypically different. This is normally carried out by visual inspection, and the selected parameters are often colony size, color, texture, edge, and elevation, according to the colony morphology protocol emitted by the American Society for Microbiology [3].

In a previous work, a software capable of semi-automatically quantifying the number of colonies in Petri plates from a digital image was developed [4]. This method did not, however, automatically distinguish different colony types. Thus, in the present work, we attempted to include this distinguishing characteristic. Therefore, three bacterial species (*Escherichia coli*, *Pseudomonas aeruginosa*, and *Staphylococcus aureus*) that represent the predominant pathogenic microorganisms in a variety of settings—food [5], clinical [6] and

Citation: Rodrigues, P.M.; Ribeiro, P.; Tavaria, F.K. Distinction of Different Colony Types by a Smart-Data-Driven Tool. *Bioengineering* **2023**, *10*, 26. https://doi.org/10.3390/bioengineering10010026

Academic Editor: Cornelia Kasper

Received: 22 November 2022
Revised: 12 December 2022
Accepted: 19 December 2022
Published: 24 December 2022

environmental [7]—were used to evaluate and develop our solution/software to support colony discrimination. Table 1 shows the the current state-of-art on colony-distinguishing methods based on machine-learning (ML) models.

Table 1. State-of-the-art papers.

Ref.	Year	ML Model	Comparison Group	Accuracy
[8]	2021	SVM	*E. coli* vs. *S. aureus* vs. *S. Typhimurium* vs. *E. faecium* vs. *P. aeruginosa*	93.3%
[9]	2017	CNN	33 bacteria comparison (all the bacteria used in this study are included)	97.24%
[10]	2019	CNN	33 bacteria comparison (all the bacteria used in this study are included)	98.22%
[11]	2022	Linear Discriminant	*E. coli* vs. *E. coli-β* vs. *S. aureus* vs. *methicillin-resistant S. aureus* vs. *P. aeruginosa* vs. *E. faecalis* vs. *K. pneumoniae* vs. *C. albicans*	92%

2. Methodology

In this section, all the procedures are described. The microbiological analysis and the image database are presented and, after that, the deep and classical machine-learning analysis of images is explained. Figure 1 presents a summary of the whole methodology procedure.

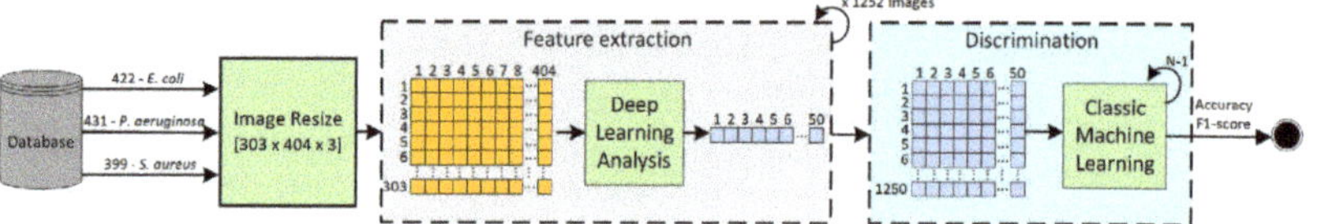

Figure 1. Methodology workflow.

2.1. Microbiological Analysis and Image Database

Plates containing *Escherichia coli*, *Pseudomonas aeruginosa* and *Staphylococcus aureus* isolates from our center's internal collection were cultivated aerobically at 37 °C, for 24 h, in Trypto-Casein Soy Agar™ (TSA, BIOKAR Diagnostics, Allonne, France) using the spread-plate technique (0.1 mL of the diluted samples). All experiments were carried out in triplicate. Colony enumeration was performed and the number of colonies was recorded and posteriorly attributed to each image of the database.

The final dataset [12] consists of about 1252 labeled Petri images with 422 colonies of *Escherichia coli*, 431 of *Pseudomonas aeruginosa* and 399 of *Staphylococcus aureus*. The color images were acquired by a smartphone camera with 12 megapixels [3024 × 4032 × 3]. For more details, consult the previous authors' published paper [4].

2.2. The Deep and Classical Machine-Learning Analysis

To verify the suitability of the Image dataset for building deep-learning models that can obtain a total of 50 features from each colony for image-based microorganism recognition, we evaluated the performance of the following standard, pre-trained 31 CNN keras models [13]: Xception; VGG16; VGG19; ResNet50; ResNet50V2; ResNet101; ResNet101V2; ResNet152; ResNet152V2; InceptionV3; InceptionResNetV2; MobileNet; MobileNetV2; DenseNet121; DenseNet169; DenseNet201; EfficientNetB0; EfficientNetB1; EfficientNetB2; EfficientNetB3; EfficientNetB4; EfficientNetB5; EfficientNetB6; EfficientNetB7; EfficientNetV2B0; EfficientNetV2B1; EfficientNetV2B2; EfficientNetV2B3; EfficientNetV2S; EfficientNetV2M; EfficientNetV2L. For more details please check the Keras default models at https://keras.io/api/applications/, accessed on 20 November 2022.

Due to the relatively high resolution of all images, the samples were scaled down to [303 × 404 × 3] to reduce the computation time and guarantee proper aspect ratios. Thus, the patches of each neural network architecture were resized to match the default input layer size. The output layer of each used standard CNN keras models [13], and was also replaced by a dense layer with 50 units and softmax as the activation function to obtain, as output, in a blinding feature extraction process, 50 features from each colony to serve as vector inputs for several classical ML models: decision trees (DT), support-vector machines (SVM), K-nearest neighbors (KNN), multi-layer perceptron (MLP) and three ensemble classifiers (please check Table 2 for more details). The models' performance was evaluated within a leave-one-out-cross-validation procedure, a well-known process that allows for the use of all datasets for testing, without leakage between train and test sets.

In this work, the feature extraction and the classification were carried out in a cloud-based service, the Google Colaboratory. The software code was developed in Python-Jupyter Notebook for machine-learning and deep-learning operations within a virtual machine with two Intel Xeon CPUs both at 2.20 GHz, 100 GB of storing, and 13 GB of Ram.

Table 2. Used classical machine-learning classifiers and optimal parameters.

ML Model		**Optimal Parameters**
DT	Medium Tree	Maximum number of splits = 150 & criterion = "gini"
SVM	Radial Basis	Cost = 1 & gamma = 2
KNN	Balltree	Number of neighbors = 3
MLP	1 input layer	activation function = "relu"
	1 hidden layer	training algorithm = "adam" L2 regulation term = 1 fullyConnectedLayer = 3
	1 output layer	hidden layer neurons = 100
Ensemble	Random Forest (RF)	Maximum number of splits = 100 & criterion = "gini"
	Bagged Trees (BagT)	Maximum number of splits = 150 & criterion = "gini"
	XGBoost	boosted trees to fit = 150 learning rate = 0.1 max depth of the tree = 6 L2 regulation term = 1

The evaluation metric for colony detection was based on the *Accuracy* and *F1-score* [14]. *Accuracy* shows how many cases were correctly labelled out of all the cases, and is defined as,

$$Accuracy = \frac{TruePositives + TrueNegatives}{TruePositives + TrueNegatives + FalsePositives + FalseNegatives} \times 100\% \quad (1)$$

where a *TruePositive* is an outcome in which the MP model correctly predicts a positive class, a *TrueNegative* is an outcome where the model correctly predicts the negative class, a *FalsePositive* is an outcome where the model incorrectly predicts the positive class and, finally, *FalseNegative* is an outcome where the model incorrectly predicts the negative class [14].

The *F1-score* is the harmonic mean of *precision* and *recall* and can be defined as,

$$F1\text{-}score = 2 \times \frac{precision \times recall}{precision + recall} \times 100\% \quad (2)$$

where *precision* and *recall* are, respectively,

$$precision = \frac{TruePositives}{TruePositives + FalsePositives} \tag{3}$$

and

$$recall = \frac{TruePositives}{TruePositives + FalseNegatives} \tag{4}$$

Thus, if the *F1-score* is high, both the precision and recall of the classifier indicate good results [14].

3. Results and Discussion

By analyzing Table 3, some considerations regarding the classification results between pairs of study groups are revealed. *Accuracies* higher than 84% were obtained for all pairs, with at least one combination of deep and classical machine-learning methods. The combination of classifiers MobileNet-XGBoost provided the best results for all study pair classifications; in this way, it was shown to be a good candidate combination for differentiating colonies. The XGBoost was shown to be the most effective classical machine-learning classifier, as 81% (82 of 93) of the best combinations of deep and classical machine-learning have XGBoost as a classifier. The group pairs comparisons that involved *Staphylococcus aureus* achieved high *Accuracy* and *F1-score* rates, above 91%. One of the explanations for these results is that *Staphylococcus aureus* produces yellow colonies [15] on a plate, which are very typical and differentiated from the *Escherichia coli* and *Pseudomonas aeruginosa* that produce beige colonies on a plate [16,17]. As *Escherichia coli* and *Pseudomonas aeruginosa* colonies are both beige on a plate, the problem of differentiating each becomes more difficult for the classifiers. Even so, the proposed methods achieved good ratios of *Accuracy* and *F1-score* ≈ 84% on *Escherichia coli* vs. *Pseudomonas aeruginosa* discrimination. The graphic of Figure 2 shows the best discrimination results between the study groups. The results are in line with those found in the state-of-art literature (please check Table 1) and provides us with a good indication that, if we continue to improve and refine the algorithm, we can build an even more helpful, powerful, and robust tool for this purpose.

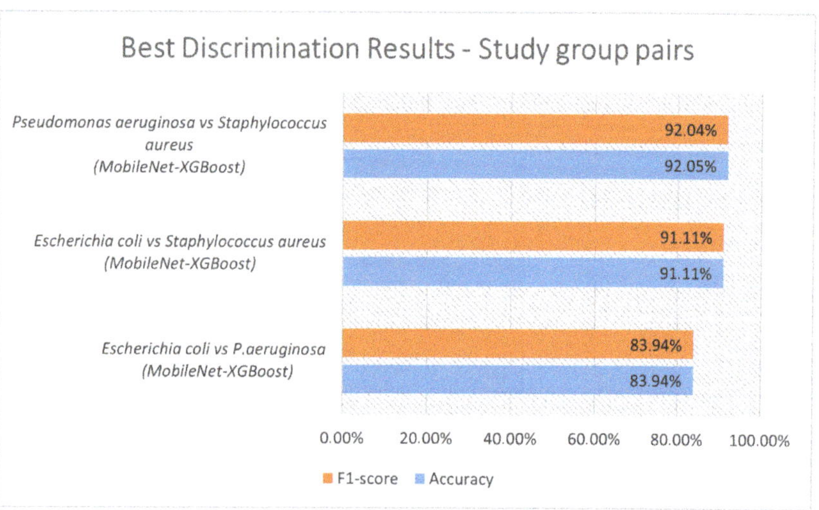

Figure 2. Best discrimination results between study group pairs.

Table 3. Summary of the best discrimination results between study group pairs.

Escherichia coli vs. *Pseudomonas aeruginosa*			*Escherichia coli* vs. *Staphylococcus aureus*			*Pseudomonas aeruginosa* vs. *Staphylococcus aureus*		
Classifiers	*Accuracy*	*F1-Score*	**Classifiers**	*Accuracy*	*F1-Score*	**Classifiers**	*Accuracy*	*F1-Score*
Xception-DT	76.79%	76.76%	Xception-XGBoost	81.49%	81.47%	Xception-XGBoost	81.33%	81.26%
VGG16-XGBoost	77.26%	77.26%	VGG16-XGBoost	84.90%	84.89%	VGG16-XGBoost	84.70%	84.67%
VGG19-XGBoost	71.86%	71.85%	VGG19-XGBoost	84.04%	84.04%	VGG19-XGBoost	84.94%	84.93%
ResNet50-XGBoost	77.96%	77.95%	ResNet50-XGBoost	86.97%	86.97%	ResNet50-XGBoost	86.75%	86.74%
ResNet50V2-XGBoost	76.20%	76.17%	ResNet50V2-XGBoost	82.10%	82.09%	ResNet50V2-XGBoost	87.11%	87.11%
ResNet101-BagT	76.91%	76.89%	ResNet101-XGBoost	85.51%	85.49%	ResNet101-XGBoost	88.43%	88.42%
ResNet101V2-XGBoost	74.79%	74.79%	ResNet101V2-XGBoost	75.52%	75.50%	ResNet101V2-XGBoost	78.43%	78.37%
ResNet152-XGBoost	79.02%	78.99%	ResNet152-XGBoost	86.11%	86.11%	ResNet152-XGBoost	86.99%	86.99%
ResNet152V2-XGBoost	75.15%	75.15%	ResNet152V2-XGBoost	78.20%	78.19%	ResNet152V2-XGBoost	80.96%	80.94%
InceptionV3-XGBoost	75.38%	75.37%	InceptionV3-XGBoost	76.49%	76.49%	InceptionV3-RF	77.83%	77.68%
InceptionResNetV2-XGBoost	74.91%	74.91%	InceptionResNetV2-XGBoost	74.30%	74.30%	InceptionResNetV2-XGBoost	79.28%	79.24%
MobileNet-XGBoost	**83.94%**	**83.94%**	**MobileNet-XGBoost**	**91.11%**	**91.11%**	**MobileNet-XGBoost**	**92.05%**	**92.04%**
MobileNetV2-XGBoost	78.90%	78.88%	MobileNetV2-XGBoost	85.75%	85.75%	MobileNetV2-XGBoost	88.55%	88.54%
DenseNet121-KNN	79.60%	79.60%	DenseNet121-KNN	83.80%	83.77%	DenseNet121-XGBoost	86.51%	86.49%
DenseNet169-XGBoost	79.48%	79.48%	DenseNet169-KNN	84.17%	84.15%	DenseNet169-KNN	84.82%	84.76%
DenseNet201-XGBoost	79.60%	79.58%	DenseNet201-XGBoost	84.41%	84.41%	DenseNet201-XGBoost	86.14%	86.15%
EfficientNetB0-XGBoost	68.35%	68.24%	EfficientNetB0-XGBoost	74.91%	74.91%	EfficientNetB0-XGBoost	80.84%	80.78%
EfficientNetB1-XGBoost	70.57%	70.54%	EfficientNetB1-XGBoost	78.93%	78.93%	EfficientNetB1-KNN	83.13%	83.06%
EfficientNetB2-XGBoost	72.22%	72.22%	EfficientNetB2-XGBoost	82.10%	82.09%	EfficientNetB2-XGBoost	81.57%	81.53%
EfficientNetB3-XGBoost	67.76%	67.75%	EfficientNetB3-XGBoost	69.79%	69.77%	EfficientNetB3-XGBoost	75.90%	75.82%
EfficientNetB4-XGBoost	76.55%	76.55%	EfficientNetB4-XGBoost	78.81%	78.80%	EfficientNetB4-XGBoost	83.73%	83.71%

Table 3. *Cont.*

Escherichia coli vs. *Pseudomonas aeruginosa*			*Escherichia coli* vs. *Staphylococcus aureus*			*Pseudomonas aeruginosa* vs. *Staphylococcus aureus*		
Classifiers	*Accuracy*	*F1-Score*	**Classifiers**	*Accuracy*	*F1-Score*	**Classifiers**	*Accuracy*	*F1-Score*
EfficientNetB5-XGBoost	71.51%	71.51%	EfficientNetB5-XGBoost	80.63%	80.63%	EfficientNetB5-BagT	83.49%	83.45%
EfficientNetB6-XGBoost	66.47%	66.47%	EfficientNetB6-XGBoost	71.86%	71.87%	EfficientNetB6-XGBoost	76.39%	76.31%
EfficientNetB7-XGBoost	75.62%	75.61%	EfficientNetB7-XGBoost	84.77%	84.77%	EfficientNetB7-XGBoost	87.83%	87.82%
EfficientNetV2B0-XGBoost	75.38%	75.38%	EfficientNetV2B0-XGBoost	83.68%	83.67%	EfficientNetV2B0-XGBoost	86.63%	86.60%
EfficientNetV2B1-XGBoost	75.85%	75.83%	EfficientNetV2B1-XGBoost	84.04%	84.03%	EfficientNetV2B1-XGBoost	87.47%	87.45%
EfficientNetV2B2-XGBoost	75.85%	75.85%	EfficientNetV2B2-KNN	80.63%	80.52%	EfficientNetV2B2-XGBoost	84.10%	84.05%
EfficientNetV2B3-XGBoost	79.95%	79.95%	EfficientNetV2B3-XGBoost	83.68%	83.68%	EfficientNetV2B3-XGBoost	86.51%	86.50%
EfficientNetV2S-XGBoost	70.93%	70.92%	EfficientNetV2S-XGBoost	75.03%	75.01%	EfficientNetV2S-XGBoost	77.47%	77.41%
EfficientNetV2M-XGBoost	65.42%	65.42%	EfficientNetV2M-XGBoost	70.89%	70.89%	EfficientNetV2M-XGBoost	67.47%	67.45%
EfficientNetV2L-BagT	63.89%	63.86%	EfficientNetV2L-XGBoost	72.59%	72.59%	EfficientNetV2L-XGBoost	72.41%	72.31%

4. Conclusions

This work introduced a preliminary method that combines standard CNN keras models and classical machine-learning models to support colony discrimination, developed in Petri-plates. In order to test and validate the system, images of three bacterial species (*Escherichia coli*, *Pseudomonas aeruginosa*, and *Staphylococcus aureus*) cultured in Petri plates were presented to the CNN models' entries to extract 50 image features to feed classical machine-learning models within a leave-one-out-cross validation procedure. The system demonstrated good *accuracy* discrimination rates between pairs of study groups: 92% for *Pseudomonas aeruginosa* vs. *Staphylococcus aureus*, 91% for *Escherichia coli* vs. *Staphylococcus aureus* and 84% *Escherichia coli* vs. *Pseudomonas aeruginosa*. The presented preliminary results showed that a combination of deep-learning models and classical machine-learning models can help to discriminate bacteria colonies in Petri-plates. Tools, such as the one developed in the present work, are really valuable in ascertaining different colony types in a single step, using a general, whole-purpose medium instead of several selective and/or differential media, rendering the process time-consuming, expensive, and prone to errors due to the increased manipulation steps required by the operator. Furthermore, differential colony counting is quite useful, since most analyzed samples in a microbiology setting are not pure-culture, but mixed cultures involving more than one bacterial species. In future work, the dataset should be extended to more bacteria colony types to evaluate the system's ability to discriminate other species and should include a set of pictures containing a mixture of colonies to evaluate the *accuracy* of the method in a mixed/complex sample. Additionally, the deep and classical machine-learning models should be refined to improve the system's performance.

Author Contributions: Conceptualization, P.M.R.; methodology, P.M.R. and P.R.; validation, P.M.R.; investigation, P.M.R. and P.R.; writing—original, P.M.R. and F.K.T.; writing—review and editing, P.M.R., P.R. and F.K.T.; supervision, P.M.R. and F.K.T.; funding acquisition, P.M.R. All authors have read and agreed to the published version of the manuscript.

Funding: This work was supported by National Funds from FCT—Fundação para a Ciência e a Tecnologia through project UIDB/50016/2020.

Institutional Review Board Statement: Not applicable.

Informed Consent Statement: Not applicable.

Data Availability Statement: The data presented in this study are openly available in FigShare at doi, reference number 10.6084/m9.figshare.20109377.v2.

Conflicts of Interest: The authors declare no conflict of interest.

References

1. Zhu, G.; Yan, B.; Xing, M.; Tian, C. Automated counting of bacterial colonies on agar plates based on images captured at near-infrared light. *J. Microbiol. Methods* **2018**, *153*, 66–73. [CrossRef] [PubMed]
2. Raju, S.; Aparna, H.G.; Krishnan, A.V.; Naryanan, D.; Gangadhran, V.; Paul, S.C. Automated counting of bacterial colonies by image analysis. *J. Multidiscip. Dent. Res.* **2020**, *5*, 19–21. [CrossRef]
3. Breakwell, D.P.; Macdonald, B.; Woolverton, C.J.; Smith, K.C.; Robison, R.A. Colony Morphology Protocol. In Proceedings of the ASM Conference for Undergraduate Educators, San Diego, CA, USA, 16–19 February 2007.
4. Rodrigues, P.M.; Luís, J.; Tavaria, F.K. Image Analysis Semi-Automatic System for Colony-Forming-Unit Counting. *Bioengineering* **2022**, *9*, 271. [CrossRef] [PubMed]
5. Farooq, U. Inhibition of *Escherichia coli*, *Pseudomonas aeruginosa*, *Staphylococcus aureus* and *Enterococcus feacalis* through Malus DomesticaExtracts to Eliminate Food Borne Illness. *Am. J. Biomed. Sci. Res.* **2019**, *3*, 391–397. [CrossRef]
6. Cleven, B.E.E.; Palka-Santini, M.; Gielen, J.; Meembor, S.; Krönke, M.; Krut, O. Identification and Characterization of Bacterial Pathogens Causing Bloodstream Infections by DNA Microarray. *J. Clin. Microbiol.* **2006**, *44*, 2389–2397. [CrossRef] [PubMed]
7. Hedge, A. Survival of *Escherichia coli*, *Pseudomona aeruginosa*, *Staphylococcus aureus* on Wood and Plastic Surfaces. *J. Microb. Biochem. Technol.* **2015**, *7*, 4. [CrossRef]
8. Kim, S.; Lee, M.H.; Wiwasuku, T.; Day, A.S.; Youngme, S.; Hwang, D.S.; Yoon, J.Y. Human sensor-inspired supervised machine learning of smartphone-based paper microfluidic analysis for bacterial species classification. *Biosens. Bioelectron.* **2021**, *188*, 113335. [CrossRef] [PubMed]

9. Zieliński, B.; Plichta, A.; Misztal, K.; Spurek, P.; Brzychczy-Włoch, M.; Ochońska, D. Deep learning approach to bacterial colony classification. *PLoS ONE* **2017**, *12*, e0184554. [CrossRef] [PubMed]

10. Khalifa, N.E.M.; Taha, M.H.N.; Hassanien, A.E.; Hemedan, A.A. Deep bacteria: Robust deep learning data augmentation design for limited bacterial colony dataset. *Int. J. Reason.-Based Intell. Syst.* **2019**, *11*, 256. [CrossRef]

11. Li, Z.; Jiang, Y.; Tang, S.; Zou, H.; Wang, W.; Qi, G.; Zhang, H.; Jin, K.; Wang, Y.; Chen, H.; et al. 2D nanomaterial sensing array using machine learning for differential profiling of pathogenic microbial taxonomic identification. *Microchim. Acta* **2022**, *189*, 273. [CrossRef] [PubMed]

12. Rodrigues, P.M.; Luis, J.; Tavaria, F.K. Petri Dishes Digital Images Dataset of *E. coli*, *S. aureus* and *P. aeruginosa*. 2022. Available online: https://figshare.com/articles/dataset/Dataset_bioengineering_17489364/20109377/2 (accessed on 20 November 2022).

13. Chollet, F. Keras. 2015. Available online: https://github.com/fchollet/keras (accessed on 20 November 2022).

14. Stehman, S.V. Selecting and interpreting measures of thematic classification accuracy. *Remote. Sens. Environ.* **1997**, *62*, 77–89. [CrossRef]

15. Missiakas, D.M.; Schneewind, O. Growth and Laboratory Maintenance of *Staphylococcus aureus*. *Curr. Protoc. Microbiol.* **2013**, *28*. [CrossRef] [PubMed]

16. Hossain, M.; Rahman, W.; Ali, M.; Sultana, T.; Hossain, K. Identification and Antibiogram Assay of *Escherichia coli* Isolated from Chicken Eggs. *J. Bio-Sci.* **2021**, *29*, 123–133. [CrossRef]

17. Agarwal, G.; Kapil, A.; Kabra, S.K.; Das, B.K.; Dwivedi, S.N. Characterization of Pseudomonas aeruginosa isolated from chronically infected children with cystic fibrosis in India. *BMC Microbiol.* **2005**, *5*, 43. [CrossRef] [PubMed]

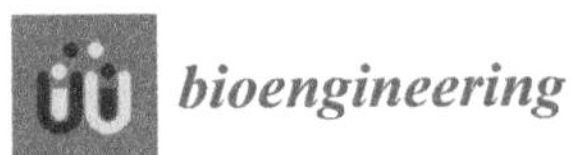

bioengineering

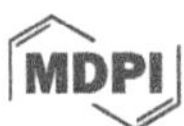

Article

Audio-Visual Stress Classification Using Cascaded RNN-LSTM Networks

Megha V. Gupta [1], Shubhangi Vaikole [2], Ankit D. Oza [3], Amisha Patel [4], Diana Petronela Burduhos-Nergis [5,*] and Dumitru Doru Burduhos-Nergis [5,*]

1   Department of Computer Engineering, New Horizon Institute of Technology and Management, University of Mumbai, Mumbai 400615, Maharashtra, India
2   Department of Computer Engineering, Datta Meghe College of Engineering, University of Mumbai, Mumbai 400708, Maharashtra, India
3   Department of Computer Sciences and Engineering, Institute of Advanced Research, Gandhinagar 382426, Gujarat, India
4   Department of Mathematics, Institute of Technology, Ahmedabad 382481, Gujarat, India
5   Faculty of Materials Science and Engineering, Gheorghe Asachi Technical University of Iasi, 700050 Iasi, Romania
*   Correspondence: diana.burduhos@tuiasi.ro (D.P.B.-N.); doru.burduhos@tuiasi.ro (D.D.B.-N.)

Citation: Gupta, M.V.; Vaikole, S.; Oza, A.D.; Patel, A.; Burduhos-Nergis, D.P.; Burduhos-Nergis, D.D. Audio-Visual Stress Classification Using Cascaded RNN-LSTM Networks. *Bioengineering* **2022**, *9*, 510. https://doi.org/10.3390/bioengineering9100510

Academic Editors: Pedro Miguel Rodrigues, João Paulo do Vale Madeiro and João Alexandre Lobo Marques

Received: 13 September 2022
Accepted: 23 September 2022
Published: 27 September 2022

Publisher's Note: MDPI stays neutral with regard to jurisdictional claims in published maps and institutional affiliations.

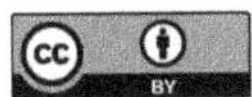

Abstract: The purpose of this research is to emphasize the importance of mental health and contribute to the overall well-being of humankind by detecting stress. Stress is a state of strain, whether it be mental or physical. It can result from anything that frustrates, incenses, or unnerves you in an event or thinking. Your body's response to a demand or challenge is stress. Stress affects people on a daily basis. Stress can be regarded as a hidden pandemic. Long-term (chronic) stress results in ongoing activation of the stress response, which wears down the body over time. Symptoms manifest as behavioral, emotional, and physical effects. The most common method involves administering brief self-report questionnaires such as the Perceived Stress Scale. However, self-report questionnaires frequently lack item specificity and validity, and interview-based measures can be time- and money-consuming. In this research, a novel method used to detect human mental stress by processing audio-visual data is proposed. In this paper, the focus is on understanding the use of audio-visual stress identification. Using the cascaded RNN-LSTM strategy, we achieved 91% accuracy on the RAVDESS dataset, classifying eight emotions and eventually stressed and unstressed states.

Keywords: stress; emotion; action units; speech; audio visual; RNN-LSTM

1. Introduction

Today, 82 percent of Indians are stressed, as per the Cigna 360 Well-being study [1]. Rising stress levels even led to India being named the world's most depressed country a few years ago. In our society, the word "stress" has become overused. There are many more people suffering from stress in India than in any Western nation, despite the fact that the issue has long been dismissed as a "western" problem. More and more Indians are experiencing stress, depression, anxiety, and other related conditions due to factors such as work pressure, life's challenges, relationships, financial stress, or mental overload. The fact that stress is one of the main factors in cardiac arrests, blood pressure increases, and an increased risk of chronic diseases at an early age is even more shocking. A recent study by the World Health Organization and the Global Burden of Disease Study found that since the COVID-19 pandemic hit, there has been an increase in stress and anxiety among people [2]. Our problems have only gotten worse as a result of the global pandemic. Experts are concerned about a recent development that suggests we may be on the verge of a terrible mental illness pandemic—not to mention the emotional and financial toll the COVID-19 crisis has taken on many. There is still a lack of mental health awareness and a continuing stigmatization of mental illnesses in our country. Despite the internet and open conversations initiated by celebrities, there are many myths, taboos, and pieces of misinformation surrounding mental health. It is important to remember that going to therapy, seeing a psychiatrist, or being open about your feelings does not make you weak or bad. Mental illnesses should not be stigmatized, and getting the right help at the right time can prevent a lot of problems.

1.1. Causes of Mental Stress

Stress is a condition of mental pressure for individuals facing problems relating to environmental and social well-being which leads to many diseases. It was discovered that academic exams, human relationships, interpersonal difficulties, life transitions, and career choices all contribute to stress. Such stress is commonly associated with psychological, physical, and behavioral issues [3].

According to Lazarus and Folkman (1984), "stress is a mental or physical phenomenon formed through one's cognitive appraisal of the stimulation and is a result of one's interaction with the environment". The existence of stress depends on the existence of the stressor. Feng (1992) and Volpe (2000) defined a stressor as "anything that challenges an individual's adaptability or stimulates an individual's body or mentality". Stress can be caused by environmental factors, psychological factors, biological factors, and social factors, as shown in Table 1.

Table 1. Major causes of stress.

	Interpersonal conflict
	Role conflict
	Career concern
Cause of Stress	Occupational demands
	Work overload
	Poor working condition
	Lack of social support
	Lack of participation in decision making

1.2. Importance of Mental Stress Detection

Human stress represents an imbalanced state [4] of an individual and is triggered when environmental demands exceed the regulatory capacity of the individual [5]. Because of its unhealthy effects [6], stress detection is an ongoing research topic among both psychologists and engineers, and has been applied to lie detection tests [7], emergency call identification [8], and the development of better human–computer interfaces [9]. People experience stress because of the requests and pressures put on them. The situation becomes more difficult when they perceive the circumstances to be overpowering and believe that it will be difficult to adapt [10]. Three levels of stress can be distinguished depending on the time of exposure to stressors. Acute stress is the innate "flight-or-fight" response in the face of short-lasting exposure to stressors, and it is not considered harmful. Episodic stress appears when stressful situations occur more frequently, but they cease from time to time. It is associated with a very stressful and chaotic life [11]. Finally, chronic stress, which is the most harmful, takes place when stressors are persistent and long-standing, such as family problems, job strain, or poverty [12]. To prevent stress reaching the highest level and help diminish the risks [13], it is necessary to detect and treat it in its earlier stages, i.e., when it is still acute or episodic stress. Stress identification has gained remarkably high attention in various fields in the last two decades. These fields include the medical sector, forensics, smart environments, teaching, learning and education, human–computer interactions, the emergency services, and of course real-time situations, which are the most crucial [14]. The identification of stress is a standout among the best research topic points for psychologists as well as engineers. Stress management should begin before stress starts to cause medical problems. This is where stress monitoring can help. In recent years, interest in artificial intelligence-aided health monitoring or psychological counseling systems has increased due to the convenience and efficiency of machine learning-based algorithms. To provide appropriate services in these areas, the mental state of the user must be detectable. Among various emotional states, we focus on a methodology to detect the user's stress status.

1.3. Role of Emotion in Stress Identification

Emotions are present in almost every decision and moment of our lives. Thus, recognizing emotions awakens interest, since knowing what others feel helps us to interact with them more effectively. Emotions are considered a psychological state [15]. In the process of detecting stress using the audio-visual approach, it is important to detect the emotional state of the person. Hence, emotion recognition should be performed to decide on the stress level. The field of emotion recognition (ER) is a part of human–computer interaction, and this field has evolved very rapidly in the last decade. Several works have been performed on emotion recognition using audio and video; however, recent work has been completed on the fusion of the different modalities. Expressing emotions while interacting with others has always been a major part of communication among humans. Emotions are reflected through voice, facial expressions, and hand gestures, and can easily transcend the boundary of languages. A lot of work has been performed over the decades on automatic emotion recognition as part of human–computer interaction.

It must be considered that emotions are subjective to an individual, i.e., each subject may experience a different emotion in response to the same stimuli. Thus, emotions can be classified into two different models—the discrete model and the dimensional model. The discrete model includes basic emotions such as happiness, sadness, fear, disgust, anger, surprise, and mixed emotions such as motivation (thirst, hanger, pain, mood), self-awareness (shame, disgrace, guilt), etc. The dimensional model is expressed in terms of two emotions, valence (disgust, pleasure) and arousal (calm, excitement). The various emotions experienced by a human can be represented through the Plutchik wheel of emotion [16], as shown in Figure 1.

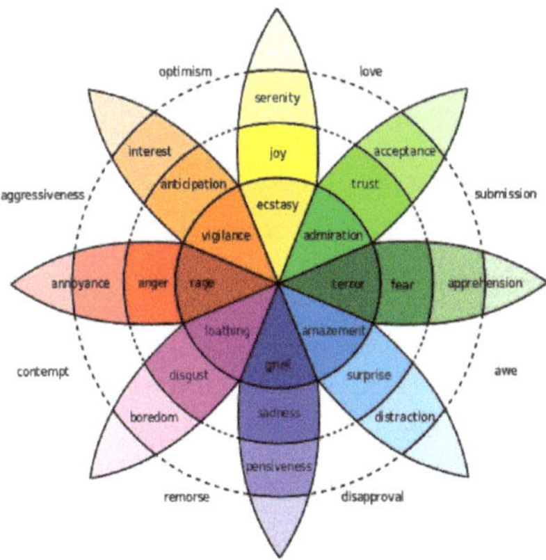

Figure 1. Plutchik wheel of emotion.

Several researchers have analyzed human stress using basic emotions. It is possible to map emotions with the stress level. Stress can be detected based on emotions obtained from the audio-visual data. Human emotions are expressed in the voice as well as on the face. The emotional state is extracted from the audio-visual data first. Positive emotions such as happiness, joy, love, pride, and pleasure can have a positive effect, such as improving daily work performance, and negative emotions such as anger, terrible, sad and, disgust can have a negative impact on the health of a person. Positive and negative emotions are represented in Figure 2. Emotional signs such as depression, terrible, unhappiness, anxiety, agitation, and anger are responsible for stress. Stress can be detected from the two emotional states of anger and disgust.

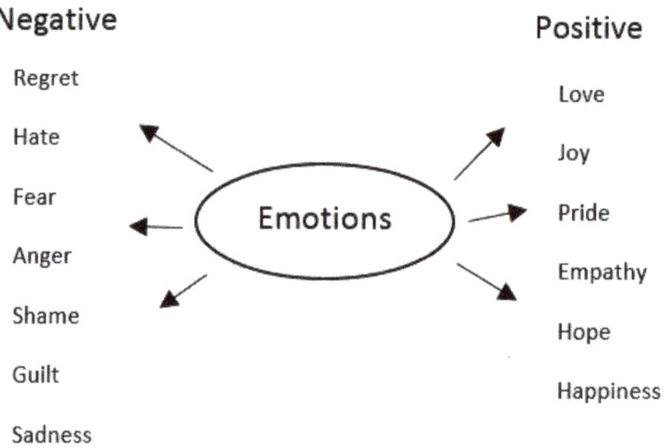

Figure 2. Positive and negative emotions.

The valence–arousal space, as illustrated in Figure 3, can be subdivided into four quadrants, namely low arousal/low valence (LALV), low arousal/high valence (LAHV), high arousal/low valence (HALV), and high arousal/high valence (HAHV) [17].

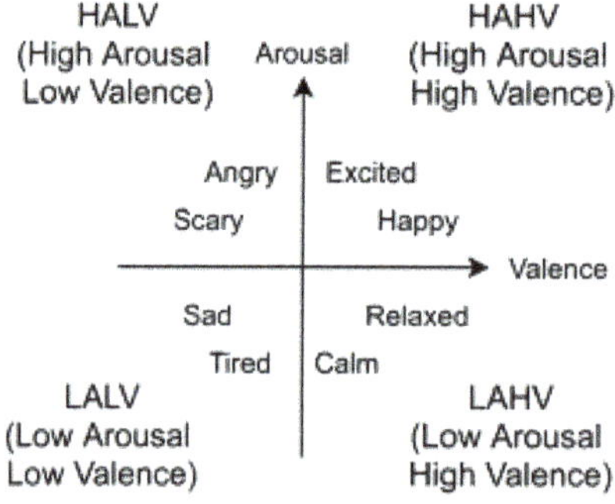

Figure 3. Arousal–valence model for emotion representation.

Our model reached an accuracy of 91% on the 'The Ryerson Audio-Visual Database of Emotional Speech and Song (RAVDESS), outperforming some of the previous solutions evaluated in similar conditions. As far as we know, our study also represents the first attempt to combine speech and facial expressions to recognize the eight emotions in RAVDESS and finally conclude on a stressed or relaxed state.

The rest of the paper is organized as follows: Section 2 describes preceding research studies related to our proposal. Section 3 presents feature extraction, elaborating on the facial action coding system (FACS) and OpenFace. Section 4 summarizes the dataset and the proposed methodology. Section 5 describes the main results obtained and performance analysis. Finally, in Section 6, we discuss the main conclusions of our study and propose future research lines.

2. Literature Review

By outlining some of the difficulties that these systems encountered, we present earlier automatic stress detection techniques here. We describe the stress-inducing stimuli that were employed, how stress was measured, the signals that were gathered, and the machine learning techniques that were applied in these studies.

2.1. Stress Detection Using Speech Signal

Stress detection from speech signals has many applications. It is used in psychology to monitor the different stress levels of patients with different stress conditions and provide necessary treatments. The safety and security of a system can be established by monitoring the different stress levels of pilots, deep sea divers and military officials undertaking law enforcement. Stress detection is also useful in speaker identification, deception detection and identification of threatening calls in a few cases of crimes [18]. In order to effectively express his or her message, a person must choose the words to use at each stage of speaking. These choices, as well as the language, syntax, and timing of speech, can all be impacted by stress [19,20]. These changes in wording, grammar, and timing can then be employed as vocal cues to indicate stress. Other changes are also brought on by stress, though. For instance, in order to create sound waves during speaking, the body modifies the tension of many muscles to push air through the vocal folds and out of the vocal tract [21]. Stress raises the breathing rate and muscle tension, which alters speech mechanics and, as a result, the way speech sounds [22,23]. A voice-based stress detection system, named StressSense [24], was implemented on Android phones to detect the stress levels from human voice. The stress model was developed in several contexts, testing various speakers and events.

Kevin Tomba et al. [25] worked on the Berlin Emotional Database (EMO-DB), the Keio University Japanese Emotional Speech Database (KeioESD) and the Ryerson Audio-Visual Database of Emotional Speech and Song (RAVDESS). SVM and ANN algorithms were used. It was found that mean energy, mean intensity, and Mel frequency cepstral coefficients proved to be good features for speech analysis. However, only audio signals were considered, and not audio-visual data. N.P. Dhole and S.N. Kale investigated RNN classification and used it on the BERLIN and HUMAINE Datasets. They also used Audacity software to build real datasets for recurrent neural network applications. Despite being effective for audio signals, the efficiency percentage was not calculated [14]. Audio-visual data were not considered. Mansouri et al. [26] used a wavelet and neural network to create and implement an emotion identification system from speech signals. EMO-DB and SAVEE were used. The accuracy was judged to be satisfactory. The procedure, however, was time-consuming. The detection of stress was not taken into account.

2.2. Stress Detection Using Audio-Visual Data

Speech and facial expression are two natural and effective ways of expressing emotions when human beings communicate with each other. During the last two decades, audio-visual emotion recognition integrating speech and facial expression has attracted extensive attention owing to its promising potential applications in human–computer interaction [27,28]. However, recognizing human emotions with computers is still a challenging task because it is difficult to extract the best audio and visual features characterizing human emotions.

G. Giannakakis et al. [29] recorded videos using a camera. The videos' facial cues were used to identify signs of anxiety and stress. This method achieved good classification accuracy. However, a 1 min video duration could yield more reliable estimates. Kah Phooi et al. [30] used the eNTERFACE and RML (RAVDESS) datasets. They used a combined rule-based and machine learning approach for emotion recognition using audio-visual data. Anupam Agrawal and Nayaneesh Kumar Mishra [31] used SAVEE and created their own dataset. They worked on emotion classification based on the fusion of audio and visual data. However, it was found that the results can be improved using deep learning techniques. Noroozi, F et al. [32] worked on audio-visual emotion recognition in video clips. The datasets used were SAVEE, eNTERFACE'05, and RML.

Audio-visual data were not considered for the stress detection, and only audio signals were used. Moreover, the accuracy of the results can be improved. Although there is much research discussing the recognition and analysis of the six basic emotions, i.e., anger, disgust, fear, happiness, sadness, and surprise, considerably less research has focused on stress and anxiety detection from audio visuals, as these states are considered as complex emotions that are linked to basic emotions (e.g., fear). The results of emotion state recognition from audio-visual data can be improved using deep learning techniques, which can be further used to detect stress.

2.3. Analysis

Overall, this seems to be an interesting area of research, and the analysis of the existing work would help in carrying out future research. Table 2 provides an overview of numerous studies reflecting the same area of interest, together with the datasets they employed, the techniques used, the pros of these techniques, and the scope for advancement.

Table 2. Analysis of earlier work in the same field of study.

Title	Datasets Used	Technique	Pros of Technique	Scope for Improvement
Stress Detection Through Speech Analysis Kevin Tomba et al. (ICETE 2018) [25]	Berlin Emotional Database (EMO-DB), the Keio University Japanese Emotional Speech Database (KeioESD), and the Ryerson Audio-Visual Database of Emotional Speech and Song (RAVDESS)	SVMs and ANNs were chosen.	MFCCs, mean energy, and the mean intensity were all demonstrated to be effective speech analysis features.	Only audio input was considered and not audio-visual data
Study of Recurrent Neural Network Classification of Stress Types in Speech Identification N.P. Dhole, S.N. Kale (IJCSE 2018) [14]	BERLIN and HUMAINE Datasets	RNN	Real time dataset was created	Efficiency percentage not calculated. Works only on audio and not audio-visual data
Designing and Implementing of Intelligent Emotional Speech Recognition with Wavelet and Neural Network Mansouri et al. (IJACSA 2016) [26]	Datasets: EMO-DB and SAVEE	Artificial neural network	Accuracy is good	Time-consuming method. Stress detection was not considered
Stress and anxiety detection using facial cues from videos G. Giannakakis et al. (Elsevier 2017) [29]	Recorded using camera	Using facial cues from the videos	Achieves good classification accuracy	1 min video duration could yield more reliable estimates
A Combined Rule-Based & Machine Learning Audio-Visual Emotion Recognition Approach Kah Phooi et al. (IEEE 2016) [30]	eNTERFACE and RML(RAVDESS)	Emotion recognition using rule-based and machine learning	Fusion of audio and visual data	Worked only on emotion using audio-visual data, stress was not detected
Fusion-based Emotion Recognition System Anupam Agrawal, Nayaneesh Kumar Mishra (IEEE 2016) [31]	SAVEE and also created own dataset	SVM for emotion classification	Fusion of audio and visual data	Results can be improved using deep learning techniques
Audio-Visual Emotion Recognition in Video Clips Noroozi, F et al. (IEEE 2016) [32]	SAVEE eNTERFACE'05 and RML	Fusion at the decision level	Comparison of results based on all 3 datasets	Stress detection was not considered

To sum up, despite the fact that other works in the literature also performed multi-modal emotion recognition on RAVDESS, such as Wang et al. [33], who used facial images to generate spectrograms, which were then used for data augmentation to improve the SER model performance in six emotions, our work is the first that, to our knowledge, detects the stressed and relaxed state using the audio-visual information of RAVDESS by means of aural and facial emotion recognition using the eight emotions.

2.4. Transition from Holistic Facial Recognition to Deep Learning Based Recognition

In the 1990s and 2000s, the face recognition community was dominated by holistic techniques. Faces are represented using holistic approaches utilising the complete facial region. Many of these approaches function by projecting facial photographs into a low-dimensional space that eliminates unimportant features and variances. PCA is one of the most prominent techniques in this field. Deep neural networks trained with extremely huge datasets have lately supplanted older approaches based on hand-crafted features and typical machine learning techniques. Deep face recognition algorithms, which employ hierarchical design to learn discriminative face representation, have significantly enhanced state-of-the-art performance and spawned a multitude of successful real-world applications. Deep learning employs many processing layers to discover data representations with numerous feature extraction levels [34,35].

3. Feature Extraction from Facial Expressions

3.1. Facial Action Coding System

Eckman and Friesen [36] created the FACS technique to analyze facial microexpressions and identify the emotions of the persons being studied. It is predicated on the notion that various facial muscle patterns can be linked to various emotions, and that the face areas where these muscles are active can be used to identify an individual's emotion. The fundamental benefit of FACS over other face analysis techniques is that it can detect concealed emotions, even when the person is attempting to imitate other emotions. People's emotions are frequently assessed using FACS.

FACS divides the face into 46 action units (AUs), as shown in Figure 4, which can be either nonadditive (an AU's activity is unrelated to the activity of other AUs) or additive (when one AU is activated, it causes another AU or group of AUs to activate). The Action units along with their pictorial representation is depicted in Table 3 below. The Facial Action Coding System (FACS) is used to classify human facial movements according to how they appear on the face. FACS encodes the movements of specific facial muscles from slight instantaneous changes in facial appearance.

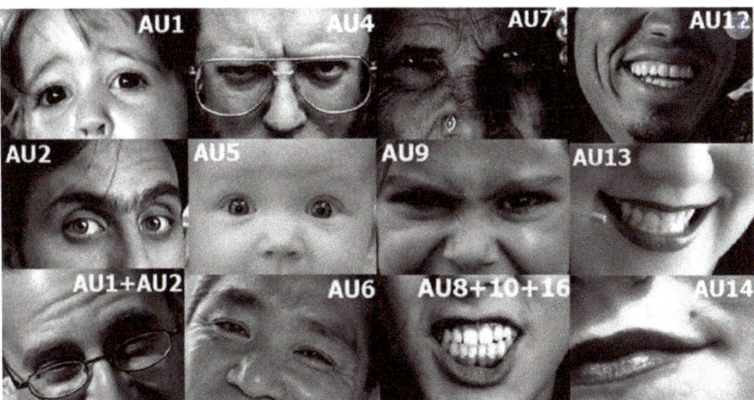

Figure 4. Action units.

Table 3. Action units.

1	Inner Brow Raiser	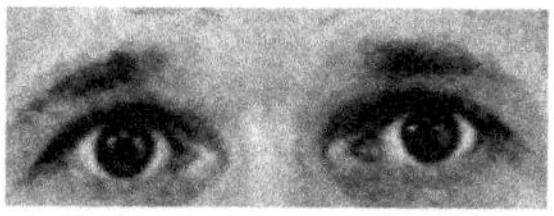
2	Outer Brow Raiser	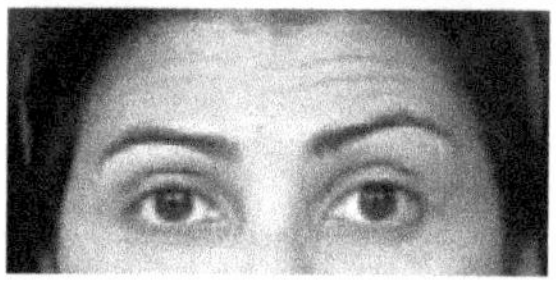
4	Brow Lowerer	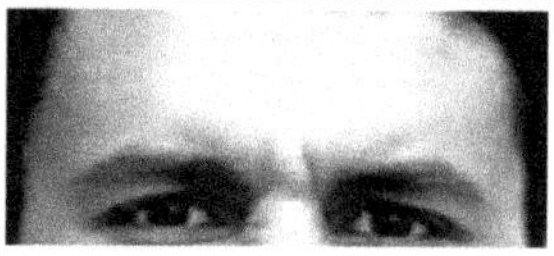
5	Upper Lid Raiser	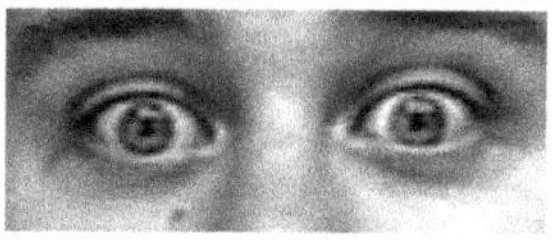
6	Cheek Raiser	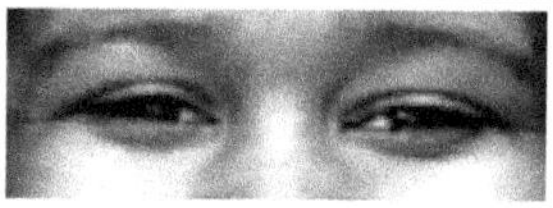
7	Lid Tightener	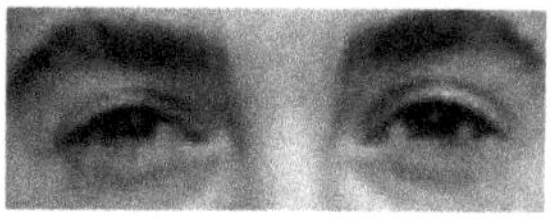
9	Nose Wrinkler	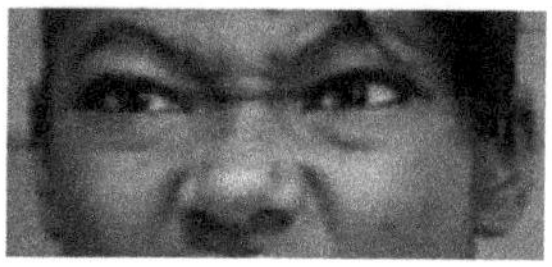
10	Upper Lip Raiser	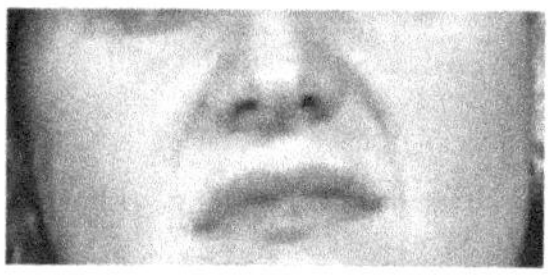
11	Nasolabial Deepener	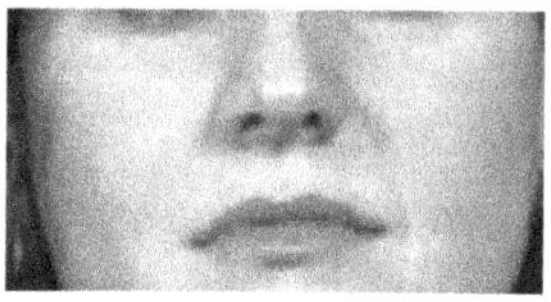

Table 3. *Cont.*

12	Lip Corner Puller 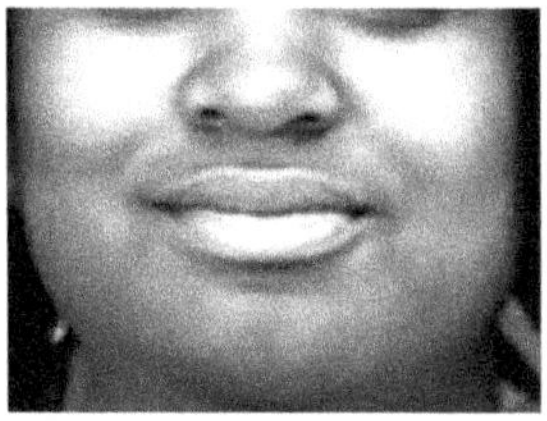
13	Cheek Puffer 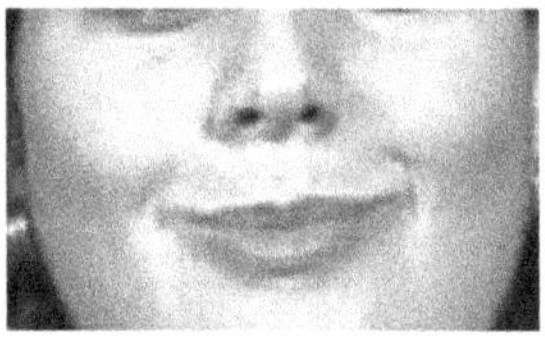
14	Dimpler 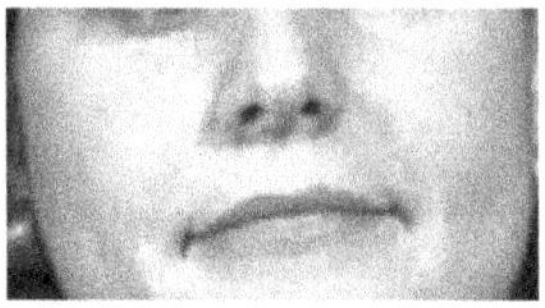
15	Lip Corner Depressor 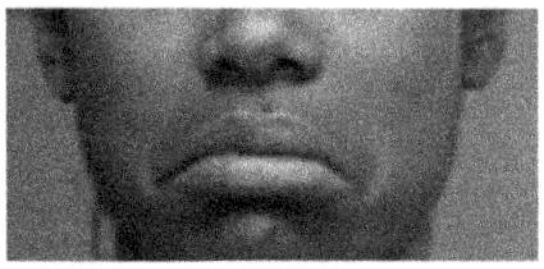
16	Lower Lip Depressor 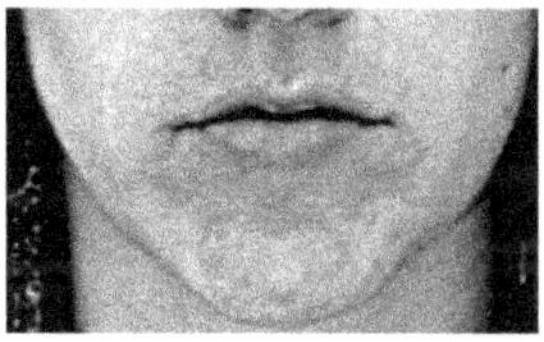
17	Chin Raiser 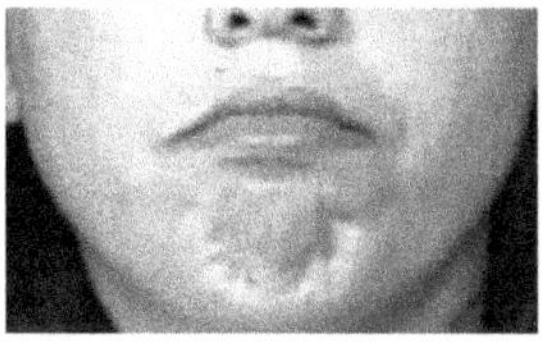
18	Lip Puckerer 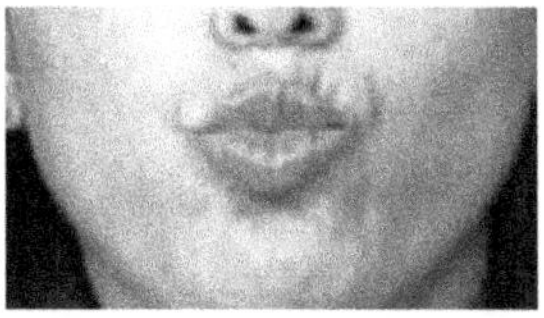
20	Lip stretcher 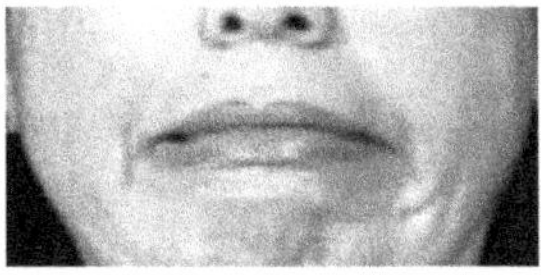

Table 3. *Cont.*

22	Lip Funneler
23	Lip Tightener
24	Lip Pressor
25	Lips part
26	Jaw Drop
27	Mouth Stretch
28	Lip Suck
41	Lid droop

Table 3. *Cont.*

42	Slit	
43	Eyes Closed	
44	Squint	
45	Blink	

Almost any anatomically conceivable facial expression can be coded using FACS, which breaks it down into the specific action units (AUs) that give rise to the expression, as shown in Table 4. FACS is a widely used method for accurately describing facial expressions. Facial expressions are considered as the signal, and emotions as the message.

Table 4. List of AUs involved in basic expressions.

Basic Expressions	Involved Action Units
Surprise	AU 1, 2, 5, 15, 16, 20, 26
Fear	AU 1, 2, 4, 5, 15, 20, 26
Disgust	AU 2, 4, 9, 15, 17
Anger	AU 2, 4, 7, 9, 10, 20, 26
Happiness	AU 1, 6, 12, 14
Sadness	AU 1, 4, 15, 23

3.2. OpenFace

OpenFace is a tool intended for computer vision and machine learning researchers, the affective computing community, and people interested in building interactive applications based on facial behavior analysis. OpenFace is the first toolkit capable of facial landmark detection, head pose estimation, facial action unit recognition, and eye-gaze estimation with available source code for both running and training the models. Specifically, OpenFace can identify AUs 1, 2, 4, 5, 6, 7, 9, 10, 12, 14, 15, 17, 20, 23, 25, 26, 28 and 45.

There are two ways to categorize AUs: intensity and presence. Presence (for instance, AU01 c) indicates whether an AU is visible on the face. On a scale of 1 to 5, intensity indicates the degree of AU intensity (min to max). Both of these scores are presented by OpenFace.

These two scores are provided by OpenFace. The output file's column AU01 c encodes 0 as not present and 1 as present for the presence of AU 1. The output file's column AU01 r has continuous values in the range of 0 (not present), 1 (present at minimum intensity), and 5 (present at maximum intensity) for the intensity of AU 1.

4. Proposed Method to Classify Mental Stress

Our proposed stress detection framework includes two systems: a speech emotion recognizer and a face emotion recognizer. The outputs of these subsystems were integrated to identify the dominant emotion and eventually result in a stressed or unstressed state. In the current research, we made a point to highlight a novel method of implementing two different algorithms to function better than any single algorithm working individually. The proposed algorithm not only improves the overall accuracy in determining emotions but also is faster than each individual algorithm, as it uses the advantages of each algorithm and eliminates the disadvantages or time-consuming processes of each of them. Further, the work may seem complicated at the first glance; however, the accuracy improvement in the field of mental stress determination is what we are looking for, and our set objectives for the research work are met through the approach.

4.1. The RAVDESS Dataset

The Ryerson Audio-Visual Database of Emotional Speech and Song (RAVDESS) is licensed under CC BY-NA-SC 4.0. The paper by Livingstone SR and Russo FA (2018) described the construction and validation of the dataset.

There are 7356 files in the RAVDESS. Each file was rated ten times for emotional validity, intensity, and authenticity. A group of 247 people who were typical untrained adult research participants from North America provided ratings. The second group of 72 people provided test–retest data. Emotional validity, interrater reliability, and test–retest intra-rater reliability were all reported to be high.

4.1.1. Description

The dataset included all 7356 RAVDESS files in their entirety (total size: 24.8 GB). The three modality formats for each of the 24 actors were audio-only (16 bit, 48 kHz.wav), audio-video (720p H.264, AAC 48 kHz,.mp4), and video-only (480p H.264, AAC 48 kHz,.mp4) (no sound). Please take note that Actor 18 did not have any song files.

4.1.2. Data

A total of 4948 samples were used for this task. Audio files were extracted from video-audio files using the "mp4 to wav" algorithm. The filenames for each of the 7356 RAVDESS files were distinctive. A seven-part numerical identifier comprised the filename (e.g., 02-01-06-01-02-01-12.mp4). These codes specified the properties of the stimulus:

The filename identifiers used are illustrated in Table 5 below.

Table 5. Identifiers of RAVDESS filenames.

Identifier	Coding Description of Factor Levels
Modality	01 = Audio-video, 02 = Video-only, 03 = Audio-only
Channel	01 = Speech, 02 = Song
Emotion	01 = Neutral, 02 = Calm, 03 = Happy, 04 = Sad, 05 = Angry, 06 = Fearful, 07 = Disgust, 08 = Surprised
Intensity	01 = Normal, 02 = Strong
Statement	01 = "Kids are talking by the door", 02 = "Dogs are sitting by the door"
Repetition	01 = First repetition, 02 = Second repetition
Actor	01 = First actor, ... 24 = Twenty-fourth actor

Taking the example of the RAVDESS filename 02-01-06-01-02-01-12.mp4:
Video-only (02)
Speech (01)
Fearful (06)
Normal intensity (01)
Statement "dogs" (02)
1st Repetition (01)
12th Actor (12)
Female, as the actor ID number is even.

4.2. Proposed System

4.2.1. Why RNN?

ANN and/or CNN have been presented before in the literature, and an accuracy of around 80% has been reported for them. In our literature review, we did not find any individual algorithm which would improve the accuracy of prediction beyond 90%. So, we needed a different approach wherein we combined two relatively less processor-heavy algorithms to work on and improve the accuracy and simultaneously work at a faster rate. However, as rightly pointed out by the reviewer, in our continued plan for our research work, we will make a point to work on ANN- and CNN-based algorithms to either present a comparative analysis or to cascade them as per our intended method to verify their performance for the said cause. Recurrent neural networks (RNNs) have been successfully applied to sequence learning issues such as action identification, scene labeling, and language processing. An RNN has a recurrent connection, unlike feed-forward networks such as convolutional neural networks (CNNs), where the previous hidden state is an input to the subsequent state. An enhanced RNN, or sequential network, called a long short-term memory network, allows information to endure. It is capable of resolving the RNN's vanishing gradient issue. Persistent memory is achieved via a recurrent neural network or RNN. Let us imagine that when reading a book or viewing a movie, you are aware of what happened in the preceding scene or chapter. RNNs function similarly; they retain the knowledge from the past and apply it to process the data at hand. Due to their inability to remember long-term dependencies, RNNs have this drawback. Long-term dependency issues are specifically avoided when designing LSTMs.

In our case, RNN is used to classify data of facial landmark position with respect to time for visual data analysis and to classify the pitch of different frequencies of the audio signal with respect to time to determine the emotions.

Speech and facial expressions are used to detect users' emotional states. These modalities are combined by employing two independent models connected by a novel approach. By merging the information from aural and visual modalities, audio-visual emotion identification is vital for the human–machine interaction system. We propose a cascaded RNN-LSTM approach for audio-visual emotion recognition through correlation analysis. The emotions will finally be categorized as a stressed mental state or a relaxed mental state. We use the RAVDESS dataset for the verification of the proposed algorithm.

4.2.2. Speech-Based Stress Detection

The flowgraph for stress recognition using speech signals is shown in Figure 5. In the proposed approach, two closely related ML algorithms viz. RNN and LSTM are cascaded together, as shown in the flowchart (Figure 6). Cascading improves the convergence time of the combined algorithm. The Mel-frequency cepstral coefficient (MFCC) is the most well-known spectral feature, since it is used to model the human auditory perception system. Here, speech signals are pre-processed and filtered using MFCC. The features of the input signal are extracted at this stage. These features are sent to 4 neurons RNN and 10 neuron LSTM working in parallel with each other. The RNN module which does not have a cell state generates the required labels for these features while the LSTM module is used for emotion prediction only. The LSTM module receives labels from the RNN module as its first input and the extracted features from MFCC as its second input. This combined approach reduces the size of the LSTM module by reducing the number of neurons required for emotion prediction, e.g., a 40-neuron LSTM module is replaced by a 10-neuron LSTM module with a 4-neuron RNN module to achieve the same result at a faster rate. Moreover, to prevent the model from overfitting, the LSTM module employs a dropout layer by randomly setting other edges of the hidden layer to zero. This reduces the convergence time to about 3/4 of the traditional approach.

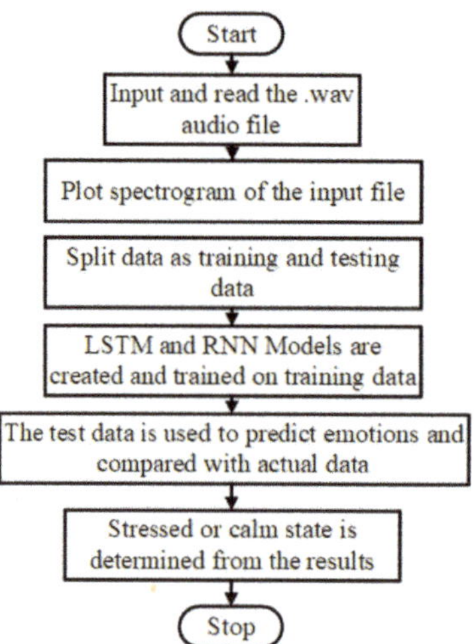

Figure 5. Flowgraph for stress recognition using speech signals.

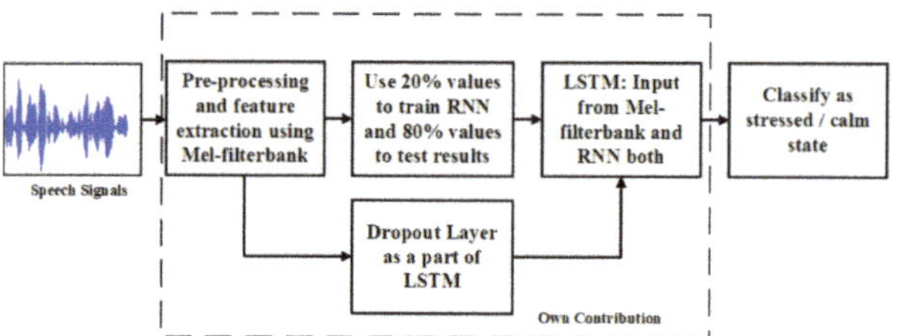

Figure 6. Speech Signals based Human Stress detection.

4.2.3. Proposed Method for Audio-Visual Based Stress Detection

Our deep learning model contains two individual input streams, i.e., the audio network processing audio signals with the cascaded RNN-LSTM model, and the visual network processing visual data with the hybrid RNN-LSTM model. The flowchart for the algorithm is in Figure 7 below.

In the proposed algorithm, audio files are extracted from the video files and processed separately. Librosa is used to process audio files while OpenFace is used to process video files. Overall, 66% of samples are used for training purposes, while the rest are used for testing the algorithm. In the algorithm, RNN and LSTM work parallelly to improve the speed of the feature extraction process. Audio signals need 20 neurons in the LSTM network while video signals need 40 neurons due to their signal processing requirements. MFCC is used as a filter for feature extraction. Dropout layers are used to prevent data from overfitting. Max pooling with convolution creates the final 8 required labels from the features. A dense sigmoid function is used for the final classification of the output with 10 neurons each. The separate outputs of both audio and video files are compared on a common platform to improve the accuracy by matching the missing labels. The following emotions are predicted in this model: "neutral": "01", "calm": "02", "happy": "03", "sad": "04", "angry": "05", "fearful": "06", "disgust": "07", "surprised": "08". Finally, 8 emotions are classified into 2 mental states—stressed and relaxed. First of all, we chose the method of comparing both audio and video files to avoid any misrepresentation of emotions due to the use of only one kind of file. In a scenario where the classification of both files is different, the average sum of scores of each signal will determine the probability of the inclination of the signals to a particular emotion. However, such a scenario has not yet occurred in our work, and hence the algorithm has not yet been validated.

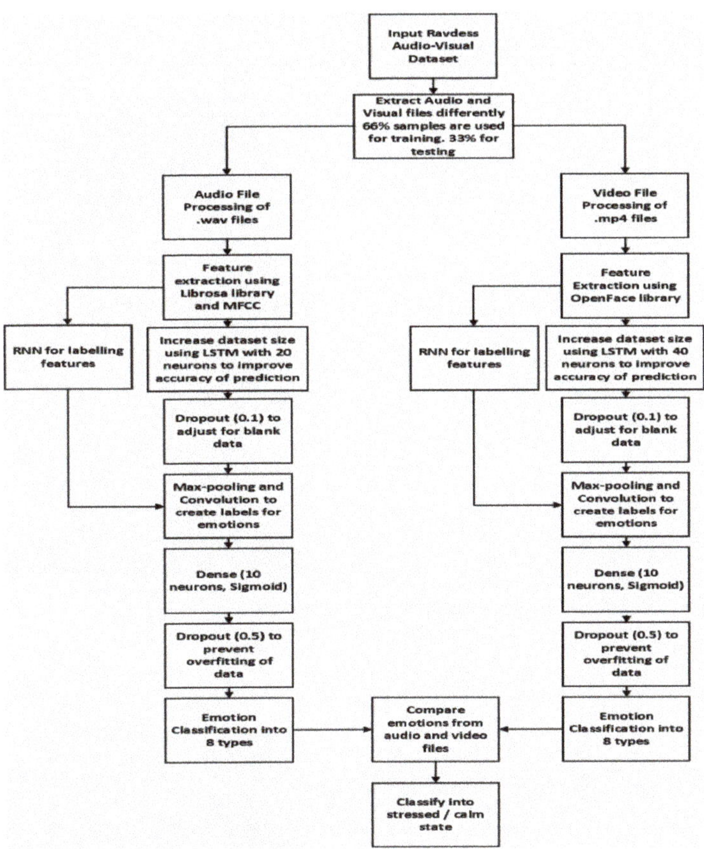

Figure 7. Proposed system workflow.

4.3. Analysis

We used the Jupyter interface to run the program. LibROSA, a python package, was used for music and audio analysis, while the OpenFace package was used for facial motion tracking.

We plotted the signal from a random file with audio and facial recognition separated as shown in Figure 8 below.

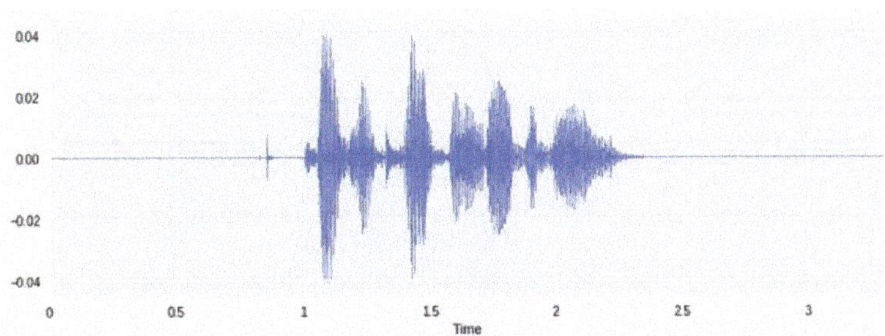

Figure 8. Audio signal.

Two facial recognition examples are illustrated in Figures 9 and 10 for frames 36 and 16 respectively.

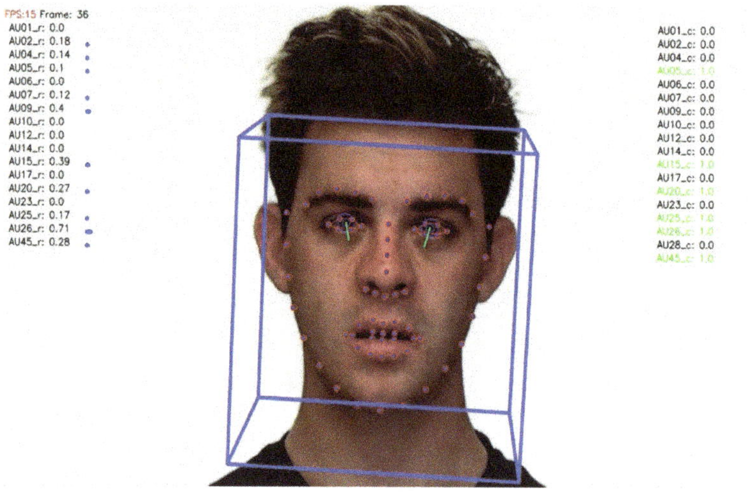

Figure 9. Facial recognition example 1.

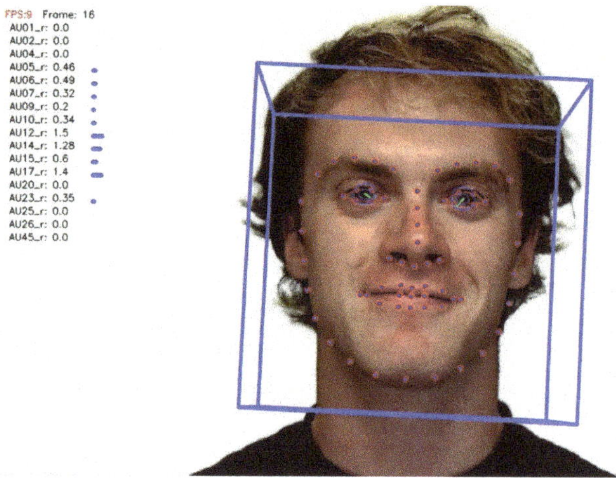

Figure 10. Facial recognition example 2.

5. Experimental Results

NumPy array was created for extracting Mel-frequency cepstral coefficients (MFCCs), while the classes for prediction were extracted from the name of the file.

To apply the cascaded RNN-LSTM method effectively, we need to expand the dimensions of our array, adding a third one using the NumPy "expand_dims" feature.

Layer (type) Output Shape Param #

===

conv1d_1 (Conv1D) (None, 40, 128) 768

activation_1 (Activation) (None, 40, 128) 0

dropout_1 (Dropout) (None, 40, 128) 0.1

max_pooling1d_1 (MaxPooling1 (None, 5, 128) 0

conv1d_2 (Conv1D) (None, 5, 128) 82,048

activation_2 (Activation) (None, 5, 128) 0

dropout_2 (Dropout) (None, 5, 128) 0.5

flatten_1 (Flatten) (None, 640) 0

dense_1 (Dense) (None, 10) 6410

activation_3 (Activation) (None, 10) 0

==
Total params: 89,226
Trainable params: 89,226
Non-trainable params: 0

The model loss of epochs based on training and test data is shown in the Figure 11 below. Figure 12 indicates the accuracy of the model.

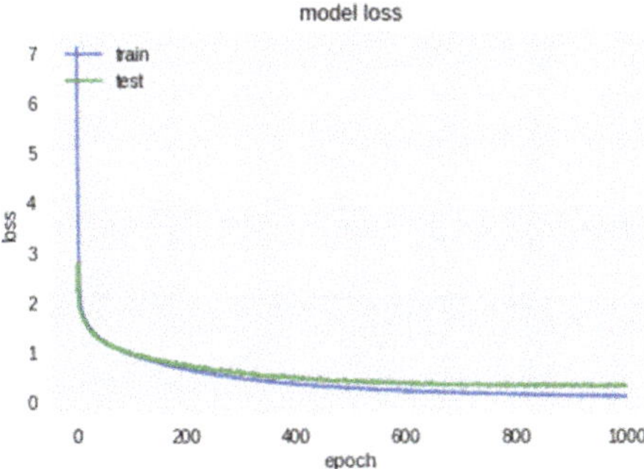

Figure 11. Loss of epochs based on training and test data.

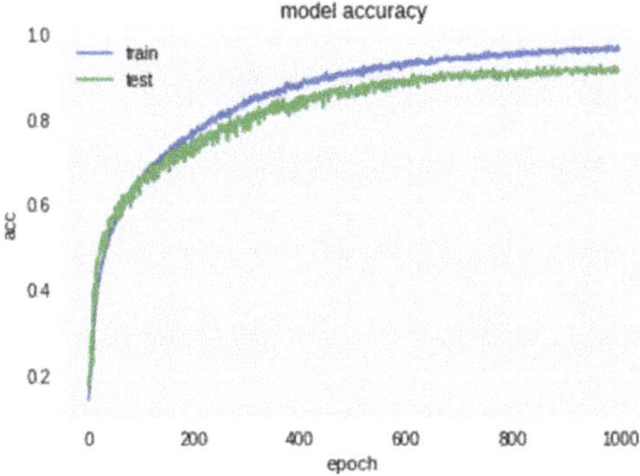

Figure 12. Accuracy of the Model.

To understand the errors of the top solution, we extracted the confusion matrix of the SVM, LSTM, and RNN-LSTM approaches with an accuracy of 76%, 82%, and 91%, respectively. The confusion matrix displayed in the Figures 13–15 below is the rounded average value of the errors and the correct predictions obtained from the folds of the 5-CV. This matrix will display an average of 288 samples (1440/5).

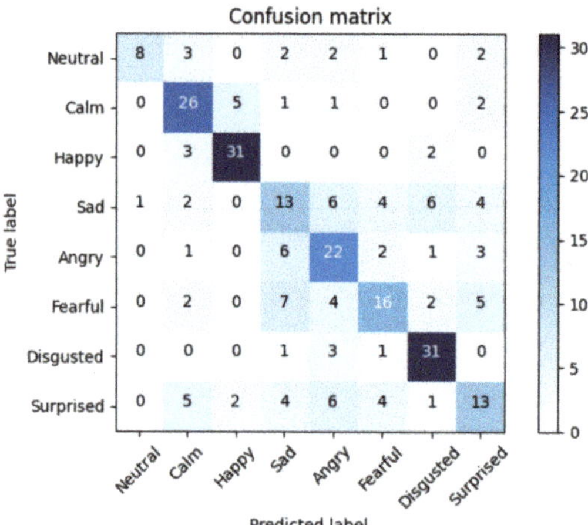

Figure 13. Average confusion matrix for the SVM algorithm. Accuracy = 76%.

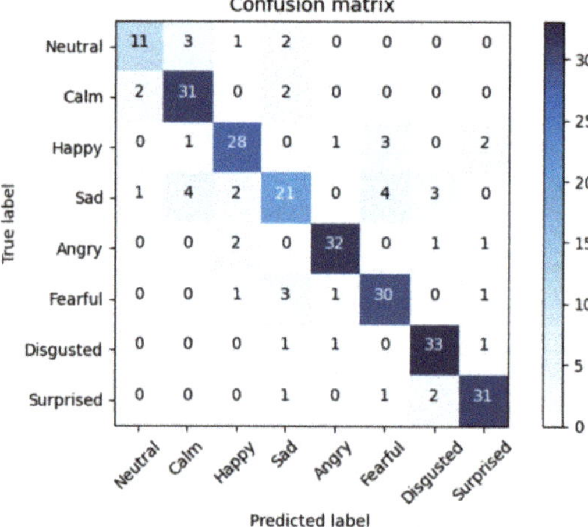

Figure 14. Average confusion matrix for the LSTM Algorithm. Accuracy = 82%.

Figure 15 reveals that the RNN-LSTM approach showed a good performance, except for some samples. The 'Sad' class contained the highest number of errors, mistaking this class in most cases for other emotions such as 'Disgusted' or 'Fearful', although it also confused this emotion with 'Calm', which may be caused by the low arousal level of both emotions.

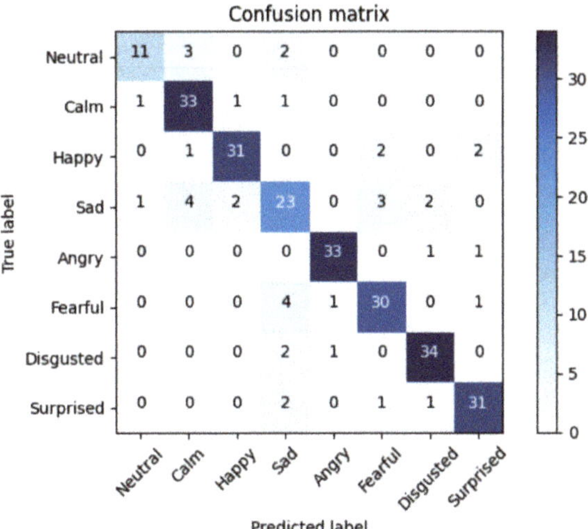

Figure 15. Average confusion matrix for RNN-LSTM approach. Accuracy = 91%.

The proposed algorithm is compared with the conventional ones and the performance analysis is presented the Table 6.

Table 6. Performance analysis of the proposed system on RAVDESS.

Classification Accuracy %	SVM	RNN	MFCC (LSTM)	MFCC(LSTM+RNN) Proposed Algorithm
Neutral	100	70	90	100
Calm	66	85	86	98
Happy	86	83	84	93
Sad	81	75	78	86
Angry	89	84	91	98
Fearful	70	72	74	87
Disgust	73	70	75	82
Surprise	60	75	78	84
Overall Accuracy	76	78	82	91

Final Output:
1633/1633 [==============================]—0s 125s/step
Accuracy: 91.00%

The existing work was focused on either audio or facial images. In audio-visual data, the separate output of audio and video files was compared on a common platform to improve accuracy by matching the missing labels. In order to enhance the accuracy further, we increased the dimensions of the dataset, as LSTM works better with more data. The accuracy for prediction for the proposed algorithm for the RAVDESS dataset is 91%.

6. Our Contributions

Only image-based classification may give polarized results in cases where the image under processing lacks the overall gesture being conveyed. Moreover, using audio and visual signals will help to improve the emotion classification accuracy, which is needed to determine whether the algorithm further needs to be fully developed for the medical determination of mental stress. Although we used well-established packages for our work, we made several changes to the algorithm to make it work and provide novelty. The changes in the algorithm include cascading or the parallel operation of algorithms (which usually runs sequentially), the addition of dropout layers to adjust the blank values and to avoid overfitting of the data, and processing of both audio and video files to compare and improve classification accuracy. We would like to state that this method of implementing the algorithm has never been reported in the literature before.

7. Conclusions and Future Scope

Detecting stress is essential before it turns chronic and leads to health issues. The current paper suggests that audio-visual data have the potential to detect stress. In our society, stress is becoming a major concern, and modern employment challenges such as heavy workloads and the need to adjust to ongoing change only make the situation worse. In addition to severe financial losses in businesses, people are experiencing health issues related to excessive amounts of stress. Therefore, it is crucial to regularly check your stress levels to detect stress in its preliminary stages and prevent harmful long-term consequences. The necessity for individuals to handle chronic stress gave rise to the concept of stress detection. The accuracy of the cascaded RNN-LSTM approach for the RAVDESS dataset is 91%. The obtained results are 15–20% better than those of other conventional algorithms. The proposed method is an excellent starting point to work towards mental health by detecting stress and improving one's quality of life.

The evaluation of the test results showed that the successful detection of stress is achieved, although further improvements and extensions can be made. The implementation of this system can be improved by using more efficient data structures and software to reduce delays and achieve real-time requirements.

Author Contributions: M.V.G. writing—original draft preparation, methodology, investigation; S.V. investigation, conceptulization, methodology; A.D.O. writing—original draft preparation, data curation, formal analysis; A.P. investigation, writing—original draft preparation; D.P.B.-N. writing—review and editing, resources, conceptulization. D.D.B.-N. writing—review and editing, resources, methodology. All authors have read and agreed to the published version of the manuscript.

Funding: This work was supported by Gheorghe Asachi Technical University of Iaşi—TUIASI-Romania, Scientific Research Funds, FCSU-2022.

Institutional Review Board Statement: The study was conducted in accordance with the Declaration of Helsinki, and approved by the Research Advisory Committee of Datta Meghe College of Engineering (protocol code RAC/006/2022 and date of approval-01/06/2022).

Informed Consent Statement: This research work has been done on the synthetic dataset. Hence no real patients are involved.

Data Availability Statement: Not applicable.

Acknowledgments: The authors would like to gratefully acknowledge the support of Datta Meghe College of Engineering, Airoli, Navi Mumbai, and New Horizon Institute of Technology and Management, Thane for facilitating a conducive environment to perform our research work.

Conflicts of Interest: The authors declare that they have no conflict of interest.

References

1. Available online: https://economictimes.indiatimes.com/wealth/personal-finance-news/82-indians-bogged-down-by-stress-cigna-360-well-being-study/articleshow/68615097.cms (accessed on 17 November 2019).
2. Mental Health and COVID-19: Early Evidence of the Pandemic's Impact, Scientific Brief by World Health Organization. Available online: https://www.who.int/publications/i/item/WHO-2019-nCoV-Sci_Brief-Mental_health-2022.1 (accessed on 19 September 2022).
3. Bhargava, D.; Trivedi, H. A Study of Causes of Stress and Stress Management among Youth. *IRA-Int. J. Manag. Soc. Sci.* **2018**, *11*, 108–117. [CrossRef]
4. Chrousos, G.P. Stress and disorders of the stress system. *Nat. Rev. Endocrinol.* **2009**, *5*, 374–381. [CrossRef]
5. Koolhaas, J.M.; Bartolomucci, A.; Buwalda, B.; de Boer, S.F.; Flügge, G.; Korte, S.M.; Meerlo, P.; Murison, R.; Olivier, B.; Palanza, P.; et al. Stress revisited: A critical evaluation of the stress concept. *Neurosci. Biobehav. Rev.* **2011**, *35*, 1291–1301. [CrossRef]
6. Lazarus, R. *Stress and Emotion: A New Synthesis*; Springer: New York, NY, USA, 2006.
7. Pavlidis, I.; Levine, J. Thermal image analysis for polygraph testing. *IEEE Eng. Med. Biol. Mag.* **2002**, *21*, 56–64. [CrossRef]

8. Lefter, L.; Rothkrantz, L.J.M.; Leeuwen, D.A.V.; Wiggers, P. Automatic stress detection in emergency (telephone) calls. *Int. J. Intell. Def. Support Syst.* **2011**, *4*, 148–168. [CrossRef]

9. Zhai, J.; Barreto, A.; Chin, C.; Li, C. Realization of stress detection using psychophysiological signals for improvement of human-computer interactions. In Proceedings of the IEEE SoutheastCon, Ft. Lauderdale, FL, USA, 8–10 April 2005; IEEE: New York, NY, USA, 2005; pp. 415–420.

10. Hunt, J.; Eisenberg, D. Mental Health Problems and Help-Seeking Behavior Among College Students. *J. Adolesc. Health* **2010**, *46*, 3–10. [CrossRef]

11. Bakker, J.; Pechenizkiy, M.; Sidorova, N. What's your current stress level? Detection of stress patterns from GSR sensor data. In Proceedings of the 2011 IEEE 11th International Conference on Data Mining Workshops, Vancouver, BC, Canada, 11 December 2011; IEEE: New York, NY, USA, 2012; Volume 1, pp. 573–580.

12. Colligan, T.W.; Higgins, E.M. Workplace Stress. *J. Work. Behav. Health* **2006**, *21*, 89–97. [CrossRef]

13. Sharma, N.; Dhall, A.; Gedeon, T.; Goecke, R. Thermal spatio-temporal data for stress recognition. *EURASIP J. Image Video Process.* **2014**, *2014*, 28. [CrossRef]

14. Dhole, N.P.; Kale, S.N. Study of Recurrent Neural Network Classification of Stress Types in Speech Identification. *Int. J. Comput. Sci. Eng.* **2018**, *6*, 2347–2693. [CrossRef]

15. Luna-Jiménez, C.; Griol, D.; Callejas, Z.; Kleinlein, R.; Montero, J.M.; Fernández-Martínez, F. Multimodal Emotion Recognition on RAVDESS Dataset Using Transfer Learning. *Sensors* **2021**, *21*, 7665. [CrossRef]

16. Plutchik, R. *Emotion, a Psychoevolutionary Synthesis*; Harper & Row: New York, NY, USA, 1980.

17. Koelstra, S.; Muhl, C.; Soleymani, M.; Lee, J.-S.; Yazdani, A.; Ebrahimi, T.; Pun, T.; Nijholt, A.; Patras, I. DEAP: A Database for Emotion Analysis; Using Physiological Signals. *IEEE Trans. Affect. Comput.* **2011**, *3*, 18–31. [CrossRef]

18. Hansen, J.; Patil, S. Speech under stress: Analysis, modeling and recognition. In *Lecture Notes in Computer Science, Müller, C., Ed.*; Springer: Berlin/Heidelberg, Germany, 2007.

19. Paulmann, S.; Furnes, D.; Bøkenes, A.M.; Cozzolino, P. How Psychological Stress Affects Emotional Prosody. *PLoS ONE* **2016**, *11*, e0165022. [CrossRef] [PubMed]

20. Scherer, K.R.; Moors, A. The Emotion Process: Event Appraisal and Component Differentiation. *Annu. Rev. Psychol.* **2019**, *70*, 719–745. [CrossRef] [PubMed]

21. Gaikwad, P.G.; Paithane, A. Novel Approach for Stress Recognition using EEG Signal by SVM Classifier. In Proceedings of the IEEE 2017 International Conference on Computing Methodologies and Communication, Erode, India, 18–19 July 2017; IEEE: New York, NY, USA, 2017.

22. Lahane, P.; Thirugnanam, M. A novel approach for analyzing human emotions based on electroencephalography (EEG). In Proceedings of the 2017 Innovations in Power and Advanced Computing Technologies (i-PACT), Vellore, India, 21–22 April 2017; IEEE: New York, NY, USA, 2018; pp. 1–6.

23. Thejaswini, S.; Kumar, K.M.R.; Vijayendra, A.; Shyam, R.; Anchan, P.D.; Gowda, E. An Algorithm to Detect Emotion States and Stress Levels Using EEG Signals. *Int. J. Latest Res. Eng. Technol.* **2017**, *3*, 5–12.

24. Lu, H.; Frauendorfer, D.; Rabbi, M.; Mast, M.S. StressSense: Detecting Stress in Unconstrained Acoustic Environments Using Smartphones. In Proceedings of the 2012 ACM Conference on Ubiquitous Computing, Pittsburgh, PA, USA, 5–8 September 2012.

25. Tomba, K.; Dumoulin, J.; Mugellini, E.; Khaled, O.A.; Hawila, S. Stress Detection Through Speech Analysis. In Proceedings of the 15th International Joint Conference on e-Business and Telecommunications (ICETE 2018), Porto, Portugal, 26–28 July 2018; Volume 1, pp. 394–398.

26. Mansouri, B.Z.; Mirvaziri, H.; Sadeghi, F. Designing and Implementing of Intelligent Emotional Speech Recognition with Wavelet and Neural Network. *Int. J. Adv. Comput. Sci. Appl.* **2016**, *7*, 26–30.

27. Hossain, M.S.; Muhammad, G.; Song, B.; Hassan, M.M.; Alelaiwi, A.; Alamri, A. Audio–visual emotion-aware cloud gaming framework. *IEEE Trans. Circuits Syst. Video Technol.* **2015**, *25*, 2105–2118. [CrossRef]

28. Gupta, R.; Malandrakis, N.; Xiao, B.; Guha, T.; Van Segbroeck, M.; Black, M.; Potamianos, A.; Narayanan, S. Multimodal prediction of affective dimensions and depression in human-computer interactions. In Proceedings of the 4th International Workshop on Audio/Visual Emotion Challenge (AVEC), Orlando, FL, USA, 7 November 2014; pp. 33–40.

29. Giannakakis, G.; Pediaditis, M.; Manousos, D.; Kazantzakis, E.; Chiarugi, F.; Simos, P.G.; Marias, K.; Tsiknakis, M. Stress and anxiety detection using facial cues from videos. *Biomed. Signal Processing Control* **2017**, *31*, 89–101. [CrossRef]

30. Seng, K.P.; Ang, L.-M.; Ooi, C.S. A Combined Rule-Based & Machine Learning Audio-Visual Emotion Recognition Approach. *IEEE Trans. Affect. Comput.* **2018**, *9*, 3–13.

31. Agrawal, A.; Mishra, N.K. Fusion based Emotion Recognition System. In Proceedings of the 2016 International Conference on Computational Science and Computational Intelligence, Las Vegas, NV, USA, 15–17 December 2016; IEEE: New York, NY, USA, 2017.

32. Noroozi, F.; Marjanovic, M.; Njegus, A.; Escalera, S.; Anbarjafari, G. Audio-visual emotion recognition in video clips. *IEEE Trans. Affect. Comput.* **2017**, *10*, 60–75. [CrossRef]

33. Wang, S.; Wu, Z.; He, G.; Wang, S.; Sun, H.; Fan, F. Semi-supervised classification-aware cross-modal deep adversarial data augmentation. *Future Gener. Comput. Syst.* **2021**, *125*, 194–205. [CrossRef]

34. Available online: https://viso.ai/deep-learning/deep-face-recognition/ (accessed on 19 September 2022).

35. Moret-Tatay, C.; Fortea, I.B.; Sevilla, M.D.G. Challenges and insights for the visual system: Are face and word recognition two sides of the same coin? *J. Neurolinguistics* **2020**, *56*, 100941. [CrossRef]
36. Eckman, P.; Friesen, W.V. *Facial Action Coding System: Investigator's Guide*; Consulting Psychologists Press: Palo Alto, CA, USA, 1978.

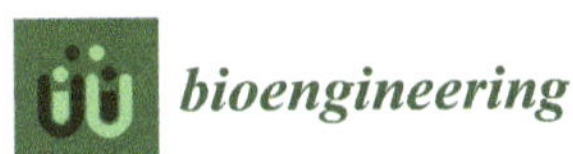

Article

Early Diagnosis of Intracranial Internal Carotid Artery Stenosis Using Extracranial Hemodynamic Indices from Carotid Doppler Ultrasound

Xiangdong Zhang [1,2,†], Dan Wu [1,*,†], Hongye Li [3], Yonghan Fang [3], Huahua Xiong [3,*] and Ye Li [1,*]

[1] Shenzhen Institute of Advanced Technology, Chinese Academy of Sciences, Shenzhen 518055, China
[2] Department of Mathematics, University of Macau, Macao 999078, China
[3] Department of Ultrasound, The First Affiliated Hospital of Shenzhen University, Shenzhen Second People's Hospital, Shenzhen 518035, China
*   Correspondence: dan.wu@siat.ac.cn (D.W.); dennis8710@163.com (H.X.); ye.li@siat.ac.cn (Y.L.)
†   These authors contributed equally to this work.

Abstract: Atherosclerotic intracranial internal carotid artery stenosis (IICAS) is a leading cause of strokes. Due to the limitations of major cerebral imaging techniques, the early diagnosis of IICAS remains challenging. Clinical studies have revealed that arterial stenosis may have complicated effects on the blood flow's velocity from a distance. Therefore, based on a patient-specific one-dimensional hemodynamic model, we quantitatively investigated the effects of IICAS on extracranial internal carotid artery (ICA) flow velocity waveforms to identify sensitive hemodynamic indices for IICAS diagnoses. Classical hemodynamic indices, including the peak systolic velocity (PSV), end-diastolic velocity (EDV), and resistive index (RI), were calculated on the basis of simulations with and without IICAS. In addition, the first harmonic ratio (FHR), which is defined as the ratio between the first harmonic amplitude and the sum of the amplitudes of the 1st–20th order harmonics, was proposed to evaluate flow waveform patterns. To investigate the diagnostic performance of the indices, we included 52 patients with mild-to-moderate IICAS (<70%) in a case–control study and considered 24 patients without stenosis as controls. The simulation analyses revealed that the existence of IICAS dramatically increased the FHR and decreased the PSV and EDV in the same patient. Statistical analyses showed that the average PSV, EDV, and RI were lower in the stenosis group than in the control group; however, there were no significant differences ($p > 0.05$) between the two groups, except for the PSV of the right ICA ($p = 0.011$). The FHR was significantly higher in the stenosis group than in the control group ($p < 0.001$), with superior diagnostic performance. Taken together, the FHR is a promising index for the early diagnosis of IICAS using carotid Doppler ultrasound methods.

Keywords: atherosclerosis; Doppler ultrasound; internal carotid artery; hemodynamic modeling; stroke

Citation: Zhang, X.; Wu, D.; Li, H.; Fang, Y.; Xiong, H.; Li, Y. Early Diagnosis of Intracranial Internal Carotid Artery Stenosis Using Extracranial Hemodynamic Indices from Carotid Doppler Ultrasound. *Bioengineering* **2022**, *9*, 422. https://doi.org/10.3390/bioengineering9090422

Academic Editors: Pedro Miguel Rodrigues, João Paulo do Vale Madeiro and João Alexandre Lobo Marques

Received: 26 July 2022
Accepted: 18 August 2022
Published: 29 August 2022

Publisher's Note: MDPI stays neutral with regard to jurisdictional claims in published maps and institutional affiliations.

1. Introduction

Atherosclerotic intracranial internal carotid artery stenosis (IICAS) is a leading cause of stroke across different races [1–3]. IICAS is normally diagnosed using cerebral digital subtraction angiography (DSA), computed tomography angiography (CTA), magnetic resonance angiography (MRA), or transcranial Doppler (TCD) ultrasound. DSA is the gold standard method for the quantitative evaluation of IICAS; however, this method is invasive and expensive [4]. CTA and MRA are less invasive than DSA; however, contrast agents are still needed, which may increase the risk of allergies and the deterioration of renal function [5]. Ultrasound is safer and less expensive; nevertheless, TCD ultrasound may have problems in locating arteries in some individuals [6]. Therefore, it is not widely applied compared with CTA/MRA/DSA. The early diagnosis of IICAS is crucial in preventing strokes and in reducing mortality. However, due to the disadvantages of these traditional methods, few asymptomatic patients in the early stage undergo these medical imaging examinations. The early diagnosis of IICAS thus remains challenging.

Because arterial stenosis may have complicated effects on blood flow velocities from a distance, correlations between invisible stenosis and hemodynamic indices measured using Doppler ultrasound, such as the peak systolic velocity (PSV), end-diastolic velocity (EDV), and resistive index (RI), have been widely investigated [7–11]. In addition, the Doppler spectrum waveform pattern may contain information on stenosis in other arterial locations [12]. Sakima et al. [13] divided left vertebral artery (VA) waveforms into five subtypes and found a significant correlation between the waveforms and the degree of left subclavian artery (SCA) stenosis. Chan et al. [14] proposed a new hemodynamic index (i.e., stenosis index (SI)) to quantitatively study the Doppler waveform patterns of the renal arteries. The index is calculated from the ratio between high- and low-frequency powers after applying the fast Fourier transform (FFT) to the waveforms. Their simulation results indicated that the SI may be a more effective diagnostic index for stenosis. In a subsequent study on the detection of significant transplant hepatic arterial stenosis, the SI outperformed the traditional RI and pulsatile index [15]. These studies indicate the possibility of detecting intracranial stenosis, which can only be imaged using CTA/MRA/DSA, from different arterial locations, such as the extracranial carotid arteries, using hemodynamic indices measured on ordinary Doppler ultrasound. Moreover, compared with CTA/MRA/DSA, Doppler ultrasound is a safer, low-cost, and easy-to-operate method that can be widely applied in physical examinations to facilitate the early diagnosis of IICAS.

Hemodynamic simulation is a powerful tool for quantitatively investigating the effects of stenosis on flow velocities and hemodynamic indices, which may facilitate the identification of effective hemodynamic indices for IICAS diagnosis. One-dimensional (1D) modeling of the arteries is a fast and effective modeling method for simulating pressure and flow-wave propagation in the human cardiovascular system [16]; it can fit Doppler ultrasound-measured flow waveforms well in actual patients [17]. Based on the 1D modeling of coronary arteries with stenosis, Yin et al. [18] developed a predictive probabilistic model of fractional flow reserve for coronary artery disease assessment. Their simulation analyses validated the efficiency of 1D models. Similar studies have validated the accuracy of 1D models with stenosis [19–21].

In this study, we developed a 1D patient-specific hemodynamic model and simulated extracranial internal carotid artery (ICA) waveforms with and without IICAS to quantitatively investigate the effects of IICAS on upstream ICA waveforms. Hemodynamic indices in the time and frequency domains were analyzed to identify sensitive indices for IICAS diagnoses. Two groups of patients with and without mild-to-moderate IICAS (<70%) were recruited to measure the Doppler waveforms at the extracranial segment of the ICA. Statistical analysis was performed to compare different hemodynamic indices, and their diagnostic performance was evaluated.

2. Materials and Methods

2.1. One-Dimensional Hemodynamic Model of the Human Cardiovascular System

In this study, we developed a patient-specific hemodynamic model of the cardiovascular system to simulate ICA blood flow velocity waveforms based on the validated modeling method in our previous work [17]. The model could simulate personalized dynamic variations in the blood pressure, flow velocity, and vessel diameter at every arterial location. As shown in Figure 1, the model consisted of a systemic artery tree (Figure 1A) combined with a cerebral artery network (Figure 1B). The governing equations for each point in each artery segment were the 1D incompressible viscous flow equations [17] coupled with the thick-wall linear elastic circular tube equation [22].

$$\frac{\partial}{\partial t}\begin{bmatrix} A \\ U \end{bmatrix} + \frac{\partial}{\partial z}\begin{bmatrix} UA \\ \frac{U^2}{2} + \frac{P}{\rho} \end{bmatrix} = \begin{bmatrix} 0 \\ -K_R\frac{U}{A} \end{bmatrix} \tag{1a}$$

$$P - P_0 = \frac{E(r_1^2 - r_0^2)}{1.5 r_1^2} \cdot \frac{r - r_0}{r_0} \tag{1b}$$

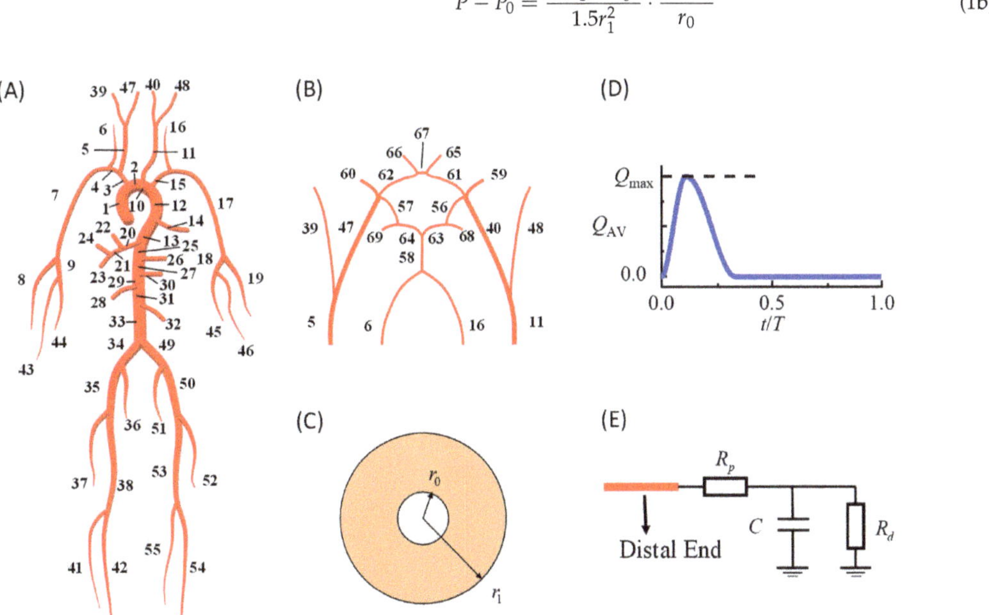

Figure 1. Hemodynamic simulation model of the human cardiovascular system: (**A**) 1D model of the systemic artery tree; (**B**) 1D model of the Willis circle; (**C**) cross-section of the artery model; (**D**) prescribed flow rate curve at the inlet of the ascending aorta; (**E**) peripheral vessel model at the outlets of the artery networks; 1D, one-dimensional.

In the above equations, A is the artery cross-sectional luminal area; r is the inner radius of the artery ($2\pi r^2 = A$); P is the corresponding pressure; E is the elastic modulus; U is the area-averaged flow velocity. R_0 and r_0 represent the inner and outer radii of the vessel when the pressure is P_0, respectively (Figure 1C). The blood density is denoted by ρ and set at 1.06 g/cm^3. K_R is the friction force term and equals $8\pi\nu$, assuming a parabolic flow velocity profile on the cross-sections [23], where ν denotes the dynamic viscosity and is set to 4.43 s^{-1}cm^2.

At the inlet of the ascending aorta (segment no. 1 in Figure 1A), a prescribed volumetric flow rate curve was modeled as the boundary condition (Figure 1D), and the area under the curve was equal to the stroke volume. At the distal ends of the arteries, widely used three-element RCR Windkessel models were used to model peripheral vessels (Figure 1E). More details regarding the modeling methods and numerical schemes can be found in the article by Zhang et al. [17]. The default parameters of each artery segment, including the diameter, wall thickness, and elastic modulus, were taken from the literature [24,25].

2.2. Patient-Specific Hemodynamic Modeling

The major parameters of the cardiovascular system model were the stroke volume, heart rate, artery diameter, artery wall elasticity, peripheral resistance, and peripheral compliance. To develop a patient-specific model, we recruited patients from the Second People's Hospital in Shenzhen, China. MRA showed that the patients had a single stenosis (43%) in the left intracranial ICA and an intact Willis circle. The stroke volume and heart rate were measured noninvasively using B-mode and M-mode ultrasound methods. B-mode ultrasound was used to measure the diameters of the ICA (nos. 40 and 47 in Figure 1A), common carotid artery (nos. 5 and 11), external carotid artery (nos. 39 and 48), VA (nos. 6 and 16), brachiocephalic artery (no. 3), and SCA (nos. 4 and 15). We also measured the diameters at several locations of the aorta, including the ascending aorta (no. 1), aortic arch (no. 10), thoracic aorta (no. 12), and abdominal aorta (no. 31), and the remaining diameters were determined via linear scaling. The geometry of the left IICAS, including the length and degree of stenosis, was estimated from MRA images. The elastic modulus, peripheral resistance, and compliance of the relevant vessels were tuned automatically to match the simulated ICA waveforms with the measured waveforms based on the Levenberg–Marquardt optimization algorithm. The measured and tuned parameters are shown in the Supplementary Data. The measurement procedures were approved by the Institutional Review Board of the Second People's Hospital of Shenzhen. The entire procedure was explained to the patients, and written consent was obtained. More details regarding the personalized modeling method can be found in the article by Zhang et al. [17].

To study the effects of IICAS on upstream hemodynamic indices, we compared the simulation results of the patient-specific model in two different cases—with and without a developed IICAS. In the normal case, we removed the geometrical narrowing in the model and reduced the local vessel's wall stiffness by 50% because increased local carotid stiffness is believed to be associated with the presence of atherosclerosis [26], while the other parameters of the cardiovascular system model remained unchanged. The PSV, EDV, and RI of proximal ICA flows were calculated for each case based on the simulated ICA blood-flow velocity waveforms. The RI was calculated using the following formula: RI = (PSV-EDV)/PSV.

In addition to the typical hemodynamic indices in the time domain, features in the frequency domain were also considered. The amplitudes of each harmonic frequency were obtained by applying the FFT to a single-period digitalized flow waveform. According to Chan et al. [14], high-frequency waves may be dampened in stenotic vessels. Therefore, in this study, we propose a new index named the first harmonic ratio (FHR), which is the ratio between the first harmonic amplitude and the sum of amplitudes from the 1st to the 20th order in order to investigate the possible high-frequency damping effect:

$$\mathrm{FHR} = \frac{AMP_1}{\sum\limits_{i=1}^{20} AMP_i} \tag{2}$$

where AMP_i denotes the amplitude of the ith order harmonic. We set the maximum order to 20 because most features of the frequency spectrum can be included in this frequency range, and the amplitudes of the higher orders are close to zero. Theoretically, when high-order harmonics are dampened, the FHR should be elevated.

2.3. Measurement of the Hemodynamic Indices in the Patient Groups

We identified patients who underwent both carotid ultrasound and cerebral CTA/MRA or DSA at the Second People's Hospital of Shenzhen (in 1 month) from 1 January 2019 to 31 December 2020. The cohort was divided into two groups: with and without mild-to-moderate IICAS (<70%). The degree of stenosis was calculated using the North American Symptomatic Carotid Endarterectomy Trial criteria [27], in which 70% is the cutoff value between severe and moderate stenosis. The following patients were excluded from the study: patients with severe stenosis, extracranial or intracranial stenosis at other locations, or heart or kidney disease or those who had undergone cardiovascular surgery. Finally, 52 and 24 patients were included in the stenosis and control groups, respectively. In the stenosis group, 14 patients had a single stenosis in the left ICA; 12 patients had a single stenosis in the right ICA; 26 patients had stenosis on both sides. There were no significant differences in the average age, sex ratio, hypertension rate, and hyperlipidemia rate between the two groups. However, the difference in the diabetes rate was relatively significant ($p < 0.05$), probably because diabetes is a major risk factor for atherosclerotic stenosis [28]. Detailed information on the two groups is presented in Table 1.

Table 1. Participant information.

	Stenosis	Normal	*p* Value
Total Number	52	24	-
Male Gender	29 (56%)	14 (58%)	0.837
Hypertension	32 (62%)	11 (46%)	0.204
Diabetes	20 (38%)	3 (13%)	0.022
Hyperlipidemia	17 (33%)	5 (21%)	0.296
Age	65.4 ± 7.9	62.8 ± 8.7	0.210

Left and right ICA flow waveforms were measured using the linear array ultrasound transducer L12-3 (3–9 MHz) of Philips EPiQ-7C. The measuring point was located at the distal segment of the extracranial ICA within the detectable range (Figure 2A). IICAS was identified from the CTA/MRA/DSA images (Figure 2B). The PSV, EDV, and RI were recorded (Figure 2C). The original Doppler waveform images containing envelop curves were saved to obtain digitalized waveform data (Figure 2D), and the amplitudes of the different orders in the frequency domain were acquired by applying the FFT to the digitalized velocity waveforms (Figure 2E). Thereafter, the index FHR in the frequency domain was calculated for each patient. This study was approved by the Institutional Review Board of the Second People's Hospital of Shenzhen.

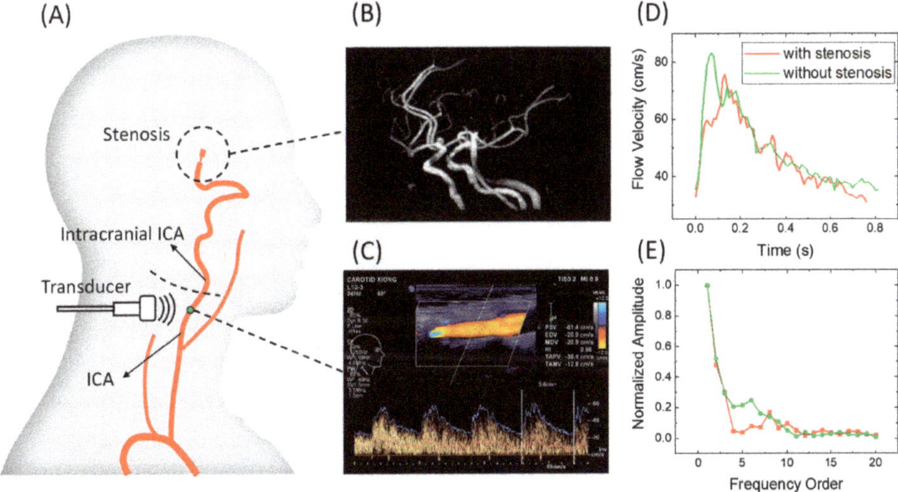

Figure 2. Schematic images of the measurement procedure: (**A**) schematic diagram of a stenosis location and the Doppler ultrasound measurement location; (**B**) magnetic resonance angiography image of a patient with IICAS; (**C**) original image of ICA flow waveforms and measurements of the PSV, EDV, and RI; (**D**) typical digitalized single-period flow velocity waveforms of a patient with IICAS and a patient without IICAS; (**E**) normalized harmonic amplitudes of waveforms in (**D**). ICA, internal carotid artery; IICAS, intracranial internal carotid artery stenosis; PSV, peak systolic velocity; EDV, end-diastolic velocity; RI, resistive index.

2.4. Statistical Analysis

To determine the differences between the hemodynamic indices of the two groups, we calculated the average value ± standard deviation of the PSV, EDV, RI, and FHR. Differences between the two groups were quantitatively evaluated using *t*-tests. Multivariate regressions were performed to investigate multiple risk factors for IICAS diagnosis and multiple contributing factors for hemodynamic index variations. Receiver operating characteristic (ROC) curves of sensitive index were analyzed, and the area under the ROC curve (AUC) value was calculated for each index to evaluate diagnostic performance. For an index with a high AUC value (AUC value of >0.8), the optimized critical value was calculated on the basis of the maximum Youden index [29].

3. Results

3.1. Patient-Specific Simulation of the ICA Waveforms

The simulated left ICA waveforms of the personalized hemodynamic model were compared to the measured waveforms in Figure 3B. The total converged mean squared error between the measured and simulated waveforms was 3.5 $(cm/s)^2$. Based on the figure, the 1D artery network model fits the Doppler waveforms well with similar major features, which indicates that the parameters are properly individualized. During the diastolic period, the measured Doppler waveforms showed small fluctuations, which may have been caused by turbulence, vortices, or measurement errors.

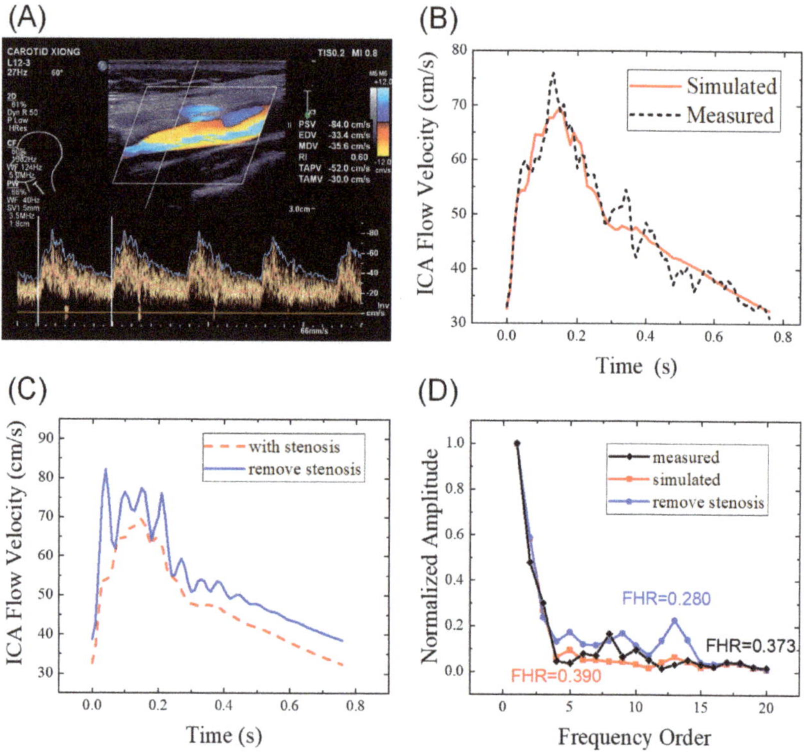

Figure 3. ICA flow waveforms of a patient: (**A**) original Doppler ultrasound data; (**B**) comparison of the measured data and simulated results from the hemodynamic model; (**C**) comparison of the simulated waveforms with and without stenoses; (**D**) comparison in the frequency domain. ICA, internal carotid artery; FHR, first harmonic ratio. The patient ID is 18 in the Supplementary Data.

We compared the simulated ICA waveforms of patients with and without IICAS while the other system parameters remained unchanged, as shown in Figure 3 and Table 2. Based on the figure, the stenosis will decrease both the PSV (-12.6 cm/s) and EDV (-6.1 cm/s), with a slightly lower amplitude (PSV-EDV) in the stenosis case. The RI remained unchanged (0.53). When the stenosis was removed, the FHR decreased dramatically from 0.390 to 0.280. Meanwhile, the simulated ICA waveform without stenosis showed typical features of ordinary individuals, with a steep upstroke and the following high platform. Therefore, we infer that IICAS tends to decrease the PSV and EDV slightly while increasing the FHR significantly. Thus, the FHR may be a promising index for IICAS diagnosis.

Table 2. Hemodynamic indices of a patient.

	PSV	EDV	RI	FHR
Measured	75.9	33.0	0.57	0.373
Simulated (with stenosis)	69.6	32.6	0.53	0.390
Simulated (without stenosis)	82.2	38.7	0.53	0.280

The mechanism of FHR elevation in the presence of developed stenosis may result from the characteristics of wave propagation in the arteries. In a fluid-filled elastic tube, wave propagations occur not only in the fluid but also in the elastic wall [30]. Because of the viscous effect, waves in the blood flow are dominated by low-frequency waves, whereas elastic waves are dominated by high-frequency reflected waves. When the wall thickness or stiffness increases, the amplitude of the elastic waves decays due to the reduced radius changes, which may lead to FHR elevations.

3.2. Diagnostic Performance of the Hemodynamic Indices

The left and right ICA flow waveforms with and without IICAS were analyzed separately. As shown in Table 3, the average PSV, EDV, and RI were lower in the stenosis group than in the control group; however, there was no significant difference between the EDV and RI on both sides ($p > 0.05$). The average right PSV in the stenosis group was significantly different from that in the control group ($p < 0.05$); however, the difference in the left PSV between the two groups was lower ($p = 0.067$). All AUC values of the PSV, EDV, and RI were below 0.8, indicating poor performance in stenosis diagnosis.

Table 3. Comparison of the hemodynamic indices between the patients with and without intracranial internal carotid artery stenosis.

	Stenosis	Control	*p* Value	AUC	95%CI
N (left)	40	24			
L. PSV	72.4 ± 19.9	82.7 ± 23.4	0.067	0.637	0.495–0.779
L. EDV	25.4 ± 8.1	28.5 ± 10.1	0.180	0.580	0.437–0.722
L. RI	0.642 ± 0.086	0.653 ± 0.087	0.598	0.566	0.420–0.711
L. FHR	0.380 ± 0.045	0.336 ± 0.033	<0.001	0.838	0.721–0.954
N (right)	38	24			
R. PSV	67.9 ± 15.6	78.9 ± 16.8	0.011	0.696	0.556–0.837
R. EDV	26.2 ± 8.9	27.1 ± 9.3	0.712	0.521	0.375–0.668
R. RI	0.612 ± 0.102	0.653 ± 0.102	0.132	0.605	0.463–0.747
R. FHR	0.372 ± 0.038	0.323 ± 0.035	<0.001	0.836	0.729–0.942

In contrast to the classical indices, the FHR showed a superior diagnostic performance. The t-test results showed a significant difference between the two groups on both sides ($p < 0.001$). The AUC values of the left and right sides were 0.838 and 0.836, respectively. The best cutoff value for the left FHR was 0.363, with a sensitivity of 70% and a specificity of 91.7%. The best cutoff value for the right FHR was 0.351, with a sensitivity of 76.3% and a specificity of 79.2%.

The FHR of both sides is plotted as a scatter plot in Figure 4A, where the labeled IDs correspond to the IDs in the Supplementary Data. Based on the figure, most negative cases are located in the lower left quarter, separated from the positive cases. A relatively high maximum FHR on both sides usually indicates stenosis in the left or right intracranial ICA. Therefore, a more accurate diagnosis with higher sensitivity and specificity may be realized by considering measurements from both sides, regardless of the stenosis location. Therefore, we conducted a statistical analysis to determine whether the maximum FHR can distinguish patients with and without IICAS on either or both sides. The results demonstrated a significant difference between the two groups ($p < 0.001$). The AUC value was 0.888, which was higher than that of the single-side diagnosis. The best cutoff value was 0.360, with a sensitivity of 88.5% and a specificity of 83.3%, as shown by the ROC curve in Figure 4B. Multivariate logistic regression was further performed to investigate possible confounding effects of age, gender, and basic diseases. As shown in Table 4, diabetes is a significant risk factor ($p < 0.05$) for IICAS, and the FHR remains significant after considering multiple factors.

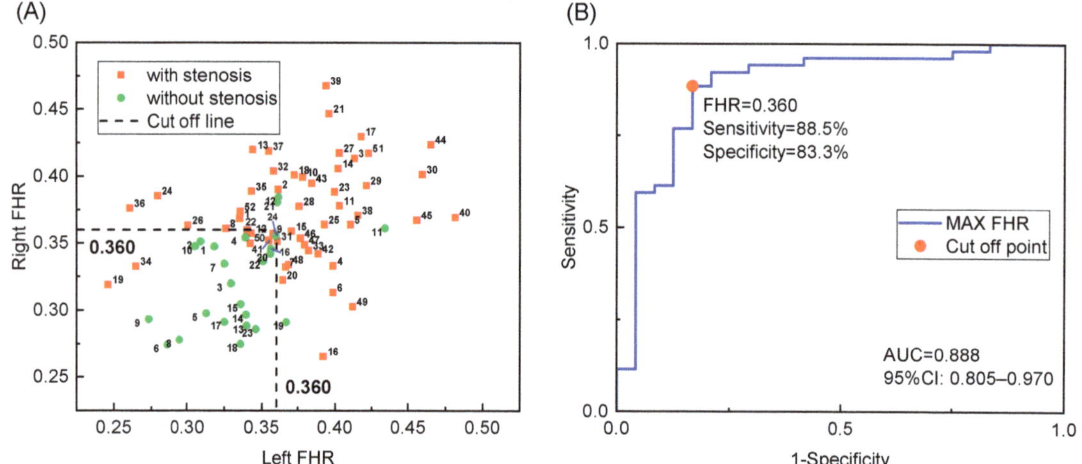

Figure 4. Diagnosis of the patients with and without IICAS: (**A**) FHR data of both sides; (**B**) receiver operating characteristic curve of IICAS diagnosis using the maximum FHR of both sides. FHR, first harmonic ratio; IICAS, intracranial internal carotid artery stenosis; AUC, area under the receiver operating characteristic curve; CI, confidence interval.

Table 4. Results of the logistic regression (N = 76).

	Coefficient	Standard Error	*p* Value	Odds Ratio
intercept	−28.052	7.810	<0.001	-
age	0.012	0.040	0.763	1.012
100× max FHR	0.726	0.197	<0.001	2.066
male gender	1.128	0.802	0.160	3.088
hypertension	0.345	0.748	0.644	1.413
diabetes	1.948	0.947	0.040	7.016
hyperlipidemia	0.668	0.840	0.426	1.951

3.3. Multiple Contributing Factors for Hemodynamic Index Variations

The simulation results indicated that the existence of IICAS will lead to significant FHR elevations, and we inferred that the mechanism of FHR elevations is caused by increased artery wall stiffness. In addition to the development of stenosis, other factors may also contribute to FHR variations and have some effects on IICAS diagnosis. Multivariate linear regression was performed to investigate the relations between the FHR and multiple factors. As shown in Table 5, stenosis remains the leading cause of FHR elevations. Moreover, gender also has significant effects on the FHR, with females tending to have higher FHR than males. Therefore, we inferred that females tend to have higher arterial stiffness and more severe atherosclerotic stenosis, which is consistent with recent studies [31–33].

Table 5. Relations between the maximum First Harmonic Ratio and multiple factors (N = 76).

	Coefficient	Standard Error	*p* Value
Intercept	0.3285	0.0302	<0.001
Age	0.0004	0.0005	0.371
Male Gender	−0.0204	0.0078	0.011
Hypertension	0.0002	0.0081	0.980
Diabetes	−0.0017	0.0088	0.852
Hyperlipidemia	0.0033	0.0087	0.704
Stenosis	0.0487	0.0086	<0.001

In addition to the above factors, medications may also lead to hemodynamic index variations. We collected information on drug use in 50 subjects in this study and performed multivariate regressions to investigate the impact of medications. The drugs were classified into five categories: (1) calcium channel blockers (CCBs, e.g., Amlodipine); (2) cerebral vasodilators (e.g., Betahistine mesylate); (3) angiotensin receptor blockers (ARBs, e.g., Valsartan) and other vasodilators; (4) hypoglycemic drugs (e.g., Metformin); (5) hypolipidemic drugs (e.g., Atorvastatin). The vasodilators were classified into three sub-categories based on different hemodynamic effects: CCBs may decrease the arterial stiffness of large arteries by blocking calcium ions into smooth muscle cells; cerebral vasodilators may reduce cerebral vascular resistance; ARBs and other vasodilators may decrease system vascular resistance. Table 6 demonstrates that the maximum FHR is insensitive to medications.

Table 6. Relations between the maximum First Harmonic Ratio and medications (N = 50).

	Coefficient	Standard Error	*p* Value
Intercept	0.3435	0.0145	<0.001
CCBs	0.0142	0.0113	0.214
Cerebral Vasodilators	0.0032	0.0132	0.811
ARBs et al.	0.0118	0.0118	0.321
Hypoglycemic Drugs	−0.0040	0.0143	0.781
Hypolipidemic Drugs	0.0081	0.0107	0.454
Stenosis	0.0528	0.0123	<0.001
Male Gender	−0.0210	0.0105	0.053

Regressions about other hemodynamic indices reveal that the left PSV is significantly affected by the usage of cerebral vasodilators, the EDV is affected by age and hyperlipidemia, and the RI is affected by age. Details of the regression results can be found in the Supplementary Data.

4. Discussion

In this study, we quantitatively investigated the effects of mild-to-moderate IICAS on proximal ICA flow waveforms using hemodynamic simulations and statistical analyses in a group of patients. The pattern of the entire waveform was quantitatively evaluated using the FHR proposed in this study, which is the ratio between the amplitudes of the low- and high-frequency waves. A 1D patient-specific hemodynamic model was developed to simulate ICA waveforms with and without stenoses. Based on the results, the removal of the stenosis will lead to an increase in the PSV and EDV and a dramatic decrease in the FHR. Statistical analysis was performed on actual patient groups to test the diagnostic performance of these indices. We found that the patients with IICAS tended to have a lower PSV, lower EDV, and significantly higher FHR than those without IICAS. Moreover, the FHR showed a good performance in IICAS diagnosis, with a sensitivity of 88.8% and a specificity of 83.3%, during dual-side carotid ultrasounds.

The diagnostic performances of the classical hemodynamic indices (PSV, EDV, and RI) in this study are poor compared with those reported in previous studies [8–10] in which severe stenosis is usually considered, and the distance between the stenosis and probe location is close despite some of the indices, such as the PSV, showing differences between the two groups to some extent. The probable cause of this phenomenon is that the classical indices may not be sensitive to mild-to-moderate stenosis from a relatively long distance, which was considered in this study. In addition, the simulated results with stenosis had a lower EDV (-6.1 cm/s) than the difference between the averaged group values (-3.1 cm/s). Hence, we infer that the compensatory vasodilation of the peripheral vessels [34,35] may also occur in narrowing the differences, because the parameters of the peripheral vessels remain unchanged in the simulation, while compensatory peripheral resistance reduction may occur in actual patients as stenosis develops.

In contrast to the classical indices, which usually use one or two single values in the Doppler waveforms, the FHR proposed in this study use information on the entire waveform, potentially making the index more sensitive to small variations induced by mild-to-moderate stenosis. The diagnosis of mild-to-moderate stenosis is more clinically significant than that of severe stenosis because severe stenosis is usually accompanied by symptoms, whereas early diagnosis and therapy of IICAS can effectively prevent severe diseases, such as strokes. Moreover, multivariate regressions reveal that the classical indices may be easily influenced by age, hyperlipidemia, and cerebral vasodilators, while the FHR is insensitive to age, basic diseases, and drug usage.

The AUC value of the single-sided FHR was 0.838 for the left ICA and 0.836 for the right ICA, while the AUC value for the maximum FHR obtained from both sides was 0.888; this finding indicates that FHR-based diagnosis is more accurate in distinguishing patients with or without IICAS than in identifying the stenosis location. Accordingly, the FHR is a promising diagnostic index for the early diagnosis of IICAS. This diagnostic method can be applied in ordinary physical examinations to identify possible patients with IICAS in the early stages, and cerebral CTA/MRA can be further applied to locate the stenosis. In addition, FHR-based diagnosis may be effective in other arteries where it is difficult to locate the stenosis directly using ultrasound images.

A personalized hemodynamic model was used to investigate the effects of IICAS on the complicated cardiovascular system. The simulation analyses demonstrated that the 1D artery network model was capable of simulating Doppler ultrasound waveforms precisely, making it a potentially useful tool in other Doppler ultrasound-related studies. In addition, personalized cardiovascular function assessment is possible by solving the inverse problem of identifying parameters from the measured Doppler waveforms. For example, the risk of atherosclerotic stenosis may be evaluated using the quantitative analysis of vascular stiffness at different arterial sites.

5. Limitations

In addition to age, gender, basic diseases and medications collected in this study, other contributing factors may also affect the results. The abnormal bending of ICA (or "Dolichocarotids") is a significant risk factor for cardiovascular events [36], and artery curvatures may have complicated effects on blood flow. However, because cerebral images usually focus on intracranial regions, parts of ICA segments are missing in many images. Scopes of the cerebral images should be adjusted to obtain complete ICA segments in future studies, and the effects of Dolichocarotids should be investigated.

A total of 76 participants were included in this study; however, the sample size was not large enough to test the diagnostic efficacy of the FHR, and the sizes of the two groups were not well balanced because the positive cases outnumbered the negative cases in the hospital. Multi-center studies should be conducted in the future to expand the sample's size. Another limitation of the statistical study is the lack of gold standard cerebral images; only two patients were diagnosed using DSA in this study because CTA/MRA is less invasive and expensive. One of the cases had different diagnostic conclusions from CTA and DSA, as shown in Figure 5. Due to a locally insufficient contrast agent, IICAS was misdiagnosed in the CTA scan. In contrast, the gold standard DSA showed no stenosis in that region. Interestingly, the FHR of the patient was within the normal range (below

0.360 on both sides), which was in accordance with the DSA diagnosis. If there are more similar cases in the positive group, the actual diagnostic performance of the FHR may be of higher quality. Therefore, more data labeled with DSA images should be collected in the future.

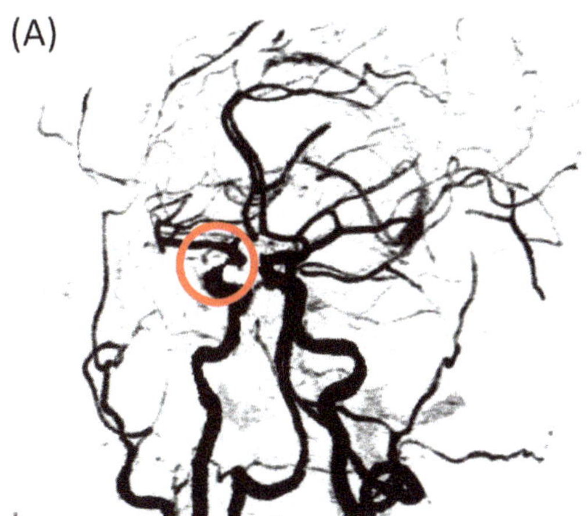
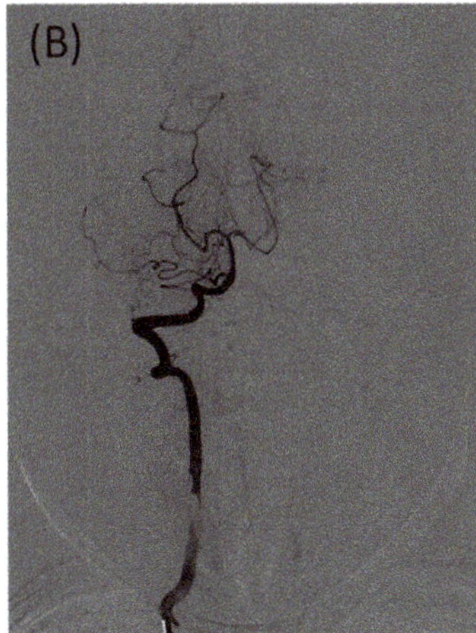

Figure 5. Incorrectly labeled case in the CTA scan due to an insufficient contrast agent, with the FHR in the normal range: (**A**) CTA image of the intracranial arteries of the patient, with the misdiagnosed intracranial internal carotid artery stenosis indicated in the red circle; (**B**) gold standard intracranial digital subtraction angiography image of the same patient showing no stenosis in the arteries, which is consistent with the FHR-based diagnosis. CTA, computed tomography angiography; FHR, first harmonic ratio.

6. Conclusions

The effects of IICAS on the extracranial hemodynamic indices were quantitatively investigated using a 1D patient-specific hemodynamic model of the human cardiovascular system. A significant dampening of high-order harmonics was found in the extracranial ICA flow waveforms in the presence of IICAS. Therefore, we proposed a new index called the FHR to quantitatively evaluate this effect. Using carotid Doppler ultrasound measurements, we further conducted a case–control study including 76 patients; we found that the FHR had a superior diagnostic performance for mild-to-moderate IICAS (<70%) and that the classical indices showed no significant differences between the stenosis and control groups. Multivariate regressions revealed that the classical indices were susceptible to age, hyperlipidemia, and cerebral vasodilators, while IICAS remained the dominant factor for FHR elevations. FHR measurements using carotid Doppler ultrasound may facilitate the early diagnosis of IICAS.

Supplementary Materials: All data involved in this study can be found at: https://www.mdpi.com/article/10.3390/bioengineering9090422/s1.

Author Contributions: X.Z. performed data analysis and hemodynamic modeling and wrote the article; D.W. participated in the data analysis and study design; H.L. and Y.F. participated in the data collection; H.X. designed the study; Y.L. critically reviewed the manuscript. All authors have read and agreed to the published version of the manuscript.

Funding: This study was supported by the National Natural Science Foundation of China (no. U1913210), Strategic Priority CAS Project (no. XDB38040200), Shenzhen Second People's Hospital Clinical Research Fund of Guangdong Province High-Level Hospital Construction Project (no. 20213357016), Guangdong Natural Science Funds (no. 2020B1515120061), Shenzhen Innovation Founding (no. KJYY20180703165202011), Sanming Project of Medicine in Shenzhen (no. SZSM201612027),

Science and Technology Planning Project of Shenzhen Municipality (no. JCYJ20180703145202065), and Shenzhen Key Medical Discipline Construction Fund (no. SZXK052).

Institutional Review Board Statement: This study was approved by the Institutional Review Board of the Second People's Hospital of Shenzhen (no. 20200727001) and complied with the Declaration of Helsinki.

Informed Consent Statement: Informed consent was obtained from all participants of the study.

Data Availability Statement: All the data involved in this study can be found in Supplementary Materials.

Conflicts of Interest: The authors declare no conflict of interest.

References

1. Bos, D.; van der Rijk, M.J.M.; Geeraedts, T.E.A.; Hofman, A.; Krestin, G.P.; Witteman, J.C.M.; van der Lugt, A.; Ikram, M.A.; Vernooij, M.W. Vernooij. Intracranial carotid artery atherosclerosis: Prevalence and risk factors in the general population. *Stroke* **2012**, *43*, 1878–1884. [CrossRef] [PubMed]
2. Hua, Y.; Jia, L.; Xing, Y.; Hui, P.; Meng, X.; Yu, D.; Pan, X.; Fang, Y.; Song, B.; Wu, C.; et al. Distribution pattern of atherosclerotic stenosis in Chinese patients with stroke: A multicenter registry study. *Aging Dis.* **2019**, *10*, 62–70. [CrossRef] [PubMed]
3. Bos, D.; Portegies, M.L.P.; van der Lugt, A.; Bos, M.J.; Koudstaal, P.J.; Hofman, A.; Krestin, G.P.; Franco, O.H.; Vernooij, M.W.; Ikram, M.A. Intracranial carotid artery atherosclerosis and the risk of stroke in whites: The Rotterdam Study. *JAMA Neurol.* **2014**, *71*, 405–411. [CrossRef] [PubMed]
4. Holmstedt, C.A.; Turan, T.N.; Chimowitz, M.I. Atherosclerotic intracranial arterial stenosis: Risk factors, diagnosis, and treatment. *Lancet Neurol.* **2013**, *12*, 1106–1114. [CrossRef]
5. Andreucci, M.; Solomon, R.; Tasanarong, A. Side effects of radiographic contrast media: Pathogenesis, risk factors, and prevention. *Biomed. Res. Int.* **2014**, *2014*, 741018. [CrossRef]
6. Mohr, J.P.; Wolf, P.A.; Moskowitz, M.A.; Mayberg, M.R.; von Kummer, R.; Grotta, J.C. *Stroke: Pathophysiology, Diagnosis, and Management*, 5th ed.; Elsevier: Philadelphia, PA, USA, 2011.
7. Guido, R.; Dario, A.; Claudio, C.; Debora, M.; Ferrara, M.; Picco, A.; Famà, F.; Colombo, B.M.; Nobili, F. Correlation between Doppler velocities and duplex ultrasound carotid cross-sectional percent stenosis. *Acad. Radiol.* **2011**, *18*, 1485–1491.
8. Gunduz YAkdemir, R.; Ayhan, L.T.; Keser, N. Can Doppler flow parameters of carotid stenosis predict the occurrence of new ischemic brain lesions detected by diffusion-weighted MR imaging after filter-protected internal carotid artery stenting? *Am. J. Neuroradiol.* **2014**, *35*, 760–765. [CrossRef]
9. Koga, M.; Kimura, K.; Minematsu, K.; Yamaguchi, T. Diagnosis of internal carotid artery stenosis greater than 70% with power Doppler duplex sonography. *Am. J. Neuroradiol.* **2001**, *22*, 413–417.
10. Rafati, M.; Havaee, E.; Moladoust, H.; Sehhati, M. Appraisal of different ultrasonography indices in patients with carotid artery atherosclerosis. *EXCLI J.* **2017**, *16*, 727–741.
11. Zhao, L.; Barlinn, K.; Sharma, V.K.; Tsivgoulis, G.; Cava, L.F.; Vasdekis, S.N.; Teoh, H.L.; Triantafyllou, N.; Chan, B.P.L.; Sharma, A.; et al. Velocity criteria for intracranial stenosis revisited: An international multicenter study of transcranial Doppler and digital subtraction angiography. *Stroke* **2011**, *42*, 3429–3434. [CrossRef]
12. Ginat, D.T.; Bhatt, S.; Sidhu, R.; Dogra, V. Carotid and vertebral artery Doppler ultrasound waveforms: A pictorial review. *Ultrasound Q.* **2011**, *27*, 81–85. [CrossRef] [PubMed]
13. Sakima, H.; Wakugawa, Y.; Isa, K.; Yasaka, M.; Ogata, T.; Saitoh, M.; Shimada, H.; Yasumori, K.; Inoue, T.; Ohya, Y.; et al. Correlation between the degree of left subclavian artery stenosis and the left vertebral artery waveform by pulse Doppler ultrasonography. *Cerebrovasc. Dis.* **2011**, *31*, 64–67. [CrossRef] [PubMed]
14. Chan, S.; McNeeley, M.F.; Le, T.X.; Hippe, D.S.; Dighe, M.; Dubinsky, T.J. The sonographic stenosis index: Computer simulation of a novel method for detecting and quantifying arterial narrowing. *Ultrasound Q.* **2013**, *29*, 155–160. [CrossRef]
15. Le, T.X.; Hippe, D.S.; McNeeley, M.F.; Dighe, M.K.; Dubinsky, T.J.; Chanet, S.S. The sonographic stenosis index: A new specific quantitative measure of transplant hepatic arterial stenosis. *J. Ultrasound Med.* **2017**, *36*, 809–819. [CrossRef] [PubMed]
16. Jin, W.; Alastruey, J. Arterial pulse wave propagation across stenoses and aneurysms: Assessment of one-dimensional simulations against three-dimensional simulations and in vitro measurements. *J. R. Soc. Interface* **2021**, *18*, 20200881. [CrossRef]
17. Zhang, X.; Wu, D.; Miao, F.; Liu, H.; Li, Y. Personalized hemodynamic modeling of the human cardiovascular system: A reduced-order computing model. *IEEE Trans. Biomed. Eng.* **2020**, *67*, 2754–2764. [CrossRef]
18. Yin, M.; Yazdani, A.; Karniadakis, G.E. One-dimensional modeling of fractional flow reserve in coronary artery disease: Uncertainty quantification and Bayesian optimization. *Comput. Methods Appl. Mech. Eng.* **2019**, *353*, 66–85. [CrossRef]
19. Hoque, K.E.; Ferdows, M.; Sawall, S.; Tzirtzilakis, E.E.; Xenos, M.A. Hemodynamic characteristics expose the atherosclerotic severity in coronary main arteries: One-dimensional and three-dimensional approaches. *Phys. Fluids* **2021**, *33*, 121907. [CrossRef]
20. Ghigo, A.R.; Taam, S.A.; Wang, X.; Lagrée, P.-Y.; Fullana, J.-M. A one-dimensional arterial network model for bypass graft assessment. *Med. Eng. Phys.* **2017**, *43*, 39–47. [CrossRef]

21. Gognieva, D.; Gamilov, T.; Pryamonosov, R.; Betelin, V.; Ternovoy, S.K.; Serova, N.S.; Abugov, S.; Shchekochikhin, D.; Mitina, Y.; El-Manaa, H.; et al. One-Dimensional Mathematical Model-Based Automated Assessment of Fractional Flow Reserve in a Patient with Silent Myocardial Ischemia. *Am. J. Case Rep.* **2018**, *19*, 724–728. [CrossRef]

22. Kim, K.; Weitzel, W.F.; Rubin, J.M.; Xie, H.; Chen, X.; O'Donnell, M. Vascular intramural strain imaging using arterial pressure equalization. *Ultrasound Med. Biol.* **2004**, *30*, 761–771. [CrossRef] [PubMed]

23. Liu, H.; Liang, F.; Wong, J.; Fujiwara, T.; Ye, W.; Tsubota, K.-I.; Sugawara, M. Multi-scale modeling of hemodynamics in the cardiovascular system. *Acta Mech. Sin.* **2015**, *31*, 446–464. [CrossRef]

24. Wang, J.J.; Parker, K.H. Wave propagation in a model of the arterial circulation. *J. Biomech.* **2004**, *37*, 457–470. [CrossRef] [PubMed]

25. Alastruey, J.; Parker, K.H.; Peiró, J.; Byrd, S.M.; Sherwin, S.J. Modelling the circle of Willis to assess the effects of anatomical variations and occlusions on cerebral flows. *J. Biomech.* **2006**, *40*, 1794–1805. [CrossRef] [PubMed]

26. Boesen, M.E.; Singh, D.; Menon, B.K.; Frayne, R. A systematic literature review of the effect of carotid atherosclerosis on local vessel stiffness and elasticity. *Atherosclerosis* **2015**, *243*, 211–222. [CrossRef]

27. U-King-Im, J.M.; Trivedi, R.A.; Cross, J.J.; Higgins, N.J.; Hollingworth, W.; Graves, M.; Joubert, I.; Kirkpatrick, P.J.; Antoun, N.M.; Gillard, J.H. Measuring carotid stenosis on contrast-enhanced magnetic resonance angiography: Diagnostic performance and reproducibility of 3 different methods. *Stroke* **2004**, *35*, 2083–2088. [CrossRef]

28. Wu, D.; Cui, G.; Huang, X.; Chen, Y.; Liu, G.; Ren, L.; Li, Y. An accurate and explainable ensemble learning method for carotid plaque prediction in an asymptomatic population. *Comput. Methods Programs Biomed.* **2022**, *221*, 106842. [CrossRef]

29. Youden, W.J. Index for rating diagnostic tests. *Cancer* **1950**, *3*, 32–35. [CrossRef]

30. Gautier, F.; Gilbert, J.; Dalmont, J.-P.; Vila, R.P. Wave propagation in a fluid filled rubber tube: Theoretical and experimental results for Korteweg's wave. *Acta Acust. United Acustica* **2007**, *93*, 333–344.

31. Kim, J.Y.; Park, J.B.; Kim, D.S.; Kim, K.S.; Jeong, J.W.; Park, J.C.; Oh, B.H.; Chung, N. KAAS investigators Gender Difference in Arterial Stiffness in a Multicenter Cross-Sectional Study: The Korean Arterial Aging Study (KAAS). *Pulse* **2014**, *2*, 11–17. [CrossRef]

32. DuPont, J.J.; Kenney, R.M.; Patel, A.R.; Jaffe, I.Z. Sex differences in mechanisms of arterial stiffness. *Br. J. Pharmacol.* **2019**, *176*, 4208–4225. [CrossRef] [PubMed]

33. Łoboz-Rudnicka, M.; Jaroch, J.; Kruszyńska, E.; Bociąga, Z.; Rzyczkowska, B.; Dudek, K.; Szuba, A.; Łoboz-Grudzień, K. Gender-related differences in the progression of carotid stiffness with age and in the influence of risk factors on carotid stiffness. *Clin. Interv. Aging* **2018**, *13*, 1183–1191. [CrossRef]

34. Kaesemann, P.; Thomalla, G.; Cheng, B.; Treszl, A.; Fiehler, J.; Forkert, N.D. Impact of severe extracranial ICA stenosis on MRI perfusion and diffusion parameters in acute ischemic stroke. *Front. Neurol.* **2014**, *5*, 254. [CrossRef] [PubMed]

35. Bokkers, R.P.; Wessels, F.J.; van der Worp, H.B.; Zwanenburg, J.J.; Mali, W.P.; Hendrikse, J. Vasodilatory capacity of the cerebral vasculature in patients with carotid artery stenosis. *AJNR Am. J. Neuroradiol.* **2011**, *32*, 1030–1033. [CrossRef] [PubMed]

36. Ciccone, M.M.; Sharma, R.K.; Scicchitano, P.; Cortese, F.; Salerno, C.; Berchialla, P.; Frasso, G.; Sassara, M.; Carbone, M.; Palmier, P. Dolichocarotids: Echo-Color Doppler Evaluation and Clinical Role. *J. Atheroscler, Thromb.* **2014**, *21*, 56–63. [CrossRef] [PubMed]

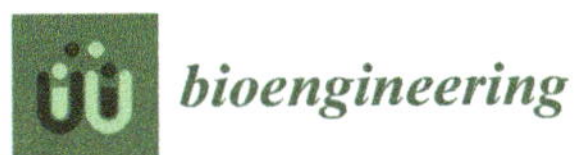

bioengineering

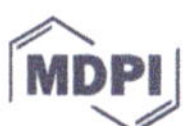

Review

Artificial Intelligence Models in the Diagnosis of Adult-Onset Dementia Disorders: A Review

Gopi Battineni [1,*], Nalini Chintalapudi [1], Mohammad Amran Hossain [1], Giuseppe Losco [2], Ciro Ruocco [1], Getu Gamo Sagaro [1], Enea Traini [1], Giulio Nittari [1] and Francesco Amenta [1]

[1] Clinical Research Centre, School of Medicinal and Health Products Sciences, University of Camerino, 62032 Camerino, Italy
[2] School of Architecture and Design, University of Camerino, 63100 Ascoli Piceno, Italy
* Correspondence: gopi.battineni@unicam.it; Tel.: +39-3331728206

Abstract: *Background:* The progressive aging of populations, primarily in the industrialized western world, is accompanied by the increased incidence of several non-transmittable diseases, including neurodegenerative diseases and adult-onset dementia disorders. To stimulate adequate interventions, including treatment and preventive measures, an early, accurate diagnosis is necessary. Conventional magnetic resonance imaging (MRI) represents a technique quite common for the diagnosis of neurological disorders. Increasing evidence indicates that the association of artificial intelligence (AI) approaches with MRI is particularly useful for improving the diagnostic accuracy of different dementia types. *Objectives:* In this work, we have systematically reviewed the characteristics of AI algorithms in the early detection of adult-onset dementia disorders, and also discussed its performance metrics. *Methods:* A document search was conducted with three databases, namely PubMed (Medline), Web of Science, and Scopus. The search was limited to the articles published after 2006 and in English only. The screening of the articles was performed using quality criteria based on the Newcastle–Ottawa Scale (NOS) rating. Only papers with an NOS score $\geq$ 7 were considered for further review. *Results:* The document search produced a count of 1876 articles and, because of duplication, 1195 papers were not considered. Multiple screenings were performed to assess quality criteria, which yielded 29 studies. All the selected articles were further grouped based on different attributes, including study type, type of AI model used in the identification of dementia, performance metrics, and data type. *Conclusions:* The most common adult-onset dementia disorders occurring were Alzheimer's disease and vascular dementia. AI techniques associated with MRI resulted in increased diagnostic accuracy ranging from 73.3% to 99%. These findings suggest that AI should be associated with conventional MRI techniques to obtain a precise and early diagnosis of dementia disorders occurring in old age.

Keywords: adult-onset dementia; Alzheimer's disease; magnetic resonance imaging; artificial intelligence; machine learning; neural networks

Citation: Battineni, G.; Chintalapudi, N.; Hossain, M.A.; Losco, G.; Ruocco, C.; Sagaro, G.G.; Traini, E.; Nittari, G.; Amenta, F. Artificial Intelligence Models in the Diagnosis of Adult-Onset Dementia Disorders: A Review. *Bioengineering* **2022**, *9*, 370. https://doi.org/10.3390/bioengineering9080370

Academic Editors: Pedro Miguel Rodrigues, João Alexandre Lobo Marques and João Paulo do Vale Madeiro

Received: 29 June 2022
Accepted: 2 August 2022
Published: 5 August 2022

Publisher's Note: MDPI stays neutral with regard to jurisdictional claims in published maps and institutional affiliations.

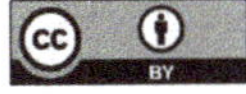

1. Introduction

Adult-onset cognitive disorders (AOCD) are characterized by a clinically significant, acquired impairment of cognitive functions [1,2]. Around 50 million people were affected by AOCD (dementia) worldwide in 2018, with a cost of approximately one trillion dollars for their care every year [3]. There is an impairment in daily functioning caused by multiple cognitive deficits. The main symptoms of AOCD are dementia, delirium, and mild cognitive impairment (MCI). A person with dementia has severe impairments in memory, language, problem solving, and other thinking abilities [4]. In most cases, delirium is defined as a state of acute disturbance of consciousness accompanied by a change in cognition during the day [5,6], whereas MCI is characterized by loss of memory and other cognitive abilities in individuals [7].

The impairment of neurocognitive function is associated with several neurological conditions, including Alzheimer's disease (AD), frontotemporal dementia, Lewy body disease, Parkinson's disease (PD), Huntington's disease, Prion disease, traumatic brain injury, and others [8–11]. A pathophysiological correlation has been demonstrated between the progression of AD and nerve cell loss, neuro-fibrillary tangles, and senile plaques [12–14]. However, amyloid levels do not correlate directly with the progression of AD, affecting primarily the hippocampal, entorhinal cortex, neocortex, and other brain regions [12]. Neurofibrillary degeneration has been observed hierarchically among brain regions, and a pattern of progression of lesions is generally accepted [15].

Neurocognitive tests, brain imaging, and cerebrospinal fluid (CSF) tests are currently used to diagnose AD [16]. By improving diagnostics, biomarkers can facilitate early AD detection and treatment [17]. Studies have demonstrated the importance of early diagnostics, pharmacological interventions, lifestyle changes, and decreasing cardiovascular risk factors in suppressing the progression of the disease [18–20]. Therefore, it is imperative to diagnose clinical conditions that can potentially progress into dementia as early as possible [21,22].

In this 21st century, artificial intelligence (AI) composed of both machine learning (ML) and deep learning (DL) is rapidly revolutionizing the field of medicine [23]. ML involves an AI algorithm that selects the most suitable model based on a set of alternatives. For complex applications, ML algorithms have several advantages, including nonlinearity, fault tolerance, and real-time operation. Although the ML models incorporate information not ordinarily available to clinicians, such as advanced neuroimaging, genetic testing, and cerebrospinal fluid biomarkers, they can be applied to specialist and research settings [24].

Recent studies demonstrated the effectiveness of ML algorithms in neuroimaging and cognitive testing for the early detection of neurodegenerative diseases such as AD [25,26]. Patients with dementia will benefit from high-quality care when these diverse and strategic resources are utilized effectively. Therefore, ML is a crucial component in achieving this goal, and there is evidence that ML knowledge from clinical data can be used to plan care for people at risk of different dementia forms [27–31]. Review articles on the use of AI in the brain sciences analyze the opportunities and challenges associated with its implementation [32,33]. Neurogenerative disorders are poorly understood due to a lack of systematic analysis of AI technologies.

This systematic review examines the involvement of AI applications in AOCDs. In this study, all performance metrics of the AI model for the early diagnosis of neurogenerative disorders such as dementia are presented. It provides a comprehensive overview of the state-of-the-art for machine learning about health informatics in dementia care. As we deal with big health data, we compile and review existing scientific methodologies. It has been demonstrated that ML can contribute to the analysis of neuroimaging data in dementia care. However, a relatively small effort has been made to apply advanced ML approaches to integrated heterogeneous data, which demonstrates the future potential and directions in dementia informatics.

2. Methods

2.1. Document Search

The review was conducted based on the guidelines of the Preferred Reporting Items for Systematic Reviews and Meta-Analyses (PRISMA) 2020. The document search was performed based on available literature from the databases PubMed, Web of Science (WoS), and Scopus. The document search was performed between the years 2006 and 2022. Articles before 2006 were excluded because of the limited literature on the topic of AI techniques in the diagnosis of neurogenerative diseases. Search keywords used were "artificial intelligence, "machine learning, "deep learning, "dementia", "Alzheimer"s disease", and "MRI". The search queries were carefully framed using Medical Subject Headings (MeSH) for different databases, which are further listed in Table 1. The document distribution of each database can be found in Figure 1.

Table 1. Search queries for three adopted databases.

Database	Query
PubMed	English AND ("Artificial Intelligence" [Title/Abstract/MeSH] OR "Machine Learning"[Title/Abstract/MeSH]) OR "Deep learning" AND ("diagnosis"[Title/Abstract] OR "detection"[Title/Abstract] OR "identification"[Title/Abstract] OR "recognition"[Title/Abstract]) OR "interpretation"[Title/Abstract]) AND ("dementia"[All Fields] AND "MRI"[All Fields]) AND "PET" [All Fields]) AND "image data"[All Fields]) NOT "classification" [Title/Abstract/MeSH] NOT "ranking"[Title/Abstract/MeSH] NOT "grouping"[Title/Abstract/MeSH] NOT Review[ptyp] NOT books and Documents [ptyp] NOT conference [ptyp]
WoS	("AI" AND "Artificial Intelligence" AND "Machine Learning" AND "Deep Learning") AND ("Diagnosis" OR "Identification" OR "recognition") AND ("dementia" OR "Alzheimer's disease" OR "MRI" OR "PET" OR "medical imaging" OR "neuro") NOT "segmentation" NOT "functional" NOT "connectivity") AND LANGUAGE: (English) AND DOCUMENT TYPES: (Review OR Proceedings Paper)
Scopus	TITLE-ABS-KEY ("Artificial Intelligence" AND "Machine Learning" AND "Deep Learning") AND ("Diagnosis" OR "Identification" OR "recognition" OR "interpretation) AND ("neurological diseases" OR "neurogenerative disorders" OR "dementia" OR "MRI" OR "PET") AND LIMIT-TO (LANGUAGE, "English") AND (LIMIT-TO (EXACT KEYWORD, "dementia")

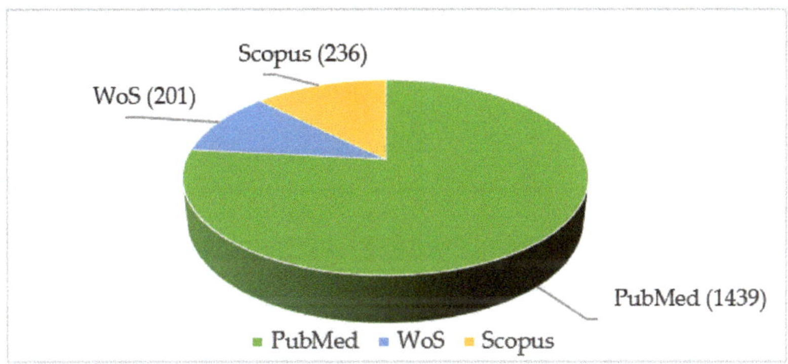

Figure 1. Document distribution of each database.

2.2. Inclusion and Exclusion Criteria

We included all articles focused on AI use in dementia diagnosis or early-stage identification. The articles handling the data of patients with different types of dementia and those in the English language met the basic requirements of the inclusion criteria. The adoption of AI-related ML and DL model outcomes with 2×2 confusion matrix outcomes was considered. Papers published before 2006 and works not reporting the training and testing data split or not providing information on validation approaches were excluded. Papers published in languages other than English and dealing with animals were not considered either. Conference papers or proceedings with insufficient data on patients' information, lack of information on the used model type, and validation approaches were excluded.

2.3. Quality Assessment

Once the literature search was carried out, the four authors independently assessed each article in two phases. In the first phase, similar or duplicate documents extracted from the three databases were eliminated by reading the abstracts. This analysis was conducted with the conventional approach of reading the article title and abstract. The inclusion and exclusion criteria of the filters were applied, and the evolution of the quality of each selected element was carried out based on the Newcastle–Ottawa scale (NOS), which varied from 0 to 9 [34]. The NOS defines each study in three ways: Poor (0–4), Moderate (5–6), and Good (7–9). These scores are based on some filters, such as study selection, comparability, and outcome. Various quality parameters, such as demonstration, coherence, risk factors, and others, are considered. The quality scores of selected articles depend on these parameters. These scores were recorded in an Excel sheet to calculate whether the selected study was suitable for final consideration or not.

3. Results

3.1. Search Outcomes

With a literature search, 1876 documents were identified in the period mentioned. Overall, 1195 documents were excluded due to duplication, ineligibility, and other reasons. This resulted in 681 documents being screened. Based on the title and abstract, 424 papers were excluded from further analysis as they were not consistent with the study objectives. At the end of the preliminary assessment, 257 works were considered for further review. For quality assessment, 76 documents were selected after applying inclusion and exclusion criteria. To perform multiple screenings, authors were given the selected documents and asked to note down quality scores anonymously for each work. In the absence of a high-quality score, items outside the review objectives were not further analyzed. We included 29 studies and summarized their findings in tabular form (Figure 2).

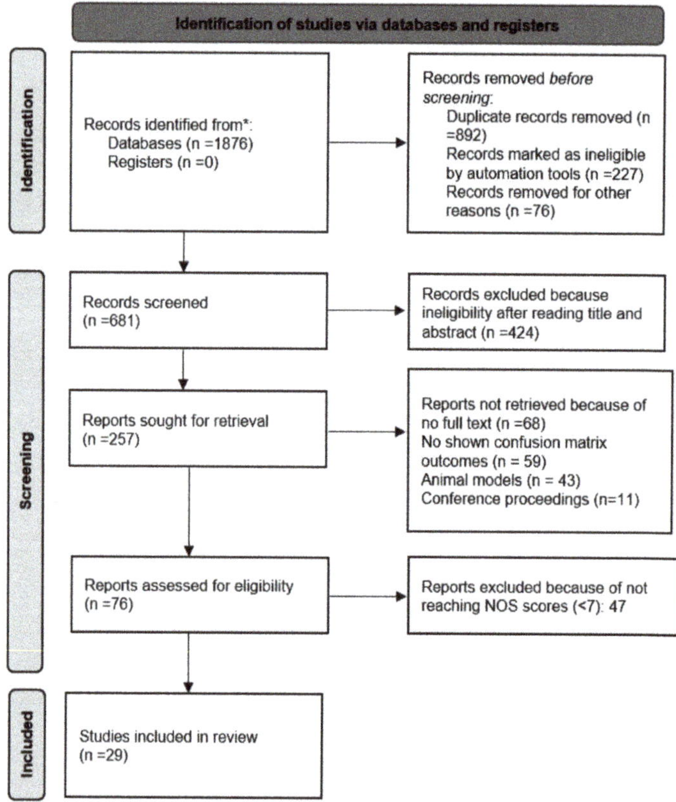

Figure 2. PRISMA 2020 flow chart for new systematic reviews with databases and registry search (*records extracted from only mentioned databases).

In terms of AI classifiers, 28.6% of the reported number of studies developed models using support vector machines (SVMs), and the models achieved accuracy ranging between 77.17% and 95.0%. In addition, two studies used Random Forest (RF) whereas the remaining eight studies used multiple AI classifiers [34,35]. In this review, we have found that AI models were used in five studies to diagnose AD, and six studies to diagnose other sorts of dementia.

In most of the studies, AD detection is considered the highest priority. All these works are associated with neuroimage data such as MRI data with dual modes (demographic or image), positron emission tomography (PET), and other cognitive datasets. Studies with deep learning neural networks produced a maximum accuracy of 98.3% [35–37]. As shown in [38], the authors used neural network modeling to verify performance, and their results showed that DenseNet-121 generated accuracy of 90.22%, which is higher than Inception-V1, V2, and Residual Networks [39]. A simple classification model based on a decision tree with hyperparameter tuning produced 99% accuracy [40].

Two studies developed an AI model for diagnosing Parkinson's disease. In one of these works, a CNN was trained and validated to detect PD from whole slide images (WSI). Model results show high accuracy, sensitivity, and specificity of 99%. Another paper developed an ML model for predicting Parkinson's disease using the MRI method [41]. The model achieved 88% accuracy. The use of AI to diagnose and determine the prognosis of dementia was explored in three studies [42–44].

3.2. Study Characteristics

The main characteristics of the selected papers (investigated country, study type, dementia category, AI models and validation approaches, and performance metrics such as accuracy, sensitivity, and specificity) are summarized in Table 2. Among 29 selected works, a major part (22) of the studies are retrospective types, and the remaining seven are prospective cohort studies. Moreover, 17 works combine the involvement of MRI data coupling with AI modeling as a means of facilitating dementia and AD diagnosis [45–51]. Furthermore, electroencephalogram (EEG) sensors and clinical data can predict the risk of other dementia types, such as MCI, PD, and frontotemporal [52–58]. On other hand, it has been observed that nine studies appeared from the USA, which was followed by the UK (3), India (3), and Canada (2).

Various AI algorithms are used to assist in identifying different forms of dementia. Results mention that the common cause of neurocognitive disorders is AD, whose main features are progressive memory loss and multidomain cognitive decline. AD represents 60% of all neurocognitive disorders [59]. AOCDs are a major cause of disability in the general population. Current data and prospects make dementia treatment a pivotal topic in the planning of national health systems, recognizing it as a major challenge for proposing sustainable choices for health and social assistance [60].

In terms of AI classifiers, 28.6% of studies applied SVM models and achieved accuracy in between 77.17% and 95.0% [49,50,56,58]. In addition, two studies used RF algorithms [45,51], whereas the remaining eight used multiple AI classifiers [46–48,52–55,57]. The present review found that five studies used AI models in AD diagnosis [45–47,52,56], and six studies to diagnose other dementia types [48–50,53,57].

Two studies developed an AI model for PD diagnosis [41,61]. A Boutet et al. developed an ML model for PD prediction using the MRI method [41], and M Signaevsky et al. trained and validated a CNN to detect PD from whole slide images (WSI) [61]. Results show high accuracy, sensitivity, and specificity. CI and MCI were classified with 81% and 96.6% of accuracy with recurrent neural networks (RNN) and artificial neural networks (ANN), respectively [43,62]. A study using multi-layer perceptrons (MLP) with cognitive data showed that 92.98% of AD cases were accurately diagnosed [63]. The mini-mental state examination (MMSE) and clinical dementia ratio (CDR) tests were also used to further classify AD stages with ResNet and DenseNet, which resulted in 99% accuracy [64,65].

Table 2. Characteristics of papers included in the review.

N	Country	Study Cohort	Dementia Category	AI Model	AI Modality	Validation Methods	Accuracy	Sensitivity	Specificity	Ref.
1	Canada	Prospective	AD	RUSRF	PET, MRI	Independent test set	84%	70.8%	86.5%	[39]
2	UK, China	Retrospective	MCI, Dementia	MobileNet, SVM	Facial expressions	5-fold cross-validation	73.3%	N/A	N/A	[42]
3	India	Retrospective	AD	DNN, Inception-V1, V2, V3, Residual Networks, DenseNet	MRI	Independent test set	90.22%	N/A	N/A	[38]
4	India	Retrospective	AD	CNN	MRI	Independent test set	98.3%	97%	N/A	[35]
5	India	Retrospective	AD	DTC-HPT	MRI	Independent test set	99%	99.10%	N/A	[40]
6	Egypt	Retrospective	AD	CNN	MRI	10-fold cross-validation	97%	95%	N/A	[36]
7	USA	Retrospective	AD	ResNet-50, GBM	MRI	10-fold cross-validation	99%	N/A	N/A	[64]
8	USA	Retrospective	AD	MLP	Cognitive data	Independent test set	92.98%	93.75%	92.68%	[63]
9	Canada	Retrospective	AD	CNN	MRI	5-fold cross-validation	84%	N/A	N/A	[37]
10	South Korea	Retrospective	MCI, Dementia	ANN	NPT data	10-fold cross-validation	96.66%	96%	96.8%	[43]
11	USA	Prospective	Dementia	LSTM, CNN	Voice Data	5-fold cross-validation	74%	66.3%	84.7%	[44]
12	USA	Prospective	PD	CNN	WSI	Cross-validation	99%	99%	99%	[61]
13	USA	Prospective	AD	RNN	MRI	5-fold cross-validation	81%	84%	80%%	[62]
14	Lithuania	Retrospective	AD	ResNet18, DenseNet201	MRI	Cross-validation	98.86%	98.89%	N/A	[65]
15	Canada	Prospective	PD	ML model	MRI	Independent test set/ 5-fold cross-validation	88%	N/A	N/A	[41]
16	Spain	Retrospective	AD	RF	MRI	Cross-validation	94.4%	N/A	N/A	[45]

Table 2. *Cont.*

N	Country	Study Cohort	Dementia Category	AI Model	AI Modality	Validation Methods	Accuracy	Sensitivity	Specificity	Ref.
17	Greece	Retrospective	AD and Frontotemporal Dementia	DT, RF, ANN, SVM, Naïve Bayes, and KNN	EEG	10-fold and leave-one-patient-out cross-validation	80% (DT)–99.1% (RF)	94% (NB)–98.6% (RF)	58% (NB)–99% (RF)	[52]
18	Italy	Retrospective	AD	Gradient boosting, SVM, LR, RF, AdaBoosting, NB	MRI	Cross-validation	95.96% (NB)–97.58% (GB)	95%–96%	N/A	[46]
19	UK	Retrospective	Dementia	RF and XGBoost	Clinical data	5-fold cross-validation	85% (RF)–87% (XGB)	73% (RF)–76% (XGB)	99% (RF) and (XGB)	[53]
20	USA	Retrospective	PD	Classification tree, Gaussian Kernel, LDA, Ensemble, KNN, LR, Naive Bayes, SVM, RF	Clinical data	Leave-one-subject-out cross-validation	74.1% (SVM)–84.5% (KNN)	70.6% (SVM)–88.5% (KNN)	79.2% (SVM)–84.6% (LR)	[54]
21	USA	Retrospective	AD	KNN, SVM, DT, RF, DL	MRI, SNP, clinical data	Internal cross-validation and an external test set	68% (KNN)–89%(DL)	N/A	N/A	[47]
22	Italy	Retrospective	PD	SVM, KNN, LDA, LR	Clinical data	10-fold cross-validation	90.1% (LDA)–91.8% (SVM)	68.4% (SVM)–87.5% (SVM optimized cost)	N/A	[55]
23	UK	Retrospective	Dementia	NB, LD, SVM, and KNN	MRI	10-fold cross-validation	77% (NB)–93% (C-SVM)	72.5% (CNN)–99% (KNN)	67% (KNN)–95% (SVM)	[48]
24	Netherlands	Retrospective	Dementia	Linear SVM	MRI, PET	LOO cross-validation and four-fold cross-validation	89% (voxel)–90% (Region)	83% (Region)–85% (voxel)	79% (voxel)–90% (Region)	[49]
25	Finland	Prospective	Dementia	SVM	MRI/CT, clinical data	5-fold cross-validation	95%	93%	99%	[50]
26	Japan	Retrospective	Dementia	XGBoost, RF, LR	Clinical data	-	86.3% (XGBoost)–89.3% (LR)	85.7% (XGBoost)–96.4% (LR)	80.0% (RF)–89.3% (LR)	[57]

Table 2. *Cont.*

N	Country	Study Cohort	Dementia Category	AI Model	AI Modality	Validation Methods	Accuracy	Sensitivity	Specificity	Ref.
27	USA	Retrospective	MCI and AD	SVM	Clinical data	5-fold cross-validation	91%	N/A	N/A	[56]
28	USA	Prospective	MCI	SVM	Clinical data	5-fold cross-validation	77.17%	81.97%	67.74%	[58]
29	Korea	Retrospective	AD and PD	RF	MRI	5-fold cross-validation	73.3%	78.0%	70.0%	[51]

4. Discussion

Our study reviewed the research literature on the application of AI models in the early detection of dementia in adults. A review of outcome data has shown that AI or ML models can greatly influence any subspecialty within AOCD at every treatment stage. To predict dementia types in advance, ANN, MRI data, and labeling segments have been most frequently used.

4.1. AI for Diagnostic Purposes

Currently, the treatment of AOCDs is limited to symptomatic therapies available, and drugs used in the treatment of dementias have very limited therapeutic value. For this reason, advanced computing techniques such as AI, ML, and deep learning have been directed toward the search for non-pharmacological approaches and support for caregivers [18]. It is now widely accepted that the phase of overt dementia in AD is preceded by a long preclinical phase, sometimes lasting several decades, that evolves through a continuum, from the initial preclinical stages to MCI up to the overt clinical stage of dementia [66,67]. People with advanced dementia have similar outcomes with psychosocial interventions as with pharmacological interventions. It has been demonstrated that cognitive stimulation improves cognition as well as the self-reported quality of life (QOL) and wellbeing. Computer-assisted exercise has been linked to better QOL for people with disabilities; however, not much research has been conducted. A pilot study examined whether computer-assisted exergaming interventions, utilizing exergaming technology (Able-X), could improve QOL, including cognitive and physical functioning, in 10 dementia patients, in addition to existing therapies and activities [68]. The role of AI algorithms in effectively detecting the different AOCD types was explained further.

A.   MCI detection

MCI is considered a transitional phase between normal aging and dementia [7]. When compared with nondepressed patients with MCI, individuals with MCI and depression perform less well on immediate and delayed memory tasks. MCI patients who experience sub-syndromic symptoms of depression have been found to have poorer function and quality of life, as well as a higher risk of dementia progression. Therefore, those who are cognitively impaired must undergo appropriate screening strategies for depression and depressive symptoms. This will enable clinicians to identify the causes of cognitive, functional, and behavioral impairments. It is thought that, in this phase, it is possible to intervene and slow the progression versus overt dementia during this stage. In this systematic review, four studies employed ML models to detect MCI [42,43,58]. An SVM model was the most incorporated algorithm in the detection of MCI and produced accuracy ranging from 73% to 91% [56,58]. Advanced ML models such as ANN can have the ability to detect MCI with 96.66% accuracy [43].

B.   AD diagnosis

AD is a brain neurodegenerative disorder occurring mainly in diseases commonly affecting elderly people, although it is not a normal part of aging. As AD progresses, memory loss, personality changes, and changes in brain function gradually worsen. AD is the most common adult-onset dementia. In this review, we found that 16 studies out of 29 (55%) used AI models to diagnose AD. According to these studies, AI models performed well in detecting AD, with an accuracy range of 73.33–99%, a sensitivity range of 70.8–90.10%, and a specificity range of 70–90%. A total of 11 studies (70%) utilized AI in conjunction with magnetic resonance imaging (MRI) to diagnose AD. Two studies analyzed clinical data, one along with MRI. One study used positron emission tomography (PET) and MRI. The remaining research used EEG and cognitive data to diagnose AD with AI models.

C.   Frontotemporal (FTD) and Lewy bodies (LBD) dementia

To target interventions and treatments for frontotemporal dementia (FTD), an accurate differential diagnosis is vital [69]. There are studies suggesting that deep learning techniques can be used to solve the differential diagnosis problem for FTD, AD, and normal controls (NCs), but their performance is still unknown. A third issue is that existing DL-assisted diagnostic studies are still reliant on expert-level preprocessing based on hypotheses. Some ML tools help to distinguish the AD and FTD symptoms with genetic algorithms [70]. It has been demonstrated that a data-centric perspective helps to understand AD and FTD disorders by allowing the results to be interpreted.

While LBD is a dementia-type syndrome with many clinical similarities, it can be difficult to diagnose clinically, especially in the advanced stages. To identify these disorders with a high prognosis, researchers proposed an ML algorithm based solely on non-invasive and easily collectable predictors [71]. The ImageNet dataset and ADNI database were used to reduce model complexity based on two-stage transfer learning technology [72,73]. Using the medical experience as a concatenation layer in the deep learning model, the AI model can automatically extract features corresponding to regulation and domain knowledge. Using this approach, the deep learning model gains better training efficiency and identifies more significant features in differentiating AD and LBD.

D.   PD diagnosis

PD is a neurological disease characterized by shaking, stiffness, and difficulties in walking, balance, and coordination. Symptoms usually develop gradually. People may have trouble walking and talking as the disease progresses. In addition, they may have psychological changes, sleeping problems, depression, and memory issues. In this systematic review, five studies associated PD detection with AI algorithms with MRI, clinical data, and WSI. They reported an accuracy range of 74–99%, a sensitivity range of 68.4–99%, and a specificity range of 70–99% for their developed AI models in PD diagnosis.

4.2. Model Assessment

Various AI algorithms are used to assist in identifying different forms of dementia in this section. There were two groups of AI algorithms, including ML and DL, reviewed in this work. Eighteen studies employed traditional ML classifiers, among which four utilized SVM, with accuracy ranging from 77.17% to 95.0% [49,50,56,58]. In addition, two studies applied RF [45,51], and one study employed Random Under-Sampling RF (RUSRF) [39], with an accuracy range of 73.3% to 94.4%. ML models were employed by G. Lee et al. [62], without mentioning any particular algorithm's name, and showed 88% accuracy. Using multilayer perceptron (MLP) modeling, AD classification with 92.98% of accuracy was achieved [63]. In [40], the authors developed a model using the decision tree classifier with hyperparameter tuning (DTC-HPT) and observed high accuracy of 99% for identifying AD. On the other hand, the remaining eight studies applied multiple ML classifiers [46–48], and they performed extremely well, with an accuracy range of 68% to 99.1% [52–55,57].

DL classifiers were used in nine (31%) of the 29 studies reviewed. Four of the selected studies employed conventional neural networks (CNNs) [35–37,61], reaching the highest accuracy of 99% and the lowest accuracy of 84%. ANN [43] and RNN [62] were used in two studies, with results of 96.66% and 81%, respectively. Three of the remaining studies compared multiple DL models [38,44,65], with accuracy ranging from 59.8% to 98.86%. Two studies were associated with both ML and DL classifiers [38,64]. A model using SVM and a second using a combination of MobileNet and Block 11 addition and SVM were noted [42]. In terms of accuracy, the combined model had the highest accuracy of 88.7%, while the SVM model had the lowest accuracy of 73.3%. A gradient-boosting model (GBM) as well as a Residual Neural Network (ResNet-50) have been designed by authors [64] and showed 91.3% and 98.99% accuracy.

4.3. Research Implications

Dementia is not a specific disease—it is a group of symptoms severely affecting memory loss, thinking, decision making, and social abilities so as to interfere with daily life. Several diseases can cause dementia. The prevalence of dementia increases with age, but it is not a normal part of aging. Symptoms vary according to the type of dementia. In this analysis, there were ten studies (33%) that developed different types of AI models to detect dementia by analyzing MRI data (40%), EEG facial expressions, NPT, and clinical and voice records. The performance of the AI model was evaluated in terms of accuracy (range of 74–99.1%), sensitivity (range of 66.3–99%), and specificity (58–99%). It is now widely accepted that the phase of overt dementia in AD is preceded by a long preclinical phase, sometimes lasting several decades, that evolves through a continuum, from the initial preclinical stages to MCI up to the overt clinical stage of dementia [66,67].

Current AI algorithms are recognized with measurable consistencies in large datasets and are routinely utilized across a scope of different domains, including disease diagnosis, but these models lack the power and generalizability related to human learning. If AI procedures could empower computers to self-learn from fewer examples, the experimental outcomes could have comprehensive logical and cultural effects. With increased memory and increased processing power, large models can provide more sophisticated outcomes and more adaptable learning. It is becoming increasingly clear that substantially more prominent figuring assets will not suffice to produce calculations suitable for learning from a few prototypes and summing up past preparation sets. Shortly, we may be able to distinguish dementia from normal aging by using movement tests and smart environments. Future directions to improve dementia detection in its earliest stages could include AI-based smart environments and multimodal examinations.

4.4. Limitations

The current work has a few important limitations that need to be addressed. First, the database search did not capture all the related papers; thus, it could not obtain all the eligible articles as a whole. The search terms mentioned in this work could be insufficient to identify the whole literature on AI combined with dementia. We highlighted the detection of adult-onset dementia disorders and ML and DL algorithms associated with it. This led to missing studies on working life dementia. On the other hand, in this review, we adopted only three major databases. This limited the coverage of other journals that are in line with the research topic.

5. Conclusions

Medicine is undergoing a revolution because of AI and ML, which help in the diagnosis of any disease, making it easier in recent years. With a more precise diagnosis, this technology could transform healthcare. A computerized system helps doctors to diagnose patients more accurately, predict what patients' future health will look like, and recommends better treatments. In this review, we have investigated current approaches of AI in the diagnosis and early prediction of adult-onset dementia disorders. In the past, dementia diagnosis was performed solely based on correlations between symptoms and the most likely cause. The newly developed methods with AI overcome several conventional limitations by utilizing causal reasoning in their machine learning. As a result of AI, dementia screening can now be automated to an even higher degree. This is particularly appealing to epidemiology studies and public health organizations that aim to target early risk reduction interventions. In contrast to clinicians' judgment alone, AI can analyze and respond quickly to large population screenings.

Author Contributions: Conceptualization, G.B. and M.A.H.; methodology, G.B.; software, N.C.; validation, G.B., N.C. and M.A.H.; formal analysis, G.L.; investigation, G.G.S.; resources, E.T. and C.R.; data curation, M.A.H.; writing—original draft preparation, G.B.; writing—review and editing, G.B., F.A., C.R.; visualization, G.N. and N.C.; supervision, F.A.; project administration, F.A. and G.L; funding acquisition, F.A. All authors have read and agreed to the published version of the manuscript."

Funding: This paper has been produced with the financial assistance of the European Union POR MARCHE FESR 2014/2020. Asse 1, OS 2, Azione 2.1—Intervento 2.1.1—Sostegno allo sviluppo di una piattaforma di ricerca collaborativa negli ambiti della specializzazione intelligente. Thematic Area: "Medicina personalizzata, farmaci e nuovi approcci terapeutici". Project acronym: Marche BioBank www.marchebiobank.it (accessed on 27 February 2022). The content of the paper is the sole responsibility of the authors and can under no circumstances be regarded as reflecting the position of the European Union and/or Marche Region authorities.

Institutional Review Board Statement: Not applicable.

Informed Consent Statement: Not applicable.

Data Availability Statement: Not applicable.

Conflicts of Interest: The authors declare no conflict of interest.

Abbreviations

AD: Alzheimer's disease; PD: Parkinson's disease; MCI: Mild cognitive impairment; MRI: Magnetic resonance imaging; PET: Positron emission tomography; CT: Computed tomography; ML: Machine learning; AI: Artificial intelligence; NB: Naïve Bayes; RF: Random Forest; ANN: Artificial neural network; RNN: Recurrent neural network; KNN: K-Nearest Neighborhood; SVM: Support vector machine; DT: Decision tree; NN: Neural network; LR: Logistic regression; RUSRF: Random Under-Sampling Random Forest; CNN: Conventional neural network; DNN: Deep neural network; DTC-HPT: Decision tree classifier with hyperparameter tuning; ResNet: Residual Network; GBM: Gradient boosting classifier; MLP: Multilayer perception; LSTM: Long Short-Term Memory; XG-BOOST: eXtreme Gradient Boosting; LDA: Linear discriminant analysis.

References

1. Harrison, R.A.; Kesler, S.R.; Johnson, J.M.; Penas-Prado, M.; Sullaway, C.M.; Wefel, J.S. Neurocognitive dysfunction in adult cerebellar medulloblastoma. *Psycho-Oncology* **2019**, *28*, 131–138. [CrossRef] [PubMed]
2. Chang, K.J.; Zhao, Z.; Shen, H.R.; Bing, Q.; Li, N.; Guo, X.; Hu, J. Adolescent/adult-onset homocysteine remethylation disorders characterized by gait disturbance with/without psychiatric symptoms and cognitive decline: A series of seven cases. *Neurol. Sci.* **2021**, *42*, 1987–1993. [CrossRef]
3. Dubois, B.; Villain, N.; Frisoni, G.B.; Rabinovici, G.D.; Sabbagh, M.; Cappa, S.; Bejanin, A.; Bombois, S.; Epelbaum, S.; Teichmann, M.; et al. Clinical diagnosis of Alzheimer's disease: Recommendations of the International Working Group. *Lancet. Neurol.* **2021**, *20*, 484–496. [CrossRef]
4. Spiegel, D.; Lewis-Fernández, R.; Lanius, R.; Vermetten, E.; Simeon, D.; Friedman, M. Dissociative disorders in DSM-5. *Annu. Rev. Clin. Psychol.* **2013**, *9*, 299–326. [CrossRef] [PubMed]
5. Gnerre, P.; La Regina, M.; Bozzano, C.; Pomero, F.; Re, R.; Meschi, M.; Montemurro, D.; Marchetti, A.; Di Lillo, M.; Tirotta, D. Delirium: The invisible syndrome. *Ital. J. Med.* **2016**, *10*, 119–127. [CrossRef]
6. Bhat, R.; Rockwood, K. Delirium as a disorder of consciousness. *J. Neurol. Neurosurg. Psychiatry* **2007**, *78*, 1167. [CrossRef] [PubMed]
7. Smith, G.E.; Bondi, M.W. *Mild Cognitive Impairment and Dementia: Definitions, Diagnosis, and Treatment*; Oxford University Press: Oxford, UK, 2013; Volume 403.
8. Vahia, V.N. Diagnostic and statistical manual of mental disorders 5: A quick glance. *Indian J. Psychiatry.* **2013**, *55*, 220–223. [CrossRef]
9. Dening, T.; Sandilyan, M.B. Dementia: Definitions and types. *Nurs. Stand.* **2015**, *29*, 37–42. [CrossRef]
10. Aarsland, D. Epidemiology and Pathophysiology of Dementia-Related Psychosis. *J. Clin. Psychiatry* **2020**, *81*, 27625. [CrossRef]
11. Ferencz, B.; Gerritsen, L. Genetics and Underlying Pathology of Dementia. *Neuropsychol. Rev.* **2015**, *25*, 113–124. [CrossRef]
12. Ingelsson, M.; Fukumoto, H.; Newell, K.L.; Growdon, J.H.; Hedley-Whyte, E.T.; Frosch, M.P.; Albert, M.S.; Hyman, B.T.; Irizarry, M.C. Early Abeta accumulation and progressive synaptic loss, gliosis, and tangle formation in AD brain. *Neurology* **2004**, *62*, 925–931. [CrossRef] [PubMed]
13. Serrano-Pozo, A.; Mielke, M.L.; Gómez-Isla, T.; Betensky, R.A.; Growdon, J.H.; Frosch, M.P.; Hyman, B.T. Reactive glia not only associates with plaques but also parallels tangles in Alzheimer's disease. *Am. J. Pathol.* **2011**, *179*, 1373–1384. [CrossRef]
14. Serrano-Pozo, A.; Frosch, M.P.; Masliah, E.; Hyman, B.T. Neuropathological Alterations in Alzheimer Disease. *Cold Spring Harb. Perspect. Med.* **2011**, *1*, a006189. [CrossRef]
15. Wisniewski, H.M.; Silverman, W. Diagnostic criteria for the neuropathological assessment of Alzheimer's disease: Current status and major issues. *Neurobiol. Aging* **1997**, *18*, S43–S50. [CrossRef]

16. McKhann, G.M.; Knopman, D.S.; Chertkow, H.; Hyman, B.T.; Jack, C.R.; Kawas, C.H.; Klunk, W.E.; Koroshetz, W.J.; Manly, J.J.; Mayeux, R.; et al. The diagnosis of dementia due to Alzheimer's disease: Recommendations from the National Institute on Aging-Alzheimer's Association workgroups on diagnostic guidelines for Alzheimer's disease. *Alzheimer's Dement.* **2011**, *7*, 263–269. [CrossRef] [PubMed]

17. Jack, C.R.; Bennett, D.A.; Blennow, K.; Carrillo, M.C.; Dunn, B.; Haeberlein, S.B.; Holtzman, D.M.; Jagust, W.; Jessen, F.; Karlawish, J.; et al. NIA-AA Research Framework: Toward a biological definition of Alzheimer's disease. *Alzheimer's Dement.* **2018**, *14*, 535–562. [CrossRef]

18. Livingston, G.; Sommerlad, A.; Orgeta, V.; Costafreda, S.G.; Huntley, J.; Ames, D.; Ballard, C.; Banerjee, S.; Burns, A.; Cohen-Mansfield, J.; et al. Dementia prevention, intervention, and care. *Lancet* **2017**, *390*, 2673–2734. [CrossRef]

19. Maki, Y.; Yamaguchi, H. Early detection of dementia in the community under a community-based integrated care system. *Geriatr. Gerontol. Int.* **2014**, *14*, 2–10. [CrossRef]

20. Arevalo-Rodriguez, I.; Smailagic, N.; Roqué-Figuls, M.; Ciapponi, A.; Sanchez-Perez, E.; Giannakou, A.; Pedraza, O.L.; Bonfill Cosp, X.; Cullum, S. Mini-Mental State Examination (MMSE) for the early detection of dementia in people with mild cognitive impairment (MCI). *Cochrane Database Syst. Rev.* **2021**, *7*, CD010783. [CrossRef]

21. Battineni, G.; Hossain, M.A.; Chintalapudi, N.; Traini, E.; Dhulipalla, V.R.; Ramasamy, M.; Amenta, F. Improved Alzheimer's Disease Detection by MRI Using Multimodal Machine Learning Algorithms. *Diagnostics* **2021**, *11*, 2103. [CrossRef]

22. Carotenuto, A.; Traini, E.; Fasanaro, A.M.; Battineni, G.; Amenta, F. Tele-Neuropsychological Assessment of Alzheimer's Disease. *J. Pers. Med.* **2021**, *11*, 688. [CrossRef] [PubMed]

23. Woźniacka, A.; Patrzyk, S.; Mikołajczyk, M. Artificial intelligence in medicine and dermatology. *Postep. Dermatol. Alergol.* **2021**, *38*, 948–952. [CrossRef]

24. James, C.; Ranson, J.M.; Everson, R.; Llewellyn, D.J. Performance of Machine Learning Algorithms for Predicting Progression to Dementia in Memory Clinic Patients. *JAMA Netw. Open* **2021**, *4*, e2136553. [CrossRef] [PubMed]

25. Herraiz, Á.H.; Martínez-Rodrigo, A.; Bertomeu-González, V.; Quesada, A.; Rieta, J.J.; Alcaraz, R. A Deep Learning Approach for Featureless Robust Quality Assessment of Intermittent Atrial Fibrillation Recordings from Portable and Wearable Devices. *Entropy* **2020**, *22*, 733. [CrossRef] [PubMed]

26. Gaubert, S.; Houot, M.; Raimondo, F.; Ansart, M.; Corsi, M.C.; Naccache, L.; Sitt, J.D.; Habert, M.O.; Dubois, B.; De Vico Fallani, F.; et al. A machine learning approach to screen for preclinical Alzheimer's disease. *Neurobiol. Aging* **2021**, *105*, 205–216. [CrossRef]

27. Tsang, G.; Xie, X.; Zhou, S.M. Harnessing the Power of Machine Learning in Dementia Informatics Research: Issues, Opportunities, and Challenges. *IEEE Rev. Biomed. Eng.* **2020**, *13*, 113–129. [CrossRef] [PubMed]

28. Kumar, S.; Oh, I.; Schindler, S.; Lai, A.M.; Payne, P.R.O.; Gupta, A. Machine learning for modeling the progression of Alzheimer disease dementia using clinical data: A systematic literature review. *JAMIA Open* **2021**, *4*, ooab052. [CrossRef]

29. Agarwal, D.; Marques, G.; De la Torre-Díez, I.; Franco Martin, M.A.; García Zapiraín, B.; Martín Rodríguez, F. Transfer Learning for Alzheimer's Disease through Neuroimaging Biomarkers: A Systematic Review. *Sensors* **2021**, *21*, 7259. [CrossRef]

30. Merkin, A.; Krishnamurthi, R.; Medvedev, O.N. Machine learning, artificial intelligence and the prediction of dementia. *Curr. Opin. Psychiatry* **2022**, *35*, 123–129. [CrossRef]

31. Landolfi, A.; Ricciardi, C.; Donisi, L.; Cesarelli, G.; Troisi, J.; Vitale, C.; Barone, P.; Amboni, M. Machine Learning Approaches in Parkinson's Disease. *Curr. Med. Chem.* **2021**, *28*, 6548–6568. [CrossRef]

32. Savage, N. How AI and neuroscience drive each other forwards. *Nature* **2019**, *571*, S15–S17. [CrossRef]

33. Fan, J.; Fang, L.; Wu, J.; Guo, Y.; Dai, Q. From brain science to artificial intelligence. *Engineering* **2020**, *6*, 248–252. [CrossRef]

34. Stang, A. Critical evaluation of the Newcastle-Ottawa scale for the assessment of the quality of nonrandomized studies in meta-analyses. *Eur. J. Epidemiol.* **2010**, *25*, 603–605. [CrossRef] [PubMed]

35. Goenka, N.; Tiwari, S. AlzVNet: A volumetric convolutional neural network for multiclass classification of Alzheimer's disease through multiple neuroimaging computational approaches. *Biomed. Signal Process. Control* **2022**, *74*, 103500. [CrossRef]

36. Helaly, H.A.; Badawy, M.; Haikal, A.Y. Deep Learning Approach for Early Detection of Alzheimer's Disease. *Cognit. Comput.* **2021**, *1*, 1–17. [CrossRef]

37. Pan, D.; Zeng, A.; Jia, L.; Huang, Y.; Frizzell, T.; Song, X. Early Detection of Alzheimer's Disease Using Magnetic Resonance Imaging: A Novel Approach Combining Convolutional Neural Networks and Ensemble Learning. *Front. Neurosci.* **2020**, *14*, 259. [CrossRef]

38. Hazarika, R.A.; Kandar, D.; Maji, A.K. An experimental analysis of different Deep Learning based Models for Alzheimer's Disease classification using Brain Magnetic Resonance Images. *J. King Saud Univ.-Comput. Inf. Sci.* **2021**. *In Press.* [CrossRef]

39. Mathotaarachchi, S.; Pascoal, T.A.; Shin, M.; Benedet, A.L.; Kang, M.S.; Beaudry, T.; Fonov, V.S.; Gauthier, S.; Rosa-Neto, P. Identifying incipient dementia individuals using machine learning and amyloid imaging. *Neurobiol. Aging* **2017**, *59*, 80–90. [CrossRef]

40. Naganandhini, S.; Shanmugavadivu, P. Effective Diagnosis of Alzheimer's Disease using Modified Decision Tree Classifier. *Procedia Comput. Sci.* **2019**, *165*, 548–555. [CrossRef]

41. Boutet, A.; Madhavan, R.; Elias, G.J.B.; Joel, S.E.; Gramer, R.; Ranjan, M.; Paramanandam, V.; Xu, D.; Germann, J.; Loh, A.; et al. Predicting optimal deep brain stimulation parameters for Parkinson's disease using functional MRI and machine learning. *Nat. Commun.* **2021**, *12*, 3043. [CrossRef]

42. Fei, Z.; Yang, E.; Yu, L.; Li, X.; Zhou, H.; Zhou, W. A Novel deep neural network-based emotion analysis system for automatic detection of mild cognitive impairment in the elderly. *Neurocomputing* **2022**, *468*, 306–316. [CrossRef]
43. Kang, M.J.; Kim, S.Y.; Na, D.L.; Kim, B.C.; Yang, D.W.; Kim, E.J.; Na, H.R.; Han, H.J.; Lee, J.H.; Kim, J.H.; et al. Prediction of cognitive impairment via deep learning trained with multi-center neuropsychological test data. *BMC Med. Inform. Decis. Mak.* **2019**, *19*, 1–9. [CrossRef] [PubMed]
44. Xue, C.; Karjadi, C.; Paschalidis, I.C.; Au, R.; Kolachalama, V.B. Detection of dementia on voice recordings using deep learning: A Framingham Heart Study. *Alzheimer's Res. Ther.* **2021**, *13*, 1–15. [CrossRef] [PubMed]
45. El-Sappagh, S.; Alonso, J.M.; Islam, S.M.R.; Sultan, A.M.; Kwak, K.S. A multilayer multimodal detection and prediction model based on explainable artificial intelligence for Alzheimer's disease. *Sci. Rep.* **2021**, *11*, 2660. [CrossRef] [PubMed]
46. Battineni, G.; Chintalapudi, N.; Amenta, F.; Traini, E. A Comprehensive Machine-Learning Model Applied to Magnetic Resonance Imaging (MRI) to Predict Alzheimer's Disease (AD) in Older Subjects. *J. Clin. Med.* **2020**, *9*, 2146. [CrossRef]
47. Venugopalan, J.; Tong, L.; Hassanzadeh, H.R.; Wang, M.D. Multimodal deep learning models for early detection of Alzheimer's disease stage. *Sci. Rep.* **2021**, *11*, 3254. [CrossRef]
48. Herzog, N.J.; Magoulas, G.D. Brain asymmetry detection and machine learning classification for diagnosis of early dementia. *Sensors* **2021**, *21*, 778. [CrossRef]
49. Bron, E.E.; Steketee, R.M.E.; Houston, G.C.; Oliver, R.A.; Achterberg, H.C.; Loog, M.; Van Swieten, J.C.; Hammers, A.; Niessen, W.J.; Smits, M.; et al. Diagnostic classification of arterial spin labeling and structural MRI in presenile early stage dementia. *Hum. Brain Mapp.* **2014**, *35*, 4916–4931. [CrossRef]
50. Pekkala, T.; Hall, A.; Lötjönen, J.; Mattila, J.; Soininen, H.; Ngandu, T.; Laatikainen, T.; Kivipelto, M.; Solomon, A. Development of a late-life dementia prediction index with supervised machine learning in the population-based CAIDE study. *J. Alzheimer's Dis.* **2017**, *55*, 1055–1067. [CrossRef]
51. Byeon, H. Application of machine learning technique to distinguish parkinson's disease dementia and alzheimer's dementia: Predictive power of parkinson's disease-related non-motor symptoms and neuropsychological profile. *J. Pers. Med.* **2020**, *10*, 31. [CrossRef]
52. Miltiadous, A.; Tzimourta, K.D.; Giannakeas, N.; Tsipouras, M.G.; Afrantou, T.; Ioannidis, P.; Tzallas, A.T. Alzheimer's disease and frontotemporal dementia: A robust classification method of eeg signals and a comparison of validation methods. *Diagnostics* **2021**, *11*, 1437. [CrossRef] [PubMed]
53. Danso, S.O.; Zeng, Z.; Muniz-Terrera, G.; Ritchie, C.W. Developing an Explainable Machine Learning-Based Personalised Dementia Risk Prediction Model: A Transfer Learning Approach With Ensemble Learning Algorithms. *Front. Big Data* **2021**, *4*, 21. [CrossRef] [PubMed]
54. Juutinen, M.; Wang, C.; Zhu, J.; Haladjian, J.; Ruokolainen, J.; Puustinen, J.; Vehkaoja, A. Parkinson's disease detection from 20-step walking tests using inertial sensors of a smartphone: Machine learning approach based on an observational case-control study. *PLoS ONE* **2020**, *15*, e0236258. [CrossRef] [PubMed]
55. Sabry, F.; Eltaras, T.; Labda, W.; Alzoubi, K.; Malluhi, Q. Machine Learning for Healthcare Wearable Devices: The Big Picture. *J. Healthc. Eng.* **2022**, *2022*, 4653923. [CrossRef]
56. Ghoraani, B.; Boettcher, L.N.; Hssayeni, M.D.; Rosenfeld, A.; Tolea, M.I.; Galvin, J.E. Detection of Mild Cognitive Impairment and Alzheimer's Disease using Dual-task Gait Assessments and Machine Learning Behnaz. *Physiol. Behav.* **2021**, *176*, 100–106. [CrossRef]
57. Shimoda, A.; Li, Y.; Hayashi, H.; Kondo, N. Dementia risks identified by vocal features via telephone conversations: A novel machine learning prediction model. *PLoS ONE* **2021**, *16*, e0253988. [CrossRef]
58. Boettcher, L.N.; Hssayeni, M.; Rosenfeld, A.; Tolea, M.I.; Galvin, J.E.; Ghoraani, B. Dual-Task Gait Assessment and Machine Learning for Early- detection of Cognitive Decline. *Physiol. Behav.* **2020**, *176*, 139–148. [CrossRef]
59. Alzheimer's Association. 2016 Alzheimer's disease facts and figures. *Alzheimer's Dement.* **2016**, *12*, 459–509. [CrossRef]
60. WHO. *Risk Reduction of Cognitive Decline and Dementia: WHO Guidelines*; WHO: Geneva, Switzerland, 2019.
61. Signaevsky, M.; Marami, B.; Prastawa, M.; Tabish, N.; Iida, M.A.; Zhang, X.F.; Sawyer, M.; Duran, I.; Koenigsberg, D.G.; Bryce, C.H.; et al. Antemortem detection of Parkinson's disease pathology in peripheral biopsies using artificial intelligence. *Acta Neuropathol. Commun.* **2022**, *10*, 21. [CrossRef]
62. Lee, G.; Nho, K.; Kang, B.; Sohn, K.A.; Kim, D.; Weiner, M.W.; Aisen, P.; Petersen, R.; Jack, C.R.; Jagust, W.; et al. Predicting Alzheimer's disease progression using multi-modal deep learning approach. *Sci. Rep.* **2019**, *9*, 1952. [CrossRef]
63. Almubark, I.; Chang, L.C.; Shattuck, K.F.; Nguyen, T.; Turner, R.S.; Jiang, X. A 5-min Cognitive Task With Deep Learning Accurately Detects Early Alzheimer's Disease. *Front. Aging Neurosci.* **2020**, *12*, 450. [CrossRef] [PubMed]
64. Fulton, L.V.; Dolezel, D.; Harrop, J.; Yan, Y.; Fulton, C.P. Classification of alzheimer's disease with and without imagery using gradient boosted machines and resnet-50. *Brain Sci.* **2019**, *9*, 212. [CrossRef] [PubMed]
65. Odusami, M.; Maskeliūnas, R.; Damaševičius, R. An Intelligent System for Early Recognition of Alzheimer's Disease Using Neuroimaging. *Sensors* **2022**, *22*, 740. [CrossRef] [PubMed]
66. Dubois, B.; Hampel, H.; Feldman, H.H.; Scheltens, P.; Aisen, P.; Andrieu, S.; Bakardjian, H.; Benali, H.; Bertram, L.; Blennow, K.; et al. Preclinical Alzheimer's disease: Definition, natural history, and diagnostic criteria. *Alzheimer's Dement.* **2016**, *12*, 292–323. [CrossRef]

67. Scheltens, P.; Blennow, K.; Breteler, M.M.B.; De Strooper, B.; Frisoni, G.B.; Salloway, S.; Van der Flier, W.M. Alzheimer's disease. *Lancet* **2016**, *388*, 505–517. [CrossRef]
68. Drury-Ruddlesden, J.; Health, I. Rehabilitation in Advanced Dementia through Computer-Assisted Exergaming with Able-X: A Collective Case Study. Ph.D. Thesis, Victoria University of Wellington, Wellington, New Zealand, 2017. [CrossRef]
69. Hu, J.; Qing, Z.; Liu, R.; Zhang, X.; Lv, P.; Wang, M.; Wang, Y.; He, K.; Gao, Y.; Zhang, B. Deep Learning-Based Classification and Voxel-Based Visualization of Frontotemporal Dementia and Alzheimer's Disease. *Front. Neurosci.* **2021**, *14*, 1468. [CrossRef]
70. García-Gutierrez, F.; Díaz-Álvarez, J.; Matias-Guiu, J.A.; Pytel, V.; Matías-Guiu, J.; Cabrera-Martín, M.N.; Ayala, J.L. GA-MADRID: Design and validation of a machine learning tool for the diagnosis of Alzheimer's disease and frontotemporal dementia using genetic algorithms. *Med. Biol. Eng. Comput.* **2022**, *1*, 1–20. [CrossRef]
71. Bougea, A.; Efthymiopoulou, E.; Spanou, I.; Zikos, P. A Novel Machine Learning Algorithm Predicts Dementia With Lewy Bodies Versus Parkinson's Disease Dementia Based on Clinical and Neuropsychological Scores. *J. Geriatr. Psychiatry Neurol.* **2022**, *35*, 317–320. [CrossRef]
72. Galvin, J.E.; Chrisphonte, S.; Cohen, I.; Greenfield, K.K.; Kleiman, M.J.; Moore, C.; Riccio, M.L.; Rosenfeld, A.; Shkolnik, N.; Walker, M.; et al. Characterization of dementia with Lewy bodies (DLB) and mild cognitive impairment using the Lewy body dementia module (LBD-MOD). *Alzheimer's Dement.* **2021**, *17*, 1675–1686. [CrossRef]
73. Ni, Y.C.; Tseng, F.P.; Pai, M.C.; Hsiao, I.T.; Lin, K.J.; Lin, Z.K.; Lin, C.Y.; Chiu, P.Y.; Hung, G.U.; Chang, C.C.; et al. The Feasibility of Differentiating Lewy Body Dementia and Alzheimer's Disease by Deep Learning Using ECD SPECT Images. *Diagnostics* **2021**, *11*, 2091. [CrossRef]

MDPI
St. Alban-Anlage 66
4052 Basel
Switzerland
www.mdpi.com

Bioengineering Editorial Office
E-mail: bioengineering@mdpi.com
www.mdpi.com/journal/bioengineering

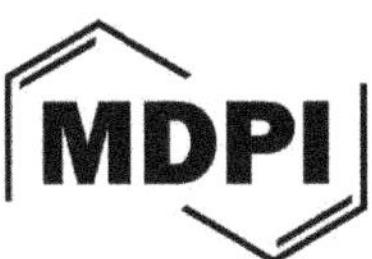

www.ingramcontent.com/pod-product-compliance
Lightning Source LLC
LaVergne TN
LVHW071242170726
843515LV00006BA/1304